Cervical, Breast and Prostate Cancer

Cervical, Breast and Prostate Cancer

Publisher: iConcept Press Ltd.
Cover design: Pineapple Design Ltd.
Interior design: iConcept Press Ltd.
Typesetting and copy editing: iConcept Press Ltd. and Pineapple Design Ltd.

ISBN: 978-1-922227-87-4

Printed in the United States of America

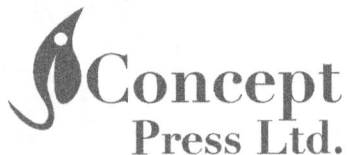

ⵎConcept
Press Ltd.

www.iconceptpress.com

Contents

Preface

Cervical cancer and breast cancer are two of the most common cancers found in women. Cervical cancer is when cancer arises from the cervix. Early on there are typically no symptoms. Later symptoms may include abnormal vaginal bleeding, pelvic pain or pain during sex. Breast cancer is when cancer develops from breast tissue. Signs of breast cancer may include a lump in the breast, a change in breast shape, dimpling of the skin, fluid coming from the nipple, or a red scaly patch of skin. Prostate cancer is when cancer develops in the prostate, a gland in the male reproductive system. It may initially cause no symptoms. In later stages it can cause difficulty urinating, blood in the urine, or pain in the pelvis, back or when urinating. This book provides some latest research and findings on breast cancer, cervical cancer and prostate cancer. The aim of this book is to serve as an important reference book for individuals working in biomedical laboratories, and for clinical professionals.

There are totally 13 chapters in this book. Chapter 1 proposes an outlook on different endoscopic surgical procedures to treat cervical cancer, using traditional laparoscopy and robotics. The chapter starts with history of radical surgery and faces with common surgical oncological problems, as fertility sparing, complications and so on. Chapter 2 reviews the clinical results of carbon ion radiotherapy (C-ion RT) for uterine cervical cancer. Carbon-ion RT has been established as a safe short-term treatment for locally advanced uterine cervical cancer. The authors show that C-ion RT has the potential to improve the treatment for locally advanced bulky squamous cell carcinoma or adenocarcinoma of the uterine cervix. Chapter 3 summarises chrysin inhibits proliferation, induces apoptosis and reduce angiogenesis in most tested cancer cells, including cervical cancer cells. The biological activities of chrysin may be improved by modification of the original structure of chrysin or combination therapy. Hence, more significant research that may help to develop ways of improving the effectiveness of chrysin in the treatment of human cancers is warranted Chapter 4 shows that involving physicians in the promotion of public health programs and initiatives is a viable option. Given the authority that physicians have with the public on health care decisions, achieving physician support of public health programs will help to increase the success and impact of these programs, and is therefore an important consideration when designing any promotion or communications campaign in support of the public's health

Chapter 5 summarizes the published findings about the controversial role of METCAM, a cell adhesion molecule, in the progression of human breast cancer. The issue is finally resolved with more scientific evidence to support the notion that METCAM plays a positive role in the progression of the cancer. Chapter 6 focuses on the biology of *neu* in breast cancer - the potential mechanisms that may contribute to tumor resistance and the numerous uncertainties that persist despite the bona-fide progress made in treating this particular subtype of breast cancer. A comprehensive discussion of novel therapeutic agents that are currently approved (or in clinical trials) for the treatment of HER2-positive breast cancer is also provided. Chapter 7 describes the mechanisms by which estrogen can exert its role in estrogenresponsive cells, focusing on specific aspects of estrogen receptor signaling. Moreover, this chapter shows how some of the proteins involved in estrogen receptor signaling can be used as predictive markers in breast cancer and describes a proposed clinical study related to the combined use of two drugs (bortezomib and tamoxifen) as therapeutic agents for estrogen receptor negative breast cancers. Chapter 8 summarizes the recent studies indicating that AngII facilitates breast cancer metastasis by contributing to the cross-talk between cancer cells and the host stroma. It provides a novel cellular model to evaluate the consequences of Angiotensin receptor (AT2) activation and blockade on breast cancer proliferation, invasion/migration, as well as on tumor growth and metastasis formation.

Chapter 9 focuses on a rationale pharmaceutical development along with a detailed understanding of biological effects so as to accelerate the incorporation of nanocarriers in breast cancer therapy. Tamoxifen-Microemulsions for tumor passive targeting, and lecithin- based nanoparticles as siRNA delivery system for silencing proteins involved in cancer progression are proposed for improving the transfer from concepts towards applications. Chapter 10 summarizes the mTOR pathway and the clinical results in breast cancer treatment, relating them to results obtained using cultured MCF-7 breast cancer tamoxifen resistant sub-lines. The authors compared the effect of mTOR inhibitor everolimus and the dual PI3K/mTOR inhibitors NVP-BEZ235 and GSK2126458 in the breast cancer cell lines model, and demonstrated synergistic effects of the combination of everolimus and NVP-BEZ235 in everolimus resistant breast cancer cell lines. Chapter 11 discusses how to develop a standard extraction method, yielding tomato products which are suitable for cell cultures, and enable product comparison of different tomato varieties, as well as compares antiproliferative potencies of products prepared in a standardized manner from five tomato varieties and broccoli. In addition, this chapter also addresses whether tomato and broccoli products substitute each other due to their common effector when administered simultaneously relative to breast and prostate cancer cells. Chapter 12 describes principles and processes that are involved in investigating biological or clinical problems with nuclear magnetic resonance (NMR) based metabolomics – an approach that involves the global analysis of metabolites. The authors use prostate cancer as a case study to outline the processes, applications and potential of metabolomics for inform scientists and clinicians.

Chapter 13 discusses the epidemiology, screening, diagnosis and treatment options of prostate cancer and its association with osteoporosis. In addition, it explores novel treatments for castration-associated osteoporosis.

Editing and publishing a book is never an easy task. Each chapter in this book has gone through a peer review, a selection and an editing process so as to guarantee its quality. Without the supports and contributions of the authors and reviewers, this book can never be able to complete. We would like to thank all of the authors in this book and all of the reviewers who participated in the reviewing process: . We hope that you, the reader, will find this book interesting and useful. Any advices please feel free and are always welcome to tell us.

iConcept Press Ltd
July 2014

Endoscopic Surgical Procedures for Cervical Cancer Treatment: A Literature Review

Andrea Tinelli, Antonio Perrone
Department of Obstetrics and Gynaecology
Vito Fazzi Hospital, Lecce, Italy

Sarah Gustapane, Giulia Pavone, Francesco Giacci
Department of Gynecology and Obstetrics
"SS. Annunziata" Hospital, Chieti, Italy

Emanuele Perrone
Department of Obstetrics and Gynecology
University of Perugia, Italy

Antonio Malvasi
Department of Obstetric & Gynecology
Santa Maria Hospital, Bari, Italy

Mykhailo V. Medvediev
Dnipropetrovsk State Medical Academy, Dnipropetrovsk, Ukraine

Marina Yu Eliseeva, Ospan A. Mynbaev
Peoples' Friendship University of Russia, Moscow, Russia

1   Introduction

Cervical cancer is the second most common cancer in women worldwide and is a leading cause of cancer-related death in women in underdeveloped countries. Worldwide, approximately 500,000 cases of cervical cancer are diagnosed each year: approximately 13,000 cases of invasive cervical cancer and in the USA 50,000 cases of cervical carcinoma in situ (i.e., localized cancer) are diagnosed yearly. In developed countries, over the last 40 years, cervical cancer death rate has decreased by more than 70% because pre-invasive lesions and cervical cancers were detected at an earlier stage (Tinelli *et al.*, 2009b).

Cervical cancer is always associated with a HPV infection, since a carcinogenic human papillomavirus (HPV) infection is necessary for the development of cervical cancer (Tinelli *et al.*, 2007). Cervical cancer risk seems to be influenced by other variables too, like smoking and immunodeficiency. Infection with other sexually transmitted viruses seems to act as a cofactor in the development of cervical cancer (Tinelli *et al.*, 2009a).

We will focus on fertility-sparing techniques such as radical trachelectomy and on the area of minimally invasive treatment of cervical cancer, since this tumor can be safely and feasibly managed from minimally invasive endoscopic radical operations, such as hysterectomy, bilateral salpingo-oophorectomy, pelvic and para-aortic lymphadenectomy for surgical treatment.

2   Cervical Cancer Staging and Radical Hysterectomy Classification

Correct staging of advanced cervical cancer is essential to optimize its oncological treatment. However, the new FIGO classification is limited to clinical findings and does not include complex imaging. The rationale is to provide a template allowing both resource-rich and resource-poor countries to compare data by stage so as to standardize management of the disease. It can be difficult to accurately assess parametrial and sidewall invasion, as well as metastases to lymph nodes, using clinical staging alone. These are the limitations of FIGO clinical staging.

The purpose of the staging system is to provide uniform terminology for better communication among health professionals and to provide appropriate prognosis for the patients resulting in treatment improvement (Pecorelli *et al.*, 2009). This is a constantly evolving process as new therapeutic modalities are being developed and new imaging and surgical approaches are applied. In those countries where medical research and more prognostic information has become available, in recent years, new knowledge has boomed.

A constantly evolving process is also being applied in surgery techniques. The term "radical" or "extended" hysterectomy encompasses various types of surgery. Since the first publications of large series of surgeries for cervical cancer by Wertheim in Austria (Wertheim, 1912) and later by Okabayashi in Japan (Okabayashi, 1921) and Meigs in the USA (Meigs, 1944), many radical procedures according with different degrees of radicality have been described and performed.

The problem with all these procedures is that they name the same anatomical structures differently and define these structures according to different anatomic interpretations. In this scenario, the Piver–Rutledge–Smith classification published in 1974 has achieved substantial popularity (Piver *et al.*, 1974). It describes five classes of radical hysterectomy (Symmonds, 1975) including a class I category, which is not radical hysterectomy, and a class V category, which is no longer used. The rationale and anatomic definitions for differentiation between class III and IV are unclear. Surgeons frequently need to define intermediate classes inbetween classes II and III (eg, II-III or II-and-a-half). The original paper does not refer to clear anatomical landmarks or international anatomical definitions. The vaginal extent of resection is systematically attached to the pericervical extent; vaginal resection is excessive—from a third to three-quarters of the vagina.

The classification by Piver *et al.* (1974) does not take into account the idea of nerve preservation that was introduced in the 1950s (Kobayashi, 1961) and subsequently refined by Japanese surgeons (Fujii *et al.*, 2007; Sakuragi *et al.*, 2005) and adopted by European surgeons (Raspagliesi *et al.*, 2004; Trimbos *et al.*, 2001). The Piver–Rutledge–Smith classification applies to open surgery only. Querleu & Morrow (2008) recently published a new radical hysterectomy classification, based, for simplification's sake, on only the lateral extent of uterine resection.

Only four types of radical hysterectomy are described, adding a few subtypes when necessary. Instead of the classification by Piver *et al.* (1974), stable anatomical landmarks are used to define the limits of resection. To make a clear distinction with the Piver–Rutledge–Smith, in the Querleu and Morrow classification (Querleu *et al.*, 2008) letters are used rather than numbers to define classes. Simple hysterectomy is not included in the classification. Lymph-node dissection, an essential part of surgical cervical cancer management, is considered separately. For lymph-node dissections, the limit between level 1 and level 2 is the bifurcation of the common iliac artery; the limit between level 2 and level 3 the bifurcation of the aorta; and the limit between level 3 and level 4 the inferior mesenteric artery.

3   History and Evolution of Surgery in Cervical Cancer

The ancient Egyptians used bamboo knives and in ancient India volcanic glass, obsidian, was used to operate on patients. Over 1,000 years later until now, steel scalpels have been used to perform surgery. Only 200 years ago, in 1809, the first documented laparotomy was performed for a gynaecological tumour by Ephraim McDowell, who removed an ovarian cyst.

Since the late nineteenth century until now, surgery, and in particular radical surgery, has taken an astonishingly conservative approach. The same technique for radical cervical surgery surgery as introduced by Wertheim in 1896 (Wertheim, 1912) is still being used today, and gynaecological oncological surgeons are very reluctant to change even minor details of this operation. Essentially, radical gynaecological surgery has remained fairly standard and unchanged. Although a first attempt at laparoscopy, on his dog, was made by Georg Kelling in 1901, it took until the 1970s for laparoscopy to be introduced into gynaecological surgery. In the beginning, it was only used for diagnostic purposes and sterilizations. As recently as 1989, the first series of 'laparoscopically assisted vaginal hysterectomy' were reported by Harry Reich (Reich & DeCaprio, 1989).

Two years earlier, Dargent (1987) had described the use of laparoscopy as 'presurgical retroperitoneal pelviscopy for Schauta's operation' in preparation for the vaginal approach for cervical cancer. In 1992, Nezhat (1992) performed the first laparoscopic radical hysterectomy with pelvic and para-aortic lymph node dissection. In 2000, Dargent *et al.* (2000) reported successful laparoscopic vaginal radical trachelectomy and pelvic lymphadenectomy for young women with cervical cancer, who wanted to preserve their fertility. In 2000, Possover *et al.* (2000) reported modified laparoscopic nerve sparing type III radical hysterectomy for cervical cancer and found that this procedure decreased postoperative bladder dysfunction incidence subsequently Pomel *et al.* (2003) evaluated, in a series of 50 consecutive patients, the feasibility, morbidity, and survival outcome of laparoscopic radical hysterectomy for carcinoma of the uterine cervix.

With technical advances and emerging devices, as well as accumulating experience in laparoscopic surgery, some surgical procedures that are difficult to carry out even by traditional open procedures can be performed successfully by laparoscopy. The major advantages associated with minimally invasive laparoscopy are, amongst others, lower intraoperative bleeding rates, less post-operative pain, a shorter recovery time and a shorter hospital stay.

In addition, the optical devices used for laparoscopic surgery feature a 10 to 15 times magnification and, therefore, provide an excellent view of pelvis anatomy.

During the past decade some reports, on a limited number of patients, have shown the feasibility of radical resection by laparoscopic surgery and have documented an equivalent number of pelvic nodes harvested by laparoscopy and open surgery (Canis *et al.*, 1995; Hsieh *et al.*, 1998; Kim *et al.*, 1998; Krause *et al.*, 1995; Pomel *et al.*, 1997; Sedlacek *et al.*, 1994; Spirtos *et al.*, 1996). Nevertheless, few long-term data on the morbidity and survival after laparoscopic radical hysterectomy are available. In gynecological oncology laparoscopic surgery does not substantially reduce tissue trauma, which makes it possible for extensive and complex operative procedures to be performed through small incisions, reducing intra-operative blood loss and impact on the body as well as common surgical complications. In addition, laparoscopic surgery is superior to conventional surgery with regard to postoperative mental rehabilitation in gynecological oncology patients.

From the original publications on this radical hysterectomy surgery, surgical technique has aimed at a re-classification including a variety of techniques via laparotomy (Averette *et al.*, 1993; Magrina *et al.*, 1999), then via laparoscopy, resulting in reasonable morbidity with similar surgical outcomes (Abu-Rustum *et al.*, 2003; Magrina, 2005). However, longer operating times, steep learning curves, and lack of training have prevented laparoscopic treatment from becoming a widely adopted surgical approach to radical hysterectomy (Boggess, 2007; Ramirez *et al.*, 2006). Although open radical hysterectomy is still considered the gold standard for the treatment of early cervical cancer (Abu-Rustum *et al.*, 2001), laparoscopic radical (LRH) and laparoscopy-assisted radical vaginal hysterectomy (LARH) are evolving as potential surgical alternatives. The principles are: to resect tumor and its surrounding tissues en bloc, to use tumor-free techniques when manipulating tumors, to preserve sufficiently incised margins, and to perform complete pelvic lymphadenectomy. Lymph node status is the most important prognostic factor in gynecologic tumor and surgical removal of the pelvic. Para-aortic lymph nodes for histological assessment are part of gynecologic malignancies staging. Hence, laparoscopic surgery is consistent with the concept of minimally invasive surgery, i.e., smaller trauma, milder pain or analgesia, better homeostasis, more accurate operative outcomes, shorter hospital stay and better psychological effects than current standard open surgery. As a technical innovation, laparoscopic techniques for gynecological oncology do not change gynecological oncological surgery fundamentally, but they have improved surgical techniques for gynecological oncology in many aspects, and enhanced the efficacy of surgical cervical cancer treatment.

Additionally, removal of bulky lymph nodes may have therapeutic benefit. According to the requirement by established FIGO classification systems, a different range of lymphadenectomy will be performed depending on the different type of tumor present. The range of lymphadenectomy, consistent with that of open abdominal surgery, depends on cervical cancer disease. Lymph nodes, para-aortic and iliac vessels are resected within the vessel sheath. Obturator and deep inguinal lymph nodes, including lymph nodes below the obturator nerve, must be resected radically.

The indication for laparoscopic surgery was similar to open surgery in cervical cancer patients. According to literature and our experience, the indication for laparoscopic radical hysterectomy (type III) and pelvic lymphadenectomy was earlier than the FIGO stage IIa in cervical cancer (Malzoni *et al.*, 2004). The indication for this surgical procedure is mainly influenced by the experience of the surgeon (Lecuru *et al.*, 1998). More recently, it was reported that stage IIb or more advanced cervical cancer may be treated with type IV radical hysterectomy under laparoscopy (Chen *et al.*, 2008; Possover *et al.*, 1998; Querleu *et al.*, 2008), as the aim of surgery is to stage and radically resect the tumor (including metastases). For certain patients, prolong survival is the objective of tumor treatment.

4   Laparoscopic and Robotic-assisted Approaches in Gynaecological Malignancies

The goal of laparoscopic surgery is to duplicate traditional open procedures via small incisions in the skin with surgical outcomes equivalent or superior to a traditional surgical approach. Laparoscopy offers multiple advantages in the management of malignancy, including smaller incisions, shorter hospital stay, quicker recovery, improved visualization, less need for postoperative analgesics, and a lower risk of complications, such as blood loss, wound infection, herniation, and ileus. These characteristics may prove particularly important in the setting of oncology where a shorter recovery period may facilitate a shorter interval to postoperative treatments such as chemotherapy or radiation. Laparoscopy also has its limitations. Disadvantages include a long learning curve, counterintuitive motions, and limited depth perception as imaging is limited to 2-dimensional views.

In an effort to overcome these limitations, multiple innovations have evolved over the last decade. Laparoscopic instrumentation has expanded to include several different vessel sealing devices with integrated cutting capabilities, endoscopic staplers, articulating instrument tips, 3-dimensional capabilities, and computer-enhanced technology in the form of robotics. Therefore, robotic surgical systems seem to be the future in gynecologic surgery, since robotic technology can improve accuracy, enhance dexterity, and provide for faster suturing and a lower training curve than laparoscopy. All of this makes gynecologic surgeons tend to perform a greater number of gynecologic procedures by robotic approach, when available. In the last five years, a large number of robotic surgery related papers have been published, both for benign and oncological cases, which is proof of the rapid spread and high acceptance of this new technology.

Gynecological oncology probably presents the optimal forum for application of robotics, given the complexity of surgical steps involved in performing radical hysterectomies for cervical cancer and lymph node sampling for endometrial cancer. Radical hysterectomy was one of the first indications for robot-assisted laparoscopy, as this made it possible to perform a complex and long procedure laparoscopically. Studies comparing the results of robot-assisted and conventional laparoscopic surgery yielded slightly different but conflicting results. Boggess *et al.* (2008) found a rate of 7.8 % for major complications after robotic surgery, compared with 16.3 % after conventional laparoscopic surgery, whereas Kruidenberg *et al.* (2011) found just the opposite, with 9.6 % and 5.5 %, respectively (statistically significant differences in both studies). Survival after both modalities seems to be similar.

5   The History of Laparoscopy in Cervical Cancer

In 1989, Querleu et al. (1989) performed the first laparoscopic pelvic lymphadenectomy for cervical cancer, then, in 1990, Canis et al. (1990) described a totally laparoscopic radical hysterectomy. In 1991, Querleu et al. (1991) reported laparoscopic pelvic lymphadenectomy and vaginal assistant radical hysterectomy for early cervical cancer. In 1992 and in 1993, Nezhat et al. (1992; 1993) reported the first case of cervical cancer treated with laparoscopic radical hysterectomy and pelvic lymphadenectomy. Since then, the techniques have been applied clinically and achieved satisfactory clinical outcomes, Vaginal radical trachelectomy and laparoscopic pelvic lymphadenectomy were done by Dargent et al. (1996).

In 2000, Possover et al. (2000) reported modified laparoscopic nerve sparing type III radical hysterectomy for the treatment of cervical cancer, and found that this procedure decreased the incidence of postoperative bladder dysfunction. In 2003, Pomel et al. (2003) reported the feasibility, morbidity, and survival outcome of the laparoscopic radical hysterectomy for carcinoma of the uterine cervix, operated between 1993 and 2001 at two cancer centers. Thirty-one patients had prior brachy therapy. The median overall operative time was 258 min. The mean number of harvested pelvic external iliac nodes was 13.22 per patient. The median postoperative hospital stay was 7.5 days. Two patients had major urinary complications; one had a bladder fistula and one ureteral stenosis. Median follow-up was 44 months. Overall 5-year survival rate of FIGO stage Ia2 and Ib1 patients was 96%. Their results demonstrated that radical hysterectomy can be performed by laparoscopy in stage IB1 or less advanced node negative cervical cancer patients without compromising survival; moreover, prior brachytherapy did not affect the feasibility of this radical procedure.

With technical advances and emerging devices, as well as accumulating experience in laparoscopic surgery, some surgical procedures that are difficult to carry out even by traditional open procedures can be performed successfully by laparoscopy. During the past decade some reports, on a limited number of patients, have shown the feasibility of a radical resection by laparoscopic surgery and have documented an equivalent number of pelvic nodes harvested by laparoscopy and open surgery (Gil-Ibáñez et al., 2013; Kho et al., 2009; Krause et al., 1995; Pomel et al., 1997; 2003; Sedlacek et al., 1994). Nevertheless, few long-term data on the morbidity and survival after laparoscopic radical hysterectomy are available. Although open radical hysterectomy is still considered the gold standard for the treatment of early cervical cancer (Spirtos et al., 1996), laparoscopic radical (LRH) and laparoscopy assisted radical vaginal hysterectomy (LARH) are evolving as potential surgical alternatives.

LRH or LARH have been established as standard procedures routinely performed as first line therapy for the treatment of early cervical cancer at specialized centers (Hatch, 1996; Kohler et al., 2004; Obermair et al., 2003; Pomel et al., 2003). The major advantages associated with minimally invasive laparoscopy are, amongst others, lower intraoperative bleeding rates, less post-operative pain, a shorter recovery time and a shorter hospital stay. In addition the optical devices used for laparoscopic surgery feature a 10 to 15 times magnification and, therefore, provide an excellent view of pelvis anatomy. Since Liang et al. reported their initial experience with 57 LRH; they have continuously improved and standardized the technique (Liang et al., 2006; Querleu, 1990). The indication for laparoscopic surgery was similar to the indication for open surgery in cervical cancer patients. According to literature and experience, the indication for laparoscopic radical hysterectomy (type III) and pelvic lymphadenectomy was earlier than the FIGO stage IIa in cervical cancer (Liang et al., 2006). However, initially, laparoscopic technique treatment of cervical cancer is associated with a high complication rate so the indication must be carefully assessed, and patients have to be counseled extensively prior to surgery. Apart from the size and stage of the tumor, the indication for this surgical procedure is mainly influenced by the experience of the surgeon (Malzoni *et al.*, 2004).

More recently, it was reported that stage IIb or more advanced cervical cancer may be treated with type IV radical hysterectomy under laparoscopy (Chen *et al.*, 2008; Lecuru *et al.*, 1998; Querleu & Morrow, 2008), as the aim of surgery is to stage and radically resect the tumor (including metastases). For certain patients, prolonged survival is the objective of tumor treatment. Through laparoscopic exploration, the feasibility and thoroughness of surgery can be evaluated, and the relative benefits of surgery for the patient can be weighed. However, it is still controversial what types or what stages of cervical cancer should be adopted for laparoscopic surgical treatment.

Another minimally invasive surgical option used for cervical cancer is laparoscopically assisted vaginal radical hysterectomy (LAVRH) or Coelio-Schauta procedure. The Coelio-Schauta procedure consists of 2 major steps, 1 laparoscopic and 1 transvaginal. Four trocars are inserted, 1 transumbilical, 2 lateral to the inferior epigastric vessels, and 1 in the right lower abdomen. Traditionally, laparoscopy has been used to develop the paravesical and pararectal spaces and to perform lymphadenectomy of iliac vessels. In the transvaginal step, the urinary bladder is dissected from the cervix, the posterior cul-de-sac is opened, and the ureters are identified before their insertion into the bladder pilar; then the uterine arteries are ligated, and the cardinal ligaments are transected 3 cm from the cervix. Ligation of the utero-ovarian ligaments (or the infudibulopelvic ligaments if ovarian preservation is not mandated) is then performed, the round ligament is resected, and the specimen is extracted (Schneider *et al.*, 1996).

A recent review of Pergialiotis *et al* (2013) on LAVRH on Medline (1966-2013) and Scopus (2004-2013), as well as on reference lists from all included studies, retrived 10 studies: including 6 retrospective cohort studies, 2 prospective cohort studies, 1 retrospective randomized trial, and a phase II randomized control trial.LAVRH provided equal recurrence-free rates when performed in patients with tumors not exceeding 2 cm in greatest diameter. Its main advantages seem to be less intraoperative blood loss and more radical pelvic lymphadenectomy. The primary disadvantages of the technique are a higher rate of disease-positive surgical margins, resulting in the need for adjuvant therapy, and the slow learning curve required for a surgeon to gain expertise.

6   Total Laparoscopic Radical Hysterectomy for Cervical Cancer

Laparoscopy can be safely and adequately used in the treatment of endometrial, ovarian and cervical cancer (Possover *et al.*, 1998). In the setting of gynecologic oncology, laparoscopic approaches have been implemented in radical hysterectomy. For gynecological oncology laparoscopic surgery is an important step forward combining scientific, technological and surgical techniques, which not only enhance the efficacy of surgical treatment of gynecological oncology, but are also superior to conventional open surgery with regard to postoperative mental rehabilitation in gynecological oncology patients. The first total laparoscopic radical hysterectomy with lymphadenectomy was reported in June 1989 by Nezhat *et al.* (1992). Since then, more than 600 cases of total laparoscopic radical hysterectomy have been reported. A recent prospective case-control series compared total laparoscopic radical hysterectomy with abdominal radical hysterectomy and found shorter hospital stays and lower blood loss as well as a statistically significantly higher nodal yield among total laparoscopic radical hysterectomy cases (Zakashansky et al., 2007).

Spirtos *et al.* (2002) described 78 patients with early-stage cervical cancer undergoing laparoscopic radical hysterectomy. In that series, 94% of the procedures were completed laparoscopical.Mean follow-up time was 67 months. Mean operative time was 205 min, and mean blood loss was 225 mL. One patient required a blood transfusion, three patients had unintended cystotomies, two patients required laparotomy to control bleeding, and one patient suffered an ureterovaginal fistula. Three patients had microscopically positive or close margins. The authors reported a cervical cancer recurrence rate of 5%.

Pomel et al. (2003) reported 50 patients with stage IA1–IB1 cervical cancer who underwent total laparoscopic radical hysterectomy. The median operating time was 258 min, and the mean number of lymph nodes harvested was 13. No conversions to laparotomy were reported. Median hospital stay was 7.5 days. The authors reported that 10 patients had early complications (within 2 months of surgery) and that three of those patients required reoperation. They also reported three patients had late complications (more than 2 months after surgery) two of them requiring reoperation. Three patients experienced recurrence with a median follow-up time of 44 months.

Frumovitz et al. (2007) compared 35 patients undergoing total laparoscopic radical hysterectomy with 54 undergoing total abdominal radical hysterectomy. Mean estimated blood loss was significantly lower in the laparoscopic-surgery group than in the open-surgery group (319 vs. 548 mL; p=0.009). Mean operative time was significantly longer with laparoscopic surgery (344 vs. 307 min; p=0.03), but median hospital stay was significantly shorter (2.0 vs. 5.0 days, pb0.001). Postoperative infections were much less common after laparoscopic surgery (18% vs. 53%; p=0.001). Notwithstanding the obvious advantages of conventional laparoscopy, recent surveys of practicing gynecologic oncologist revealed that most respondents believed minimally invasive surgery by conventional laparoscopy had only a minimal role in the management of cervical cancer (Fastrez et al., 2009).

Puntambekar et al. (2007) reported a retrospective review of 248 patients with FIGO stage Ia2 (n=32) and Ib1 (n=216) cervical cancer who underwent a TLRH (type III) with bilateral pelvic lymphadenectomy, which is the largest single-institution study. The operation was performed entirely by laparoscopy in all patients and by the same surgical team. Median operative time was 92 min. Median number of resected pelvic nodes was 18. Median blood loss was 165 ml. Median duration of hospital stay was 3 days. None of the patients required conversion to laparotomy. Seventeen patients had complications within 2 months of surgery. Seven patients had recurrences after a median 36-month follow-up. They concluded that TLRH can be performed safely, reduces morbidity associated with ARH and is an easily replicable technique.

Colombo et al. (2009) evaluated surgical outcome and oncologic results of total laparoscopic radical hysterectomy (TLRH) after neoadjuvant chemoradiation therapy (CRT) for locally advanced cervical carcinoma. All patients who underwent TLRH after CRT for stages IIB–IIA and bulky IB diseases were reviewed. The control group for this analysis was a cohort of patients treated with abdominal radical hysterectomy (ARH) after CRT for the same stage cancers. They reviewed 102 patients operated on between 2000 and 2008 (46 TLRH and 56 ARH). Mean age at diagnosis was 44 years, and mean B.M.I was 22.1. There was no difference in tumor characteristics between the two groups. Seven patients in the laparoscopic group required conversion to laparotomy (15%). Mean estimated blood loss (200 vs. 400 mL, pb0.01) and the median duration of hospital stay (5 vs. 8 days, p<0.01) were significantly lower in the laparoscopic group. Morbidity rates and urinary complications were reduced in the laparoscopic group (p=0.04). Local recurrence rates, disease-free and overall survival were comparable in the two groups. Best survival was observed for patients with pathological complete response or microscopic residual disease compared to patients with macroscopic residues (pb0.01). Authors concluded that radical hysterectomy after CRT, with significant morbidity rates, is known to be difficult and remains controversial in comparison to exclusive CRT. TLRH after preoperative CRT is feasible in 85% of the cases for patients with locally advanced cervical cancer. For these patients, TLRH compared with ARH was associated with favorable surgical outcome with comparable oncological results.

Although laparoscopic surgery has many advantages, it is also associated with a number of potential drawbacks, including limited range of intra-abdominal motion (only 4° of freedom), counterintuitive movements, amplification of tremors in prolonged cases due to the length and rigidity of the instrumentation, and reduced depth perception secondary to a two-dimensional view. Naturally, total laparoscopic radical hysterectomy is not without its risks and complications.

There are still several new challenges to be met regarding theory and enhancement of surgical skils (Persson *et al.*, 2008). Firstly, to form a laparoscopic surgical team, a lot of special requirements relating to both the team members and the equipment have to be met, thus restricting the popularization of laparoscopic radical hysterectomy. Secondly, every detail should be taken into careful consideration, risks should be balanced and benefits ascertained before performing laparoscopic procedures. Moreover, it is likely that well-known barriers to the implementation of advanced minimally invasive procedures such as association with a long learning curve, lack of training, complexity of the operations, limitation of technology and instrumentation, and the necessity of an expert assistant were responsible for this sentiment. For these reasons, only a few surgeons have adopted a laparoscopic approach to type III cervical cancer radical. There are issues with the length of the procedure, as type III laparoscopic hysterectomies take significantly longer than open cases. Furthermore, intraoperative complications of the urinary tract (for example as a result of thermal injuries) tend to be much more common in laparoscopic than in open cases (Xu *et al.*, 2007).

A recent experience of Malzoni *et al.* (2009) on 71 patients treated by total laparoscopic radical hysterectomy (type II, III) with lymphadenectomy was done between January 2000 and March 2008. The authors concluded that total laparoscopic radical hysterectomy can be considered a safe and effective therapeutic procedure for the management of early stage cervical cancer with a low morbidity, offering an alternative option for patients undergoing radical hysterectomy, although multicenter studies and long-term follow-up are required to evaluate the oncologic outcomes of this procedure.

A literature review on laparoscopic radical hysterectomy demonstrates the procedure is also safe and feasible, but is associated with an operative time range of 205 min–371 min, an estimated blood loss of 200 cc–445 cc, a nodal yield ranging from 13–25, a hospital stay ranging from 1–7.5 days, and an overall complication rate of 11%–20%, as sorted by the referenced papers who provide a good cross section of the data (Abu-Rustum *et al.*, 2003; Magrina, 2007; Pomel *et al.*, 2003; Ramirez *et al.*, 2006; Spirtos *et al.*, 1996; 2002).

7   Contra-indications to Laparoscopic Surgery for Gynecological Oncology

As previously noted, there are very few absolute contra-indications. However, with increased anesthesia ability, some of these may not be considered as absolute. Severe cardiac diseases could be a problem, since some patients may not tolerate the operation due to the deep Trendelenburg positions necessary during most operative laparoscopy in order to maintain an adequate pneumoperitoneum. Severe patient liver/renal/respiratory dysfunction, which cannot be corrected preoperatively, is also considered to be an absolute contraindication.

Surgeons may refuse laparoscopy for advanced or late stage gynecological tumor in patients with stage III or above cervical carcinoma, lymph node metastases of cervical cancer which inter-fuse and encapsulate vital vessels, and/or extensive infiltration of adjacent tissues. On the other hand, there are few relative contra-indications to laparoscopy for cervical cancer patients; for example, severe abdominal adhesions or morbid obesity and so on.

8 Total Robotic-assisted Laparoscopic Radical Hysterectomies

Today there is only one U.S. Food and Drug Administration approved device for surgical robotics. This current robotic platform is known as the "da Vinci" surgical system, developed by Intuitive Surgical, Inc. (Intuitive Surgical, Mountain View, CA, USA). The da Vinci surgical system is equipped with a 3-dimensional vision system in which double endoscopes generate two images resulting in perception of a 3D image. In addition, with the development of endowrist, it reproduces the range of motion and dexterity of the surgeon hand, providing high precision, flexibility and the ability to rotate instruments 360 degrees. Thus, the learning curve of achievement for the surgeons using the da Vinci surgical system was shortened. In 2001, a more advanced da Vinci surgical system with four robotic arms gained US FDA approval and is now being used in many surgical procedures throughout the world.

Recently, FDA-approved robotic surgery has become an option in the definitive surgical management of early stage cervical cancers. Several case series about robotic-assisted radical hysterectomies for cervical cancer have now been published (Boggess, 2007; Kim *et al.*, 2008; Magrina *et al.*, 2008; Magrina, 2007; Malzoni *et al.*, 2004; 2009).

The initial experience and the first publications on robot assistance in gynecological oncology date from recent years. In February, 2006, Boggess (2005) performed the first live telecast, demonstrating a technique for performing robotic-assisted radical hysterectomy and subsequently presented data for a series of 13 radical hysterectomies at the Society of Gynecologic Oncologists annual meeting in March of the same year. Since this initial demonstration of feasibility and technique, the interest in robotic-assisted gynecologic oncology procedures has spread rapidly.

Recently, Nezhat *et al.* (2008) prospectively compared the outcomes of 13 total robotic-assisted laparoscopic radical hysterectomies to 30 cases of traditional total laparoscopic radical hysterectomy with pelvic lymphadenectomy in patients with stage IB to IIA cervical cancer. There was no difference in operative time, hospital stay, blood loss, complications, or number of nodes retrieved. This study suggests that robotic radical hysterectomy may be a feasible alternative to total laparoscopic radical hysterectomy (unpublished data). However, there were no advantages of robotic-assisted procedures compared to traditional total laparoscopic radical hysterectomy when performed by an experienced laparoscopic gynecologic oncologist.

Fanning *et al.* (2008) reported the first series of robotic radical hysterectomy on 20 women with stage IB–IIA cervical carcinoma. Median operative time was 6.5 hours, and median blood loss was 300 mL.No complications were encountered, and all patients were discharged home on the first postoperative day. A retrospective cohort study of robotic vs. open radical hysterectomy found that the mean blood loss was significantly lower for the robotic group (81.9 vs. 665 mL, p<0.0001), but operative time was longer (4.5 vs. 3.39 hours, p=0.0002). The mean number of lymph nodes resected did not differ, and no complications were reported in the robotic assisted group (Ko *et al.*, 2008). Furthermore, laparoscopic radical hysterectomy studies, although variable, report an operating times from 92 to 350 minutes, an estimated blood loss of 165 ml, and a length of stay of three days, whereas for robotic surgery comparable figures are 190-370 minutes, 140 ml, and two days (Decloedt & Vergote, 1999; Li *et al.*, 2007; Possover *et al.*, 1998; Zakashansky *et al.*, 2007).

The first radical hysterectomy in cervical cancer with robot assistance was described by Sert and Abeler (2006). They concluded that radical dissection could be performed much more precisely than with conventional laparoscopy. In 2007, they described 15 women with early-stage cervical cancer as a pilot case–control study and compared robotic-assisted laparoscopic radical hysterectomy with conventional total laparoscopic radical hysterectomy. There was a significant difference in mean operating time (241 minutes in the robot group and 300 minutes in the conventional group). No difference in the number of lymph nodes and size of parametrial tissue was found. In the robot group, there was significant less bleeding and shorter hospital stay.

Kim *et al.* (2008) performed robotic radical hysterectomy and pelvic lymphadenectomy in ten cases and found a mean operating time of 207 minutes. The mean docking time was 26 minutes, but this was reduced significantly with experience (from 35 to 10 minutes). These small series, however, do not report the outcome of surgery in terms of lymph node yield and radicality and also lack sufficient onco-logical follow up.

Boggess *et al.* (2008) found no difference in the operating time (242 versus 240 minutes). He per-formed 13 robot-assisted radical hysterectomies and compared them with 48 open radical hysterectomies. Significantly more lymph nodes were collected in the robot group (33 versus 22). All the robotic patients were discharged within 24 hours. He also describes how to set up a robotic program in gynaecological oncology.

Recently, a study of Lowe *et al.* (2009) reported a multi-institutional experience with robotic-assisted radical hysterectomy in patients with early stage cervical cancer with respect to peri-operative outcomes. In their investigation, a multi-institutional robotic surgical consortium consisting of five board-certified gynecologist oncologists in distinct geographical regions of the United States was created, in or-der to evaluate the utility of robotics for gynecologic surgery (benign and malignant). Between April 2003 and August 2008, a total of 835 patients underwent robotic surgery for benign gynecologic disor-ders and/or gynecologic malignancies by a surgeon in the consortium. For the purpose of the study, a multi-institutional HIPPA compliant database was then created for all patients. In the results, from a da-tabase of 835 patients who underwent robotic surgery by a gynecologic oncologist they identified, a total of 42 patients who underwent a robotic-assisted type II (n=10) or type III (n=32) radical hysterectomy for early stage cervical cancer. With regard to stage, seven patients (17%) were Stage IA2, twenty-eight pa-tients (67%) were Stage IB1 and six patients (14%) were Stage IB2. There was a single patient with Stage IA1 cervical cancer with vascular space invasion who underwent type II radical hysterectomy. Overall median operative time was 215 min. Overall median estimated blood loss was 50 cc. No patient received a blood transfusion. Median lymph node count was 25. Median hospital stay was 1 day. Positive lymph nodes were detected in 12% of the patients. Pelvic radiotherapy or chemo-radiation was given to 14% of the patients based on final surgical pathology. Intraoperative complications occurred in 4.8% of the pa-tients and included one conversion to laparotomy (2.4%) and one ureteral injury (2.4%). Postoperative complications were reported in 12% of patients and included a DVT (2.4%), infection (7.2%), and blad-der/urinary tract complication (2.4%) Conversion rate to laparotomy was 2.4%. In their conclusions, Lowe *et al.* reported that robotic-assisted radical hysterectomy is associated with minimal blood loss, a shortened hospital stay, and few operative complications. Operative time and lymph node yields are acceptable. This data suggests that robotic-assisted radical hysterectomy may offer an alternative to traditional radical hysterectomy.

Persson *et al.* (2009) reported their experience in 80 robot-assisted laparoscopic radical hysterectomies to evaluate its feasibility and morbidity, from December 2005 to September 2008. They used a prospective protocol, and an active investigation policy to define adverse events, perioperative, and short and long term data. Also in their conclusions, authors showed that robot- assisted laparoscopic radical hysterectomy could be a feasible alternative to conventional laparoscopy and open surgery, even if efforts should be made to ensure proper closure of the vaginal cuff, trocar sites and to develop nerve sparing techniques.

Cantrell *et al.* (2010) assessed progression-free and overall survival for women with cervical cancer who underwent type III robotic radical hysterectomy, in a retrospective analysis of women who underwent RRH from 2005 to 2008. They were compared to a group of historical open radical hysterectomies. They analyzed seventy-one women who had undergone attempted RRH during the study period. Eight were excluded from analysis: 4 for non-cervical primary and 4 cases were aborted due to the extent of the disease. Squamous was the most common histology (62%) followed by adenocarcinoma (32%). Median patient age was 43 years. There was one intraoperative complication (asystole after induction) and two postoperative complications (ICU admission to rule out myocardial infarction and reoperation for cuff dehiscence). Of the patients who underwent RRH, 32% received whole-pelvis radiation with chemo sensitization. Median follow-up was 12.2 months (range 0.2–36.3 months). Kaplan–Meier survival analysis demonstrated 94% PFS and OS at 36 months due to recurrence and the death of one patient. As compared with a historical cohort at our institution, there was no statistically significant difference in PFS (P=0.27) or OS (P=0.47). In the conclusions, Cantrell *et al.* reported that RRH is safe and feasible and has been shown to be associated with improved operative measures. This study showed that at 3 years, RRH appears to have PFS and OS equivalent to that of traditional laparotomy. While the 5-year data are not yet available for the cohort of patients treated with robotic surgery, the 94% survival upon 3 years of performing RRH is comparable to other surgical methods and radiation.

9   The problem of Lymph-node in Endoscopic Lymphadenectomy

The limitations of FIGO clinical staging involve the possibility to detect metastases to lymph nodes, using clinical staging alone. This leads to under staging of some patients (Lagasse *et al.*, 1980; LaPolla *et al.*, 1986). Failure to detect metastasis to para-aortic nodes in patients with locally advanced cervical cancer leads to suboptimal treatment. One option consists of evaluating lymph node invasion using imaging techniques. However, as reported recently, false negative rates as high as 11% have been reported when comparing PET to lymphadenectomy in advanced cervical cancer (Mortier *et al.*, 2008). Ramirez *et al.* compared positron emission tomography (PET)/computed tomography (CT) with laparoscopic extraperitoneal staging in the evaluation of para-aortic lymph nodes. The sensitivity and specificity of PET/CT in detecting positive para-aortic nodes when nodes were negative on CT or MRI were 36% and 96%, respectively. The PPV and NPV of PET/CT for para-aortic metastasis were 71% and 83%, respectively. For the subset of patients with positive pelvic lymph nodes on preoperative PET/CT, the sensitivity of PET/CT for identifying para-aortic lymph node metastases was 45%, the specificity was 91%, the PPV was 71%, and the NPV was 78% (Pecorelli *et al.*, 2009). Therefore, another option is to perform surgical staging (Kohler *et al.*, 2004; Marnitz *et al.*, 2005; Possover *et al.*, 1998).

Laparoscopic para-aortic node sampling has been shown to be feasible in gynecological malignancies. In addition, it is associated with lower morbidity than staging using laparotomy (Dargent *et al.*, 2000; Denschlag *et al.*, 2005; Querleu *et al.*, 1993; 2000; Spiritos *et al.*, 1995; Vergote *et al.*, 2002). Its only technical limitation occurs in obese patients. However, using the classical laparoscopic approach, the surgeon is limited in the degrees of his movements. By assisted-robotic surgery, this problem could be solved. The feasibility of a robotically assisted retroperitoneal approach, to dissect lower lumbo-aortic lymph nodes, was reported recently. Simultaneously to Vergote *et al.* (2008), Fastrez *et al.* (2009), evaluated the feasibility and safety of a robot-assisted laparoscopic transperitoneal approach of the para-aortic lymph node dissection on 8 patients with advanced cervical carcinoma who were eligible for primary pelvic radiotherapy combined with concurrent cisplatin chemotherapy or pelvic exenteration and who underwent a pre-treatment robot assisted transperitoneal laparoscopic para-aortic lymphadenectomy. Authors isolated from 1 to 38 para-aortic nodes per patient and had one para-aortic node positive patient who was treated with extended doses of pelvic radiotherapy. We did not encounter any major complications and post-operative morbidity was low. In the conclusions, Fastrez reported that robot assisted transperitoneal laparoscopic para-aortic lymphadenectomy is feasible and provides the surgeon with greater precision than classical laparoscopy, even if larger prospective multicentre trials are needed to validate the generalized usefulness of this technique.

The technique of the robotic retroperitoneal para-aortic lymphadenectomy has been described by Vergote *et al.* (2008), who reported the feasibility of robot-assisted laparoscopic retroperitoneal para-aortic lymphadenectomy in five patients.

In 2008 Ramirez *et al.* (2008) described a series of patients diagnosed with invasive cervical cancer after undergoing simple hysterectomy who subsequently underwent robotic radical parametrectomy and bilateral pelvic lymphadenectomy. In their results, authors included 5 patients in analysis, with invasive squamous cell carcinoma of the cervix. There were no conversions to laparotomy. There was 1 intraoperative complication—cystotomy. No patient required blood transfusion. The mean duration of hospital stay was 1 day (range, 1 to 2). One patient experienced two postoperative complications, a vesicovaginal fistula and a lymphocyst. No patient had a residual tumor in the parametrectomy specimen, and no patient underwent adjuvant therapy. Median number of pelvic lymph nodes removed was 14 (range, 6 to 16). Median follow-up for all patients was 7.5 months (range, 1.3 to 13.8), without recurrences. In conclusion, Ramirez assessed that robotic radical parametrectomy and bilateral pelvic lymphadenectomy is feasible and safe and can be performed with an acceptable complication rate.

Robotic assistance with the Da Vinci system provides the surgeon with more precise dissection conditions, thanks to the three-dimensional visualization, instrumentation with articulating tips, that allows the surgeon's hands more mobility and decreases tremor movements. This increased precision in procedure as compared with classical laparoscopy is particularly important in the para-aortic region and may enhance safety and decrease intraoperative morbidity.

10   Fertility-sparing Surgery in Cervical Cancer

The incidences of cervical cancer are increasing in young women and women are delaying their childbearing. Available literature shows that there are interesting fertility-sparing treatment alternatives to the "golden standard" for the management of early cervical cancer in young women. So, the fertility-sparing surgery becomes an option for young women affected by cervical cancer. Fertility-sparing surgery can be offered to carefully selected patients with cervical cancer for the management of early-stage (IA or IB1) disease who wish to preserve fertility (Lange *et al.*, 2013). Simple trachelectomy (cervicectomy) and radical trachelectomy (resection of parametrial tissue with cervix) are being used in women with early stage disease. Cervical conization used in preinvasive cancer as investigative biopsy could also become a therapy. Randomized controlled trials of fertility-preserving surgery are impractical and unfeasible; however, radical trachelectomy has been retrospectively shown to have similar oncologic outcomes to radical hysterectomy in select patients with stage IB1 cervical cancer. In patients with stage IA1 cervical cancer, conization is a valid alternative. Patients with stage IA2-IB1 disease can be conservatively treated by radical trachelectomy. This is as well-established conservative approach and appears to be safe and effective in allowing a high chance of conception (Lange *et al.*, 1986).

Prematurity is the most serious issue in pregnancies following trachelectomy. Less invasive options such as simple trachelectomy or conization seem to be feasible for stages IA2-IB1, but more and better evidence is needed. Neoadjuvant therapy might allow conservative surgery to be performed, also in patients with more extensive lesions. Ovarian transposition is important when adjuvant radiation is needed (Noyes *et al.*, 2011).

Trachelectomy has been adopted by many oncological centers all over the world with good oncological and obstetric results. The selection of patients by adequate preoperative evaluation is an important process before a decision regarding conservative treatment is taken. Lesionextent is of great importance; the tumor should be small in size and confined to the cervix without parametrial invasion or spread to the uterine corpus. A 19% recurrence rate has been reported for patients with lesions >2   cm and 25% for those with lesions >2   cm and depth of invasion > 1 cm (Lambaudie *et al.*, 2010 Ramirez *et al.*, 2008).

Radical trachelectomy is performed in select patients diagnosed with early-stage cervical cancer who wish to preserve their fertility. Since the procedure was first described by Dargent *et al.* (1994), numerous reports have documented the safety and feasibility of the vaginal approach (Beiner *et al.*, 2008; Dursun *et al.*, 2007; Hertel *et al.*, 2006; Plante, 2008; Ungar *et al.*, 2005). Alternatively, the procedure may also be performed successfully via the abdominal approach. Several groups have published works on the success rate and feasibility of the abdominal approach (Geisler *et al.*, 2008; Pergialiotis *et al.*, 2013).

The first to report on robotic radical trachelectomy were Geisler *et al.* (2008), who reported on a patient with stage IB1 cervix adenosarcoma. In this case, total operative timewas 172 min, and the estimated blood loss was 100 ml. No residual tumor was found in the surgical specimen, and all lymph nodes were negative for any evidence of disease .

Persson *et al.* (2008) published on 2 patients who underwent robotic radical trachelectomy. One patient was diagnosed with a stage IB1 cervix adenocarcinoma and the other with a stage IA2 squamous cervix carcinoma. This group of investigators was the first to publish on robotic radical trachelectomy in conjunction with lymphatic mapping and sentinel node identification. In that study, console time was 387 min for the first patient and 359 min for the second. Estimated blood loss was 150 ml for the first patient and 100 ml for the second. The authors reported no intraoperative complications. Neither patient had residual cancer or evidence of lymph node disease.

Chuang *et al.* (2008) described a robotic radical trachelectomy in a young woman with cervical cancer who desired preservation of fertility; the patient had previously undergone a cervical conization procedure, with negative margins. Findings at positron emission tomography and computed tomography were normal, and there was no evidence of metastasis before surgery. The operation lasted 345 minutes, with 200 mL blood loss. Final pathologic analysis showed no evidence of residual cancer. All reported cases were completed successfully and highlight robotic-assisted laparoscopy as a useful approach to trachelectomy in appropriate patients.

As one could argue that parametrectomy is not necessary for small tumours, it is relevant that this approach allows one to tailor the extent of parametrectomy according to the size of the tumour. Potentially, this minimally invasive approach may also overcome a severe disadvantage of abdominal trachelectomy, namely that pregnancy rate is much lower than after vaginal radical trachelectomy, but series are as yet too small to assess this potential benefit.

The robotic approach also seems safe in cases where surgery follows neoadjuvant chemotherapy for locoregional extensive tumours. In a study comparing robot-assisted laparoscopy, conventional laparoscopy and laparotomy groups, there was no difference in the recurrence rate (27.3 %, 29.4 % and 30 %, respectively) (Burnett *et al.*, 2009; Dargent *et al.*, 1994).

Ramirez *et al.* (2010) described their surgical technique in a retrospective review on 4 patients who underwent robotic radical trachelectomy and bilateral pelvic lymphadenectomy from October 2008 to May 2009. Their analysis included 4 patients with early-stage squamous cell carcinoma of the cervix. The median body mass index was 27.1 kg/m2 (range, 22.7 to 39.1). Three patients had stage IA2 adenocarcinoma; 1 patient had stage IA1 adenocarcinoma with lymph-vascular space invasion. Median operative time was 339.5 min (range, 245 to 416). Median console time was 282.5 min (range, 217 to 338). Median estimated blood loss was 62.5 ml (range, 50 to 75). There were no conversions to laparotomy. There were no intraoperative complications. No patient required blood transfusion. The mean duration of hospital stay was 1.5 days (range, 1 to 2). One patient experienced a postoperative complication, transient left lower extremity sensory neuropathy. No patient had residual tumor in the trachelectomy specimen, and no patient underwent adjuvant therapy. The median number of pelvic lymph nodes removed was 20 (range, 18 to 27). The median time to a successful voiding trial was 8 days (range, 7 to 9). The median follow-up was 105 days (range, 82 to 217). There were no recurrences. Ramirez *et al.* concluded that robotic radical trachelectomy and bilateral pelvic lymphadenectomy is feasible and safe and should be considered for patients desiring fertility-sparing surgery.

There is increasing evidence in literature that not only is radical trachelectomy feasible and safe but the oncologic outcomes are similar to those of equivalent patients undergoing radical hysterectomy. In a recent article, Diaz *et al.* (2008) compared the outcomes of 40 patients with stage IB1 cervical cancer who underwent radical trachelectomy and 110 patients with stage IB1 cervical cancer who underwent radical hysterectomy. The median follow-up time was 44 months. The 5-year recurrence-free survival rate was 96% for the radical trachelectomy group compared to 86% for the radical hysterectomy group (p=NS). The authors concluded that for select patients with stage IB1 cervical cancer, fertility-sparing radical trachelectomy appears to produce oncologic outcomes similar to those after radical hysterectomy.

Recently, many studies analysed the reproductive outcome after fertility-sparing radical trachelectomy. One of these studies was performed by Kim *et al.* (2012) on 105 patients who underwent RT. 77 (73%) did not require a conversion to radical hysterectomy or postoperative treatment. Median age was 32 (range, 25-38 years). Most patients (75%) had stage IB1 disease. Sixty-six patients (63%) were nulliparous. Thirty-five women were actively attempting conception 6 months after surgery, and 23 (66%) women were successful in conceiving: there were 20 live births, 3 elective terminations, and 4 spontaneous miscarriages. Four patients had 2 pregnancies each; all delivered their second pregnancy between 32 and 36 weeks. Cerclage erosion through the vaginal wall occurred in 6 cases and was treated by transvaginal removal of protruding suture material. One of these patients experienced a second trimester miscarriage. In conclusion: the majority of women who attempted to conceive after radical trachelectomy were successful, and most of their pregnancies resulted in full-term births.

Finally, even more intriguing, recent studies have suggested that even more conservative techniques such as cervical conization, with or without pelvic lymphadenectomy, may be applicable in treatment of early-stage cervical cancer including stage IB1 (Maneo *et al.*, 2011). If the surgical community accepts the findings of these early reports, minimally invasive techniques including simple conization or trachelectomy plus lymphadenectomy may need to either become more challenging, with cases with more advanced presurgical staging, or totally lose ground as treatment alternatives. Assisted reproduction played an important role in select women. Cerclage likely contributed to a post-trachelectomy uterine ability to carry a pregnancy to the third trimester. The second post-trachelectomy pregnancy appears to be at higher risk for preterm delivery than the first pregnancy. In term of histopatological outcomes there is no evidence.

11   Comparison between Laparoscopy and Robotic in Radical Hysterectomy

There is a growing trend to practice less aggressive surgery in order to preserve fertility in young women and avoid an excess of treatment in some selected patients and nerve-sparing techniques can help to improve the quality of life. Laparoscopic robotic-assisted radical hysterectomy with nerve sparing technique is an attractive surgical approach for early invasive cervical cancer. Robotic technology allows a stereoscopic visualization of blood vessels and autonomic nerve supplies (sympathetic and parasympathetic branches) to the bladder and rectum making nerve sparing a safe and feasible procedure (Gil-Ibáñez *et al.*, 2013).

Magrina *et al.* (2008) recently presented the first prospective study comparing the perioperative results of patients undergoing radical hysterectomy and lymph node dissection by robotics, laparoscopy and laparotomy. Mean operating time for a robotic, laparoscopic and radical hysterectomy per laparotomy was 190, 220 and 167 min, respectively; mean blood loss was 133, 208 and 444 mL respectively; mean number of removed lymph nodes was 26, 26 and 28, respectively, and mean hospital stay was 1.7, 2.4 and 3.6 days, respectively. There were no significant differences in intra- or postoperative complications among the three groups and no conversions in the robotics or laparoscopic groups. At a mean follow up of 31 months, none of the patients with cervical cancer experienced a recurrence. The authors concluded that laparoscopy and robotics are preferable to laparotomy for patients requiring radical hysterectomy, with advantages like significantly shorter operating times noted for robotics over laparoscopy. Their results are in accordance with other groups, although some reported the feasibility of a more radical lymph node dissection with the robotic system when compared to conventional laparoscopy (Boggess, 2007; Kim *et al.*, 2008). Several case reports suggest that debulking surgery is a further potential application for robotics surgery in gynaecological oncology (Chavin, 2008; van Dam *et al.*, 2007).

In a recent paper, Cho and Nezhat (2009) compared robotic and laparoscopy in gynecological oncology. The objectives of their article were to review the published scientific literature about robotics and its application to gynecologic oncology to date and to summarize findings of this advanced computer enhanced laparoscopic technique. Relevant sources were identified by a search of PUBMED from January 1950 to January 2009 using the key words Robot or Robotics and Cervical cancer, Endometrial cancer, Gynecologic oncology, and Ovarian cancer. Appropriate case reports, case series, retrospective studies, prospective trials, and review articles were selected. A total of 38 articles were identified on the subject, and 27 were included in the study. The data for gynecologic cancer show comparable results between robotic and laparoscopic surgery for estimated blood loss, operative time, length of hospital stay, and complications. Overall, there were more wound complications with the laparotomy approach compared with laparoscopy and robotic-assisted laparoscopy. There were more lymphocysts, lymphoceles, and lymphedema in the robotic-assisted laparoscopic group compared with the laparoscopy and laparotomy groups in patients with cervical cancer. Overall, 126 robotic-assisted laparoscopies, 68 laparoscopies, and 136 laparotomies were performed in the cohort studies of cervical cancer, each with varying intraoperative and postoperative issues. In the robotic-assisted laparoscopy group, there were 24 complications, with lymphocysts or lymphoceles, infections, and vaginal cuff complications most commonly reported. In the traditional laparoscopy group, there were 16 complications, with lymphocysts or lymphoceles and infections most commonly reported. In the laparotomy group, there were 24 complications, with adverse wound and gastrointestinal sequelae most commonly reported.

Computer-enhanced technology may enable more surgeons to convert laparotomies to laparoscopic surgery with its associated benefits. It seems that in the hands of experienced laparoscopic surgeons, final outcomes are the same with or without use of the robot (Cho & Nezhat, 2009).

Lambaudie *et al.* (2010) compared the feasibility and efficacy of 22 robot-assisted laparoscopies with 20 traditional laparotomy and 16 conventional laparoscopy in a series of patients with locally advanced cervical cancer managed in two institutions. In the results, there was no significant difference between the three groups in terms of body mass index, FIGO stage, or tumor histology. Complication rate was similar in the three groups of patients, although there was a trend towards more lymphatic complications in the robot-assisted subgroup managed medically. There was no significant difference in the recurrence rate between the robot-assisted laparoscopy, conventional laparoscopy and laparotomy groups (27.3%, 29.4% and 30%, respectively). Authors concluded that robot-assisted laparoscopy is feasible after concurrent chemoradiation and brachytherapy in cases of locally advanced cervical cancer, reduces hospital stay, and seems to result in less severe complications than conventional laparotomy without modifying the oncological outcome.

12   Complications of Endoscopy in Cervical Cancer

Robotics, like any novel technology, has its advantages, disadvantages and reported complications. In the modern era of minimally invasive techniques, current developments in surgical robotics represent only the initial attempts to simplify complex laparoscopic procedures, providing precision in dexterity and perfection of repetitive tasks such as suturing. The current evidence shows that minimally invasive surgery is associated with less morbidity compared with open surgery and can be considered as an alternate option for surgical management of cervical cancer without compromising the oncologic outcome. There are several studies in literature, which compared laparoscopic or robotic surgeries with open method. In a majority of the studies, the operating time for laparoscopy was higher compared with the open method (Li *et al.*, 2007; Malzoni *et al.*, 2009).

In comparative studies, laparoscopic and robotic methods were associated with shorter hospital stay when compared to the open method. Mean blood loss and transfusion rates were more for the open method. In a comparative study between laparoscopic and robotic radical hysterectomy, Nezhat *et al.* (2008) showed that there is no difference between operating time, hospital stay, mean pelvic lymph node yield or intraoperative or postoperative complications between the robotic and laparoscopic method. The complication rates of robotic radical hysterectomy are lower compared to our historical cohort of radical hysterectomy by standard laparotomy.

Many authors and surgeons affirm that some complications may be associated with robotic or laparoscopic surgery per se. The frequent reported complications are on vaginal cuff (dehiscence, lymphatic leaking, infection, hematoma, vault prolapse, short vagina), on the lymphatic system (proximal lymphedema, mild distal lymphedema, severe distal lymphedema, lymphocyst), on the neural peripheral system (genitofemoral nerve injury, partial obturator nerve palsy), on the abdominal wall (port site hernia, port site muscle rupture, hematoma, port site metastases) and the vascular system (postop hemoglobin and/or transfusion, ovarian vein thrombosis and pulmonary embolism).

Symptomatic postoperative lymphocysts (SPOLs) and lower-limb lymphedema (LLL) are probably underestimated complications of lymphadenectomy for gynecologic malignancies. Adjuvant radiotherapy was significantly associated with the development of lymphedema in women who had undergone radical surgery with lymphadenectomy for FIGO stage I to stage IIA cervical cancer (odds ratio, 3.47; 95% confidence interval, 2.086-5.788; P = 0.000) (Kim et al., 2012). Moreover, there are also risks of infection by pneumonia, with pyelonephritis and/or fever of unknown origin, a risk of ureter stenosis and of uncorrected positioning, with arm/shoulder/leg pain.

In the Piver study, there were 2 deaths (one from pneumonia and one from pelvic abscess), 2 pulmonary emboli, one ureterovaginal fistula and one ureteral stricture and a total of 15 complications in 55 patients who underwent type III open radical hysterectomy (27%). Moreover, Piver et al. (1974) showed a 5-year disease-free interval of 87.5–100% in women with cervical cancers less than 3 cm treated by type III radical hysterectomy.

About the incidence of port site hernia and/or dehiscence after laparoscopic surgery and robotic assisted surgery in oncology, literature has recent evidences. The incidence of port site hernia and/or dehiscence using bladeless trocars is 0-1.2%. Robotic surgery uses additional port sites and increases manipulation of instruments, raising the concern for more complications. Authors reviewed Robotically-assisted (RA) 842 procedures performed for suspected gynecologic malignancy between 1/2006 and 12/2011. Bladeless 12mm and 8mm robotic trocars were used. Fascial closure was not routinely performed except after specimen removal through the port site. The decision to close the fascia remained at the discretion of the surgeon. RA-total laparoscopic hysterectomy (TLH)±unilateral or bilateral salpingo-oophorectomy (BSO)±lymphadenectomy (LND) accounted for 91.6% of procedures. Final pathology confirmed malignancy in 58.6% of cases, primarily endometrial cancer. In 35 cases, the specimen was removed through the port site; fascia was closed in 54.3% of them and no port site hernias or dehiscences occurred. In the study conclusion, authors affirmed that port site hernias and dehiscences are rare in RA gynecologic oncology procedures. When bladeless dilating trocars are used, routine closure of even up to a 12mm port site is unnecessary, even in cases requiring removal of the specimen through the trocar sites (Boone et al., 2013).

13   Literature Drawbacks Concerning Robotic Surgery in Gynaecological Oncology

In recent years, robotic surgery or robot assisted surgery has been developed to support a range of surgical procedures. Robotic surgery in cervical and endometrial cancer is one of the fastest growing areas.

Robotic surgical systems have been used to perform surgery for endometrial, cervical cancer and ovarian cancer. There is mounting evidence which demonstrates the feasibility and safety of robotic surgery for gynaecological oncology.

Cochrane Gynaecological Cancer Group evaluated in 2012 all randomised controlled trials (RCTs) comparing robotic assisted surgery for gynaecological cancer to laparoscopic or open surgical procedures as well as RCTs comparing different types of robotic assistants. To review authors independently screened studies for inclusion and no RCTs were identified (Lu *et al.*, 2012). The robotic approach was explored in a study by Lambaudie *et al* (2010); it seemed safe in cases where surgery follows neoadjuvant chemotherapy for locoregional extensive tumours. In a study comparing robot-assisted laparoscopy, conventional laparoscopy and laparotomy groups, there was no difference in the recurrence rate (27.3 %, 29.4 % and 30 %, respectively). Although already known to be commoner after laparoscopic hysterectomy than after laparotomy (Chan *et al.*, 2012), a particularly striking finding is a relative high number, up to 20 %, of patients with vaginal dehiscence after robot-assisted laparoscopic surgery (Persson *et al.*, 2009). This may be explained by the initial use of extensive cautery or tight suturing, causing necrosis. Although some authors reported a significant decrease in vaginal cuff dehiscence when closing the vagina vaginally instead of laparoscopically (Uccella *et al.*, 2011), others did not find a difference between the methods of closure (Hwang *et al.*, 2011).

In recent series, this complication seems to occur less prominently than in the past, maybe due to caution with cautery and the use of self-locking sutures. Published experience has suggested that the outcomes with Robotic Radical Hysterectomy (RRH) are similar to that for patients undergoing a traditional radical hysterectomy via an exploratory laparotomy (Cantrell *et al.*, 2010; Estape *et al.*, 2009; Maggioni *et al.*, 2009). These primarily single institution series have compared primarily surgical outcomes of patients undergoing RRH with Laparoscopic RH and/or Abdominal RH. Secondary to the relatively recent introduction of roboticassisted radical hysterectomies, limited information regarding oncologic outcomes specifically in terms of survival is available. Overall, these studies have suggested that robotic surgery is generally longer, with less estimated blood loss and similar nodal yield.

Lowe *et al.* (2009) reported their multi-institutional experience in a group of 42 patients undergoing Type II or III RRH. Overall 42 patients underwent either a Type II or III RRH with operative outcomes similar to other series and an overall low complication rate of 4.8%. Many authors affirmed that robotic total laparoscopic radical hysterectomy with pelvic and para-aortic lymphadenectomy is feasible and may be preferable over laparoscopic or radical abdominal hysterectomy. They reported advantages to both minimally invasive approaches, with decreased average estimated blood loss, length of stay, number of catheter days, days on pain medication, and a faster return to work in both the robotic and laparoscopic groups when compared to laparotomy.

Even with increased visualization and surgical precision, complications still may occur. A large review from Kho *et al.* (2009) at the Scottsdale Arizona Mayo Clinic of >500 patients undergoing various robotic-assisted surgical procedures noted a 4.1% (95% CI 2.3–5.8%) vaginal cuff dehiscence rate. Of these 21 patients, 9 (43%) had a pre-operative diagnosis of cancer including 3 with cervical carcinoma. This rate is similar to the 7.5% incidence seen in the cervical cancer series from Italy by Maggioni *et al.* (2009), although as they note in their follow-up letter to the editor, following a modification in surgical technique, the incidence in their patients has decreased to 1% (Sert, 2010). Although unlikely, based on the size of the predicted fascial defect, herniation of small bowel through an 8-mm robotic trocar has been reported (Seamon *et al.*, 2008).

The published data comparing different surgical approaches to radical hysterectomy, including traditional laparoscopy or laparotomy show that the robotic approach produces more favorable perioperative outcomes, such as less blood loss, abbreviated hospitalizations, and equivalent or lower rates of intraoperative and postoperative complications. While these series are relatively small and non-randomized, they consistently demonstrate safety and efficacy with respect to complications, blood loss, operative time and patient convalescence comparing robotic assisted surgery with laparoscopy (Estape *et al.*, 2009; Magrina *et al.*, 2008; Nezhat, 2008; Symmonds, 1975). Despite that these findings are consistently reproducible in larger and multi-institutional studies, there are no prospective data to resolve these unequivocal comparisons in cervical cancer patients. We hope that the prospective randomized controlled trial that is currently ongoing will provide further insight. Although robotic-assisted technology is supposedly an enhancement of conventional laparoscopy, several studies have reported conversion of the robotic approach to laparotomy, not laparoscopy. There were 6 conversions from robotic-assisted laparoscopy to laparotomy in 2 studies (Boggess *et al.*, 2008).

14   Pro and Contra of Robotic Assisted Surgery

In 2005, the first feasibility studies in both Europe and the United States were published, since robotic-assisted procedures provide several advantages. Binocular vision and 3-dimensional views permit improved depth perception, which may facilitate advanced laparoscopic procedures, such as intracorporeal suturing. The console is located away from the patient and permits the surgeon to operate in a comfortable, seated position, thus making operator positioning more ergonomic.

Tremor filtration is another benefit of robotic-assisted surgery, as the video laparoscope is no longer in a human hand, which may tire or move, but rather is fixed in position by the robotic arm. This feature permits finer surgical movements with more precise dissections. The articulating instrument tips that are utilized in traditional laparoscopy are taken to a new level with not only rotational capabilities but an independent 90-degree articulation of the tip. These features make robotic surgery more intuitive, with a shorter learning curve. Additional robotic arms have been introduced to further minimize the need for surgical assistants in institutions that may have limited staff.

Robotic-assisted procedures are not, however, without their limitations. The equipment is still very large, bulky, and expensive. The staff must be trained specifically on draping and docking the apparatus to maintain efficient operative times. Functional limitations include lack of haptic feedback, limited vaginal access, limited instrumentation, and larger port incisions requiring fascial closure. In terms of haptic feedback, visual cues become imperative to ensure that tissue manipulation is not performed with undue force. Intracorporeal knots must be tied carefully such that the suture is not avulsed by the strength imposed by the robotic arm. Limited vaginal access can be problematic in gynecologic surgery as frequent uterine or vaginal manipulation is necessary, particularly in extirpative procedures. Once the robot has ascended into place, access to the vagina becomes markedly limited. Robotic accessory trocars are 8 mm in size with a 12 mm laparoscope. These incision sizes are larger than the 5 mm accessories that are frequently used in traditional laparoscopy and also require fascial closure, with higher risks of herniation.

The robot is also limited in its instrumentation. Exchanging instruments becomes more cumbersome and requires a surgical assistant to change the instruments. Additionally, the current robotic instruments do not include endoscopic staplers or vessel sealing devices. Moreover, the trocars required for robotic procedures are larger than those used for traditional laparoscopy. In radical hysterectomy, the dissection of the uterine arteries, ureteral tunneling, and vaginal cuff closure are among the most useful indications for robotic-assisted procedures. The greater range of motion afforded by the robotic instruments permits easier maneuverability for these dissections.

These multiple optional of robotic-assisted surgery had been evaluated by literature. A recent paper on robotics has definitely been shown that robotic surgeries are more costly than regular laparoscopic approaches (Shah *et al.*, 2011). Nevertheless, one study found an additional $3000 in operative case per robot-assisted vs laparoscopic hysterectomy (Jonsdottir *et al.*, 2011). This cost differential may change with a decrease as other robotic systems come on line in the future. Moreover, another blinded, prospective randomized controlled trial comparing operative time and intra- and postoperative complications between total laparoscopic hysterectomy and robotic-assisted total laparoscopic hysterectomy, concluded that, although laparoscopic and robotic-assisted hysterectomies are safe approaches to hysterectomy, robotic-assisted hysterectomy requires a significantly longer operative time. The lengthier times in the robot group are likely due to operating room set up, docking time, troubleshooting of technical aspects that may be faulty with the robot (e.g., collision of arms, malfunctioning instrumentation), and less efficient electrosurgical vessel-sealing instrumentation for robot-assisted surgery during the time that this trial was undertaken (Paraiso *et al.*, 2013).

A recent investigation show that robotic-assisted laparoscopy is safe, effective, and successful in obese and morbidly obese patients who undergo hysterectomy for malignancy which further decreases the incidence of laparotomy in the future (Leitao *et al.*, 2012) and an American study on 1000 cases on robotic surgery (RS) in oncology from May 2006 through December 2009, analyzed patient characteristics and outcomes on a total of 377 women undergoing RS for endometrial cancer staging (ECS), compared with the historical data of 131 undergoing open ECS. Authors concluded that RS is associated with favorable morbidity and conversion rates in an unselected cohort. Compared to laparotomy, robotic ECS results in improved outcomes (Paley *et al.*, 2011). Thus, after data revision, robot-assisted hysterectomy does not confer any perioperative patient benefits over laparoscopic hysterectomy in the hands of experienced conventional laparoscopic surgeons, except in gynecological oncology, where robotics have advantages (Rodriguez, 2013).

15   Conclusions

The robotic-assisted surgery has emerged as an invaluable minimally invasive approach to comprehensive surgical staging and the treatment of cervical cancer. There is good evidence that robotic surgery facilitates laparoscopic surgery, with equivalent if not better operative time and comparable surgical outcomes, shorter hospital stay, and fewer major complications than with surgeries using the laparotomy approach. And the role of robotic-assisted surgery is still expanding (Krill & Bristow, 2013). In addition to radical hysterectomy, gynecologic oncologists are applying robotic technology to ovarian transposition, lymphadenectomy, and even tumor debulking. Some future directions that will further the scope of robotic-assisted surgery include incorporation of the robotic system in the operating room facility to permit better accessibility to the patient during the procedure as well as expansion in instrumentation. Total laparoscopic radical hysterectomy is a feasible and safe procedure that is associated with fewer intraoperative and postoperative complications than abdominal radical hysterectomy. Longer follow-up is needed, but early data are supportive of at least equivalent oncologic outcomes compared with other surgical modalities. The role of robotic-assisted surgery is continuing to expand and new promising approaches with added benefits are emerging, such as the one of the ALF-X system. Surgeons await results from additional series of radical hysterectomy performed by robo-endoscopic assisted surgery and from International prospective randomized trial evaluating outcomes in patients randomly assigned to either open or laparoscopic/robotic radical hysterectomy.

References

Abu-Rustum NR, Gemignani ML, Moore K, Sonoda Y, Venkatraman E, Brown C, et al.. Total laparoscopic radical hysterectomy with pelvic lymphadenectomy using the argon-beam coagulator: pilot data and comparison to laparotomy. Gynecol Oncol 2003;91(2):402–9.

Abu-Rustum NR, Hoskins WJ. Radical abdominal hysterectomy. Surg Clin NorthAm 2001;81:815–28.

Averette HE, Nguyen HN, Donato DM, Penalver MA, Sevin BU, Estape R, Little WA. Radical hysterectomy for invasive cervical cancer. A 25-year prospective experience with the Miami technique. Cancer 1993;71(4 Suppl):1422-37.

Beiner ME, Hauspy J, Rosen B, Murphy J, Laframboise S, Nofech-Mozes S, Ismiil N, Rasty G, Khalifa MA, Covens A. Radical vaginal trachelectomy vs. radical hysterectomy for small early stage cervical cancer: a matched case-control study. Gynecol Oncol 2008;110:168–71.

Boggess JF, Gehrig PA, Cantrell L, et al.. A case–control study of robot-assisted type III radical hysterectomy with pelvic lymph node dissection compared with open radical hysterectomy. Am J Obstet Gynecol. 2008;199:357.e1–7.

Boggess JF, Gehrig PA, Cantrell L, Shafer A, Ridgway M, Skinner EN, Fowler WC. A comparative study of 3 surgical methods for hysterectomy with staging for endometrial cancer: Robotic assistance, laparoscopy, laparotomy. Am J Obstet Gynecol 2008;199:360:1-9.

Boggess JF. Robotic surgery in gynecologic oncology: evolution of a new surgical paradigm. J Robotic Surgery 2007;1(1):31–7.

Boggess JF. Robotic-assisted radical hysterectomy for cervical cancer: National Library of Medicine Archives. 2006 [updated 2006; cited 2008 11/08/2008]; Available from: http://www.nlm.nih.gov/medlineplus/surgeryvideos.html

Boone JD, Fauci JM, Barr ES, Estes JM, Bevis KS. Incidence of port site hernias and/or dehiscence in robotic-assisted procedures in gynecologic oncology patients. Gynecol Oncol. 2013 Jul 9. doi:pii: S0090-8258(13)00915-3. 10.1016/j.ygyno.2013.06.041. [Epub ahead of print]

Burnett AF, Stone PJ, Duckworth LA. Robotic radical trachelectomy for preservation of fertility in early cervical cancer: case series and description of technique. J Minim Invasive Gynecol. 2009;16:569–72.

Canis M, Mage G, Pouly JL, Pomel C, Wattiez A, Glowaczover E, Bruhat MA. Laparoscopic radical hysterectomy for cervical cancer. Baillieres Clin Obstet Gynaecol 1995;9:675–89.

Canis M, Mage G, Wattiez A, Pouly JL, Manhes H, Bruhat MA. Does endoscopic surgery have a role in radical surgery of cancer of the cervix uteri?.J Gynecol Obstet Biol Reprod (Paris) 1990;19:921.

Cantrell LA, Mendevil A, Gehring PA, Boggess JF. Survival outcomes for women undergoing type III robotic radical hysterectomy for cervical cancer: A 3-year experience. Gynecol Oncol 2010;117:260–265.

Chan WS, Kong KK, Nikam YA, Merkur H. Vaginal vault dehiscence after laparoscopic hysterectomy over a nine-year period at Sydney West Advanced Pelvic Surgery Unit - our experiences and current understanding of vaginal vault dehiscence. Aust N Z J Obstet Gynaecol. 2012 Apr;52(2):121-7.

Chavin G. Robotic-assisted laparoscopy for the excision of a pelvic leiomyosarcoma. J Robotic Surg 2008; 1: 315–317.

Chen Y, Xu H, Li Y, Wang D, Li J, Yuan J, Liang Z. The outcome of laparoscopic radical hysterectomy and lymphadenectomy for cervical cancer: a prospective analysis of 295 patients. Ann Surg Oncol 2008;15:2847–55.

Cho JE, Nezhat FR. Robotics and Gynecologic Oncology: Review of the Literature. J Minim Invasive Gynecol 2009; 16 (6):669-681

Chuang LT, Lerner DL, Liu CS, Nezhat FR. Fertility-sparing robotic assisted radical trachelectomy and bilateral pelvic lymphadenectomy in early-stage cervical cancer. J Minim Invasive Gynecol. 2008;15:767–770.

Colombo PE, Bertrand MM, Gutowski M, Mourregot A, Fabbro M, Saint-Aubert B, Quenet F, Gourgou S, Kerr C, Rouanet P. Total laparoscopic radical hysterectomy for locally advanced cervical carcinoma (stages IIB, IIA and bulky stages IB) after concurrent chemoradiation therapy: Surgical morbidity and oncological results Gynecol Oncol 2009;114:404–409.

Dargent D, Ansquer Y, Mathevet P. Technical development and results of left extraperitoneal laparoscopic para-aortic lymphadenectomy for cervical cancer. Gynecol Oncol 2000;77:87–92.

Dargent D, Brun JL, Roy M, Remy I. Pregnancies following radical trachelectomy for invasive cervical cancer (Abstract). Gynecol Oncol 1994;52:105.

Dargent D, Martin X, Sacchetoni A, Mathevet P. Laparoscopic vaginal radical trachelectomy: a treatment to preserve the fertility of cervical carcinoma patients. Cancer 2000;88:1877–82.

Dargent D. A new future for Schauta's operation through pre-surgical retroperitoneal pelviscopy. Eur J Gynaecol Oncol. 1987;8:292–6.

Decloedt J, Vergote I. Laparoscopy in gynaecologic oncology: a review. Crit Rev Oncol Hematol 1999;31:15–26.

Denschlag D, Gabriel B, Mueller-Lantzsch C, Tempfer C, Henne K, Gitsch G, Hasenburg A. Evaluation of patients after extraperitoneal lymph node dissection for cervical cancer. Gynecol Oncol 2005;96(3):658–64.

Diaz JP, Sonoda Y, Leitao MM, Zivanovic O, Brown CL, Chi DS, Barakat RR, Abu-Rustum NR. Oncologic outcomes of fertility-sparing radical trachelectomy versus radical hysterectomy for stage IB1 cervical carcinoma. Gynecol Oncol 2008;111:255–60.

Dursun P, LeBlanc E, Nogueira MC. Radical vaginal trachelectomy (Dargent's operation): a critical review of the literature. Eur J Surg Oncol 2007;33:933–41.

Estape R, Lambrou N, Diaz R, Estape E, Dunkin N, Rivera A. A case matched analysis of robotic radical hysterectomy with lymphadenectomy compared with laparoscopy and laparotomy. Gynecol Oncol. 2009;113(3):357-61.

Fanning J, Fenton B, Purohit M. Robotic radical hysterectomy. Am J Obstet Gynecol 2008;198:649:1-4.

Fastrez M, Vandromme J, George P, Rozenberg S, Degueldre M. Robot assisted laparoscopic transperitoneal para-aortic lymphadenectomy in the management of advanced cervical carcinoma. Eur J Obstet Gynaecol Reprod Biol 2009; 147:226–229.

Frumovitz M, dos Reis R, Sun CC, Milam MR, Bevers MW, Brown J, Slomovitz BM, Ramirez PT. Comparison of total laparoscopic and abdominal radical hysterectomy for patients with early-stage cervical cancer. Obstet Gynecol 2007;110:96–102.

Frumovitz M, Ramirez PT, Greer M, Gregurich MA, Wolf J, Bodurka DC, Levenback C. Laparoscopic training and practice in gynecologic oncology among Society of Gynecologic Oncologists members and fellow-in-training. Gynecol Oncol 2004;94:746–53.

Fujii S, Tanakura K, Matsumura N, Higuchi T, Yura S, Mandai M, Baba T. Precise anatomy of the vesico-uterine ligament for radical hysterectomy. Gynecol Oncol 2007; 104: 186–91.

Geisler JP, Orr CJ, Manahan KJ. Robotically assisted total laparoscopic radical trachelectomy for fertility sparing in stage IB1 adenosarcoma of the cervix. J Laparoendosc Adv Surg Tech 2008;18:727–9.

Gil-Ibáñez B, Díaz-Feijoo B, Pérez-Benavente A, Puig-Puig O, Franco-Camps S, Centeno C, Xercavins J, Gil-Moreno A. Nerve sparing technique in robotic-assisted radical hysterectomy: results. Int J Med Robot. 2013 Sep;9(3):339-44.

Hatch KD, Hallum 3rd AV, Nour M. New surgical approaches to treatment of cervical cancer. J Natl Cancer Inst Monogr 1996:71–5.

Hertel H, Kohler C, Grund D, Hillemanns P, Possover M, Michels W, Schneider A; German Association of Gynecologic Oncologists (AGO). Radical vaginal trachelectomy (RVT) combined with laparoscopic pelvic lymphadenectomy: prospective multicenter study of 100 patients with early cervical cancer. Gynecol Oncol 2006;103:506–11.

Hsieh YY, Lin WC, Chang CC, Yeh LS, Hsu TY, Tsai HD. Laparoscopic radical hysterectomy with low paraaortic, subaortic and pelvic lymphadenectomy. Results of short-term follow-up. J Reprod Med 1998;43:528–34.

Hwang JH, Lee JK, Lee NW, Lee KW. Vaginal cuff closure: a comparison between the vaginal route and laparoscopic suture in patients undergoing total laparoscopic hysterectomy. Gynecol Obstet Invest. 2011;71(3):163-9.

Jonsdottir GM, Jorgensen S, Cohen SL, Wright KN, Shah NT, Chavan N, Einarsson JI. Increasing minimally invasive hysterectomy: effect on cost and complications. Obstet Gynecol. 2011 May;117(5):1142-9.

Kho RM, Akl MN, Cornella JL, Magtibay PM, Wechter ME, Magrina JF. Incidence and characteristics of patients with vaginal cuff dehiscence after robotic procedures. Obstet Gynecol. 2009 Aug;114(2 Pt 1):231-5.

Kim DH, Moon JS. Laparoscopic radical hysterectomy with pelvic lymphadenectomy for early, invasive cervical carcinoma. J Am Assoc Gynecol Laparosc 1998;5:411–7.

Kim JH, Choi JH, Ki EY, Lee SJ, Yoon JH, Lee KH, Park TC, Park JS, Bae SN, Hur SY. Incidence and risk factors of lower-extremity lymphedema after radical surgery with or without adjuvant radiotherapy in patients with FIGO stage I to stage IIA cervical cancer. Int J Gynecol Cancer. 2012;22(4):686-91

Kim YT, Kim SW, Hyung WJ, Lee SJ, Nam EJ, Lee WJ. Robotic radical hysterectomy with pelvic lymphadenectomy for cervical carcinoma: A pilot study. Gynecol Oncol 2008; 108:312–316.

Ko EM, Muto MG, Berkowitz RS, Feltmate CM. Robotic versus open radical hysterectomy: A comparative study at a single institution. Gynecol Oncol 2008;111:425–430.

Kobayashi T. Abdominal radical hysterectomy with pelvic lymphadenectomy for cancer of the cervix. Tokyo: Nanzando, 1961: 178.

Kohler C, Klemm P, Schau A, Possover M, Krause N, Tozzi R, Schneider A. Introduction of transperitoneal lymphadenectomy in a gynecologic oncology center: analysis of 650 laparoscopic pelvic and/or para-aortic transperitoneal lymphadenectomies. Gynecol Oncol 2004;95(1):52–61.

Kohler C, Tozzi R, Klemm P, Schneider A. "Schauta sine utero": technique and results of laparoscopic-vaginal radical parametrectomy. Gynecol Oncol 2003;91:359–68.

Krause N, Schneider A. Laparoscopic radical hysterectomy with para-aortic and pelvic lymphadenectomy. Zentralbl Gynakol 1995;117:346–8.

Krill LS, Bristow RE. Robotic surgery: gynecologic oncology. Cancer J. 2013 Mar-Apr;19(2):167-76.

Kruijdenberg CB, van den Einden LC, Hendriks JC, et al.. Robot-assisted versus total laparoscopic radical hysterectomy in early cervical cancer, a review. Gynecol Oncol. 2011;120:334–9.

Lagasse LD, Creasman WT, Shingleton HM, Ford JH, Blessing JA. Results and complications of operative staging in cervical cancer: experience of the Gynecologic Oncology Group. Gynecol Oncol 1980;9:90.

Lambaudie E, Narducci F, Bannier M. Role of robot-assisted laparoscopy in adjuvant surgery for locally advanced cervical cancer. Eur J Surg Oncol. 2010;36:409–13.

Lange S, Hurst BS, Matthews ML, Tait DL. Fertility preservation in patients with gynecologic cancer – Part I: the impact of Gynecologic Malignancies on fertility. Postgrad Obstet Gynecol 2013;33(13):1-7.

Lange S, Hurst BS, Matthews ML, Tait DL. Fertility preservation in patients with gynecologic cancer – Part II: the impact of Gynecologic Malignancies on fertility. Postgrad Obstet Gynecol 2013;33(14):1-5.

LaPolla JP, Schlaerth JB, Gaddis O, Morrow CP. The influence of surgical staging on the evaluation and treatment of patients with cervical carcinoma. Gynecol Oncol 1986;24:194.

Lecuru F, Taurelle R. Transperitoneal laparoscopic pelvic lymphadenectomy for gynecologic malignancies (II). Indications. Surg Endosc 1998;12:97–100.

Leitao MM Jr, Briscoe G, Santos K, Winder A, Jewell EL, Hoskins WJ, Chi DS, Abu-Rustum NR, Sonoda Y, Brown CL, Levine DA, Barakat RR, Gardner GJ. Introduction of a computer-based surgical platform in the surgical care of patients with newly diagnosed uterine cancer: outcomes and impact on approach. Gynecol Oncol. 2012 May;125(2):394-9.

Li G, Yan X, Shang H, Wang G, Chen L, Han Y. A comparison of laparoscopic radical hysterectomy and pelvic lymphadenectomy and laparotomy in the treatment of Ib-IIa cervical cancer. Gynecol Oncol 2007;105:176–80.

Liang Z, Xu H, Chen Y, Chang Q, Shi C.. Laparoscopic radical trachelectomy or parametrectomy and pelvic and para-aortic lymphadenectomy for cervical or vaginal stump carcinoma: report of six cases. Int J Gynecol Cancer 2006;16:1713–6.

Lowe MP, Chamberlain DH, Kamelle SA, Johnson PR, Tillmanns TD. A multi-institutional experience with robotic-assisted radical hysterectomy for early stage cervical cancer. Gynecol Oncol. 2009;113(2):191-4.

Lu D, Liu Z, Shi G, Liu D, Zhou X. Robotic assisted surgery for gynaecological cancer. Cochrane Database Syst Rev. 2012 Jan 18;1:CD008640.

Maggioni A, Minig L, Zanagnolo V, Peiretti M, Sanguineti F, Bocciolone L, Colombo N, Landoni F, Roviglione G, Vélez JI. Robotic approach for cervical cancer: comparison with laparotomy: a case control study. Gynecol Oncol. 2009 Oct;115(1):60-4.

Magrina JF, Goodrich MA, Lidner TK, Weaver AL, Cornella JL, Podratz KC. Modified radical hysterectomy in the treatment of early squamous cervical cancer. Gynecol Oncol 1999;72(2):183–6.

Magrina JF, Kho RM, Weaver AL, Montero RP, Magtibay PM. Robotic radical hysterectomy: Comparison with laparoscopy and laparotomy. Gynecol Oncol 2008;109:86–91.

Magrina JF. Outcomes of laparoscopic treatment for endometrial cancer. Curr Opin Obstet Gynecol 2005;17(4):343–6.

Magrina JF. Robotic surgery in gynecology. Eur J Gynaecol Oncol 2007; 28: 77–82.

Malzoni M, Malzoni C, Perone C, Rotondi M, Reich H. Total laparoscopic radical hysterectomy (type III) and pelvic lymphadenectomy. Eur J Gynaecol Oncol 2004;25:525–7.

Malzoni M, Tinelli R, Cosentino F, Fusco A, Malzoni C. Total laparoscopic radical hysterectomy versus abdominal radical hysterectomy with lymphadenectomy in patients with early cervical cancer: Our experience. Ann Surg Oncol. 2009;16:1316–23.

Maneo A, Sideri M, Scambia G, Boveri S, Dell'anna T, Villa M, Parma G, Fagotti A, Fanfani F, Landoni F. Simple conization and lymphadenectomy for the conservative treatment of stage IB1 cervical cancer. An Italian experience. Gynecol Oncol. 2011 Dec;123(3):557-60.

Marnitz S, Kohler C, Roth C, Fuller J, Hinkelbein W, Schneider A. Is there a benefit of pretreatment laparoscopic transperitoneal surgical staging in patients with advanced cervical cancer? Gynecol Oncol 2005;99(3):536–44.

Meigs JV. Carcinoma of the cervix—the Wertheim operation. Surg Gynecol Obstet 1944; 78: 195–98.

Mortier DG, Stroobants S, Amant F, Neven P, Van Lambergen E, Vergote I. Laparoscopic para-aortic lymphadenectomy and positron emission tomography scan as staging procedures in patients with cervical carcinoma stage IB2–IIIB. Int J Gynecol Cancer 2008;18:723–9.

Nezhat CR, Burrell MO, Nezhat FR. Laparoscopic radical hysterectomy with paraaortic and pelvic node dissection. Am J Obstet Gynecol. 1992;166:864–5.

Nezhat CR, Nezhat FR, Burrell MO, Ramirez CE, Welander C, Carrodeguas J, Nezhat CH. Laparoscopic radical hysterectomy and laparoscopically assisted vaginal radical hysterectomy with pelvic and paraaortic node dissection. J Gynecol Surg 1993;9:105–20.

Nezhat F. Minimally invasive surgery in gynecologic oncology: Laparoscopy versus robotics. Gynecol Oncol 2008; 111(2):29-32

Nezhat FR, Datta MS, Liu C, Chuang L, Zakashansky K. Robotic radical hysterectomy versus total laparoscopic radical hysterectomy with pelvic lymphadenectomy for treatment of early cervical cancer. JSLS. 2008;12:227–37

Noyes N, Knopman JM, Long K, Coletta JM, Abu-Rustum NR. Fertility considerations in the management of gynecologic malignancies. Gynecol Oncol. 2011 Mar;120(3):326-33.

Obermair A, Ginbey P, McCartney AJ. Feasibility and safety of total laparoscopic radical hysterectomy. J Am Assoc Gynecol Laparosc 2003;10:345–9

Okabayashi H. Radical abdominal hysterectomy for cancer of the cervix uteri. Surg Gynecol Obstet 1921; 33: 335–41.

Paley PJ, Veljovich DS, Shah CA, Everett EN, Bondurant AE, Drescher CW, Peters WA 3rd. Surgical outcomes in gynecologic oncology in the era of robotics: analysis of first 1000 cases. Am J Obstet Gynecol. 2011 Jun;204(6):551.e1-9.

Paraiso MF, Ridgeway B, Park AJ, Jelovsek JE, Barber MD, Falcone T, Einarsson JI. A randomized trial comparing conventional and robotically assisted total laparoscopic hysterectomy. Am J Obstet Gynecol. 2013 May;208(5):368.e1-7.

Pareja RF, Ramirez PT, Borrero MF, Angel CG. Abdominal radical trachelectomy: a case series and literature review. Gynecol Oncol 2008;111:555–60.

Pecorelli S, Zigliani L, Odicino F. Revised FIGO staging for carcinoma of the cervix. Int J Gynaecol Obstet 2009;105:107-8.

Pergialiotis V, Rodolakis A, Christakis D, Thomakos N, Vlachos G, Antsaklis A. Laparoscopically Assisted Vaginal Radical Hysterectomy: Systematic Review of the Literature. J Minim Invasive Gynecol. 2013 Jul 11. doi:pii: S1553-4650(13)00271-9. 10.1016/j.jmig.2013.04.021. [Epub ahead of print]

Persson J, Kannisto P, Bossmar T. Robot-assisted abdominal laparoscopic radical trachelectomy. Gynecol Oncol. 2008;111:564–567.

Persson J, Reynisson P, Borgfeldt C, Kannisto P, Lindahl B, Bossmar T. Robot assisted laparoscopic radical hysterectomy and pelvic lymphadenectomy with short and long term morbidity data. Gynecol Oncol 2009;113:185–190.

Piver MS, Rutledge F, Smith JP. Five classes of extended hysterectomy for women with cervical cancer. Obstet Gynecol 1974; 44: 265–72.

Plante M. Radical vaginal trachelectomy: an update. Gynecol Oncol 2008;111:S105–110.

Pomel C, Atallah D, Le Bouedec G, Rouzier R, Morice P, Castaigne D, Dauplat J.. Laparoscopic radical hysterectomy for invasive cervical cancer: 8-year experience of a pilot study. Gynecol Oncol 2003;91:534–9.

Pomel C, Canis M, Mage G, Dauplat J, Le Bouëdec G, Raiga J, Pouly JL, Wattiez A, Bruhat MA. Laparoscopically extended hysterectomy for cervix cancer: technique, indications and results. Apropos of a series of 41 cases in Clermont. Chirurgie 1997;122:133–6.

Possover M, Krause N, Kuhne-Heid R, Schneider A. Laparoscopic assistance for extended radicality of radical vaginal hysterectomy: description of a technique. Gynecol Oncol 1998;70:94–9.

Possover M, Krause N, Plaul K, Kuhne-Heid R, Schneider A. Laparoscopic paraaortic and pelvic lymphadenectomy: experience with 150 patients and review of the literature. Gynecol Oncol 1998;71(1):19–28.

Possover M, Stober S, Plaul K, Schneider A. Identification and preservation of the motoric innervation of the bladder in radical hysterectomy type III. Gynecol Oncol 2000;79:154–7.

Puntambekar SP, Palep RJ, Puntambekar SS, Wagh GN, Patil AM, Rayate NV. Laparoscopic total radical hysterectomy by the Pune technique: our experience of 248 cases. J Minim Invasive Gynecol 2007;14:682-9.

Querleu D, Dargent D, Ansquer Y, Leblanc E, Narducci F. Extraperitoneal endosurgical aortic and common iliac dissection in the staging of bulky or advanced cervical carcinomas. Cancer 2000;88:1883–91.

Querleu D, Leblanc E, Castelain B. Pelvic lymphadenectomy under celioscopic guidance. J Gynecol Obstet Biol Reprod (Paris) 1990;19:576–8.

Querleu D, Morrow CP. Classification of radical hysterectomy. Lancet Oncol 2008; 9: 297–303.

Querleu D. Laparoscopic paraaortic node sampling in gynecologic oncology: a preliminary experience. Gynecol Oncol 1993;49(1):24–9.

Querleu D. Radical hysterectomies by the Schauta-Amreich and Schauta-Stoeckel techniques assisted by celioscopy. J Gynecol Obstet Biol Reprod (Paris) 1991;20:747–8.

Ramirez PT, Jhingran A, Macapinlac HA, Euscher ED, Munsell M, Coleman RL, Soliman PT, Schmeler KM, Frumovitz M, Ramondetta LM. Laparoscopic extraperitoneal para-aortic lymphadenectomy in locally advanced cervical cancer. Cancer 2011;117: 1928–1934

Ramirez PT, Schmeler KM, Malpica A, Soliman PT. Safety and feasibility of robotic radical trachelectomy in patients with early-stage cervical cancer. Gynecol Oncol 2010; 116:512–515.

Ramirez PT, Schmeler KM, Wolf JK, Brown J, Soliman PT. Robotic radical parametrectomy and pelvic lymphadenectomy in patients with invasive cervical cancer. Gynecol Oncol 2008;111: 18–21.

Ramirez PT, Slomovitz BM, Soliman PT, Coleman RL, Levenback C. Total laparoscopic radical hysterectomy and lymphadenectomy: the M.D. Anderson Cancer Center experience. Gynecol Oncol 2006;102:252–5.

Raspagliesi F, Ditto A, Fontanelli R, Solima E, Hanozet F, Zanaboni F, Kusamura S. Nerve-sparing radical hysterectomy: a surgical technique for preserving the autonomic hypogastric nerve. Gynecol Oncol 2004; 93: 307–14.

Reich H, DeCaprio J. Laparoscopic hysterectomy. J Gynecol Surg. 1989;5:213–6.

Rodriguez AO. The logic of the robotic revolution in gynecologic oncology. Curr Opin Obstet Gynecol. 2013 Feb;25(1):1-2.

Sakuragi N, Todo Y, Kudo M, Yamamoto R, Sato T. A systematic nerve-sparing radical hysterectomy technique in invasive cervical cancer for preserving postsurgical bladder function. Int J Gynecol Cancer 2005;15: 389–97.

Schmeler KM, Frumovitz M, Ramirez PT. Conservative management of early stage cervical cancer: is there a role for less radical surgery? Gynecol Oncol. 2011 Mar;120(3):321-5.

Schneider A, Possover M, Kamprath S, Endisch U, Krause N, Nöschel H. Laparoscopy-assisted radical vaginal hysterectomy modified according to Schauta-Stoeckel. Obstet Gynecol. 1996 Dec;88(6):1057-60.

Seamon LG, Backes F, Resnick K, Cohn DE. Robotic trocar site small bowel evisceration after gynecologic cancer surgery. Obstet Gynecol. 2008 Aug;112(2 Pt 2):462-4.

Sedlacek TV, Campion MJ, Hutchins RA, Reich H. Laparoscopic radical hysterectomy: a preliminary report. J Am Assoc Gynecol Laparosc 1994;1:S32.

Sert BM, Abeler VM. Robotic-assisted laparoscopic radical hysterectomy (Piver type III) with pelvic node dissection–case report. Eur J Gynaecol Oncol 2006;27:531–3.

Sert MB. Comparison between robot-assisted laparoscopic radical hysterectomy (RRH) and abdominal radical hysterectomy (ARH): a case control study from EIO/Milan. Gynecol Oncol. 2010 May;117(2):389

Shah NT, Wright KN, Jonsdottir GM, Jorgensen S, Einarsson JI, Muto MG. The Feasibility of Societal Cost Equivalence between Robotic Hysterectomy and Alternate Hysterectomy Methods for Endometrial Cancer. Obstet Gynecol Int. 2011;2011:570464.

Spiritos NM, Schlaerth JB, Spirtos TW, Schlaerth AC, Indman PD, Kimbal RE. Laparoscopic bilateral pelvic and para-aortic lymph node sampling: an evolving technique. Am J Obstet Gynecol 1995;173:105–11.

Spirtos NM, Eisenkop SM, Schlaerth JB, Ballon SC. Laparoscopic radical hysterectomy (type III) with aortic and pelvic lymphadenectomy in patients with stage I cervical cancer: surgical morbidity and intermediate follow-up. Am J Obstet Gynecol 2002;187:340–8.

Spirtos NM, Schlaerth JB, Kimball RE, Leiphart VM, Ballon SC. Laparoscopic radical hysterectomy (type III) with aortic and pelvic lymphadenectomy. Am J Obstet Gynecol 1996;174:1763–7.

Symmonds RE. Some surgical aspects of gynecologic cancer. Cancer 1975; 36: 649–60.

Tinelli A, Leo G, Pisanò M, Leo S, Storelli F, Vergara D, Malvasi A. HPV viral activity by mRNA-HPV molecular analysis to screen the transforming infections in precancer cervical lesions. Curr Pharm Biotechnol 2009; 10 (8), 767-71.

Tinelli A, Malvasi A, Lorusso V, Martignago R, Vergara D, Vergari U, Guido M, Zizza A, Pisanò M, Leo G. An outlook on uterine neoplasms: from DNA damaging to endometrial and cervical cancer development and minimally invasive management. In: Matsumoto, A, Nakano, M. The human genome: features, variations and genetic disorders. Nova Science Publishers Editor, Hauppauge (NY), USA 2009; Chapter 12: 227-255.

Tinelli A, Vergara D, Leo G, Malvasi A, Casciaro S, Leo E, Montanari MR, Maffia M, Marsigliante S, Lorusso V. Human papillomavirus genital infection in modern gynaecology: genetic and genomic aspects. Eur Clinics Obstet Gynaecol 2007; 3:1-6.

Trimbos JB, Maas CP, Deruiter MC, Peters AA, Kenter GG. A nerve-sparing radical hysterectomy: guidelines and feasibility in Western patients. Int J Gynecol Cancer 2001; 11: 180–86.

Uccella S, Ghezzi F, Mariani A, Cromi A, Bogani G, Serati M, Bolis P. Vaginal cuff closure after minimally invasive hysterectomy: our experience and systematic review of the literature. Am J Obstet Gynecol. 2011 Aug;205(2):119.e1-12.

Ungar L, Palfalvi L, Hogg R, Siklós P, Boyle DC, Del Priore G, Smith JR. Abdominal radical trachelectomy: a fertilitypreserving option for women with early cervical cancer. Br J Obstet Gynaecol 2005;112:366–9.

van Dam PA, van Dam PJ, Verkinderen L, Vermeulen P, Deckers F, Dirix LY. Robotic-assisted laparoscopic cytoreductive surgery for lobular carcinoma of the breast metastatic to the ovaries. J Minim Invasive Gynecol 2007; 14: 746–749.

Vergote I, Amant F, Beterloot P, Van Gramberen M. Laparoscopic lower paraaortic staging lymphadenectomy in stage IB2, II, and III cervical cancer. Int J Gynecol Cancer 2002;12:22–6.

Vergote I, Pouseele B, Van Gorp T, Vanacker B, Leunen K, Cadron I, Neven P, Amant F. Robotic retroperitoneal lower para-aortic lymphadenectomy in cervical carcinoma: first report on the technique used in 5 patients. Acta Obstet Gynecol Scand 2008;87:783–7.

Wertheim E. The extended abdominal operation for carcinoma uteri. Am J Obstet Dis Women Child. 1912;66:169–232.

Xu H, Chen Y, Li Y, Zhang Q, Wang D, Liang Z. Complications of laparoscopic radical hysterectomy and lymphadenectomy for invasive cervical cancer: Experience based on 317 procedures. Surg Endosc 2007; 21: 960–964.

Zakashansky K, Chuang L, Gretz H, Nagarsheth NP, Rahaman J, Nezhat FR. A case-controlled study of total laparoscopic radical hysterectomy with pelvic lymphadenectomy versus radical abdominal hysterectomy in a fellowship training program. Int J Gynecol Cancer 2007;17:1–8.

Zapardiel I. Is robotic surgery suitable for all gynecologic procedures? Acta Obst Gynecol Scandinavica 2009;88:10,1176.

A Review of Update Clinical Results of Carbon Ion Radiotherapy for Uterine Cervical Cancer

Masaru Wakatsuki
Research Center for Charged Particle Therapy
National Institute of Radiological Sciences, Japan

Shingo Kato
Department of Radiation Oncology
Saitama Medical University International Medical Center, Japan

Kumiko Karasawa, Hirohiko Tsujii, Tadashi Kamada
Research Center for Charged Particle Therapy
National Institute of Radiological Sciences, Japan

1   Introduction

This Heavy-charged particle radiation therapy for cancer treatment started at the National Institute of R Heavy-charged particle radiation therapy for cancer treatment started at the National Institute of Radiological Sciences in June 1994 using carbon ions that were generated by the heavy-ion medical accelerator in Chiba, where all patients have been treated within prospective Phase I/II or Phase II studies. Carbon ion beams have improved the properties of dose localization, a potentiality that can produce great effects on tumors while minimizing normal tissue damage. Moreover, they possess a biological advantage due to their high relative biological effectiveness (RBE) in the Bragg Peak. Since 1994, more than 7000 patients have been treated with carbon-ion radiation therapy (C-ion RT), demonstrating the benefit of C-ion RT over other modalities for various types of tumors in terms of high local control and survival rates(Tsujii & Kamada, 2012).

Standard therapy for locally advanced cervical carcinoma is concurrent chemoradiation therapy. Recently, many researchers have reported clinical trials for locally advanced cervical carcinoma, and cisplatin-based concurrent chemoradiation therapy (CCRT) has become the standard therapy (Chemoradiotherapy for Cervical Cancer Meta-Analysis, 2008; Eifel *et al.*, 2004; Green *et al.*, 2001; Rose *et al.*, 2007). However, analyses of failure patterns following CCRT in locally advanced disease showed locoregional recurrence of 20–30% of the patients treated, and this proportion increased with increasing tumor bulk. In addition, the majority of patients included in most of the clinical trials have squamous cell histology, with adenocarcinomas representing approximately 10% of the patients enrolled (Eifel *et al.*, 2004; Green *et al.*, 2001; Rose *et al.*, 2007). However, as uterine cervical adenocarcinoma is more radioresistant and thus has poorer prognosis than squamous cell carcinoma, radiation therapy with or without chemotherapy is still unsatisfactory. This means that both locally advanced bulky cervical cancers and adenocarcinomas are in need of even more aggressive approaches. One such strategy for applying more treatment is to use drugs for radiosensitizing chemotherapy (Nagai *et al.*, 2012), and another is the use of particle therapy (Kagei *et al.*, 2003; Kato *et al.*, 2006; Nakano *et al.*, 1999). Since 1995, we have conducted several clinical trials for locally advanced squamous cell carcinoma or adenocarcinoma of the cervix, with 4 already completed, 2 have finished patient enrollment, and another is still ongoing.

2   Eligibility Criteria

There were 7 clinical trials for locally advanced squamous cell carcinoma or adenocarcinoma of the uterine cervix. Patients were eligible for these studies if they had previously untreated and histologically proven squamous cell carcinoma, adenocarcinoma or adenosquamous cell carcinoma, and International Federation of Gynecology and Obstetrics (FIGO 1994) Stage IIB, III, or IVA disease (> 4 cm in diameter for squamous cell carcinoma), and no rectal invasion. Bladder or rectal involvement was assessed by endoscopy. Eligible patients had World Health Organization performance status < 3, were aged < 80 years, and had an estimated life expectancy of > 6 months. Patients were excluded if they had severe pelvic infection, severe psychological illness, or active double cancer. Pretreatment evaluation consisted of an assessment of the patient's history, physical and pelvic examinations by gynecologists and radiation oncologists, cervical biopsy, routine blood cell counts, chemistry profile, chest X-ray, cystoscopy, and rectoscopy. CT scans of the abdomen and pelvis, magnetic resonance imaging (MRI) of the pelvis, and positron emission tomography (PET) scans were also performed for all patients. Patients were staged according to the FIGO staging system, but patients with para-aortic lymph nodes > 1 cm in minimum diameter on CT images were excluded from the studies, although those with enlarged pelvic lymph nodes only were included. Tumor size was assessed by both pelvic examination and MRI, and the dimensions of the cervical tumor were measured on T2-weighted MRI images. Staging laparotomy was not performed, and no histologic confirmation of CT-positive pelvic lymph nodes was obtained. No patient underwent lymph node resection. PET scans were supplementally used for detecting distant metastases. Tumor specimens were examined by working group pathologists. The treatment protocols for these clinical studies were reviewed and approved by the National Institute of Radiological Sciences Ethics Committee of Human Clinical Research, and all patients signed an informed consent form before the initiation of therapy.

Eligibility criteria
1. Histologically proven squamous cell carcinoma, adenocarcinoma or adenosquamous cell carcinoma
2. FIGO Stage IIB, III, or IVA disease and without rectal invasion (> 4 cm in diameter for squamous cell carcinoma)
3. World Health Organization performance status 0-3
4. No prior treatment for cervical cancer
5. No para-aortic metastases on CT-images
6. Age < 80 years
7. Expected prognosis of more than 6 months

Table 1: Eligibility criteria

3   Carbon-ion Radiation Therapy

Carbon-ion RT was given once daily, 4 days per week (Tuesday to Friday). At every treatment session, the patient was positioned on the treatment couch with immobilization devices, and the patient's position was verified with a computer-aided, on-line positioning system. To minimize internal target positional uncertainty, 100-150 mL of normal saline was infused into the bladder. Patients were also encouraged to use laxatives, if necessary, to prevent constipation throughout the treatment period. The radiation dose was calculated for the target volume and surrounding normal structures and was expressed in GyE, defined as the carbon physical dose (Gy) multiplied by a relative biologic effectiveness value of 3.0 (Ando *et al.*, 1998; Kanai *et al.*, 1999).

The treatment consisted of prophylactic whole pelvic or extended-field irradiation and local boost. Recently, planning computed tomography (CT) scan has been basically performed three times during the treatment course, and the clinical target volume (CTV) for local boost is reduced twice in accordance with tumor shrinkage. The CTV of whole pelvic irradiation include all areas of gross and potentially microscopic disease, consisting of the tumor, uterus, ovaries, parametrium, at least the upper half of the vagina, and pelvic lymph nodes (common iliac, internal iliac, external iliac, obturator and presacral lymph nodes) (CTV-1) (Figure1). The CTV of the extended-field irradiation consists of CTV of whole pelvic irradiation and the para-aortic lymph node area. After completing CTV-1 irradiation, the first reduction of CTV includes the gross tumor volume (GTV) and uterine cervix, uterine corpus, parametrium, upper half of the vagina and ovaries (=CTV-2). Finally, CTV is shrunk to GTV only (=CTV-3) (Kato *et al.*, 2006) (Figure2).

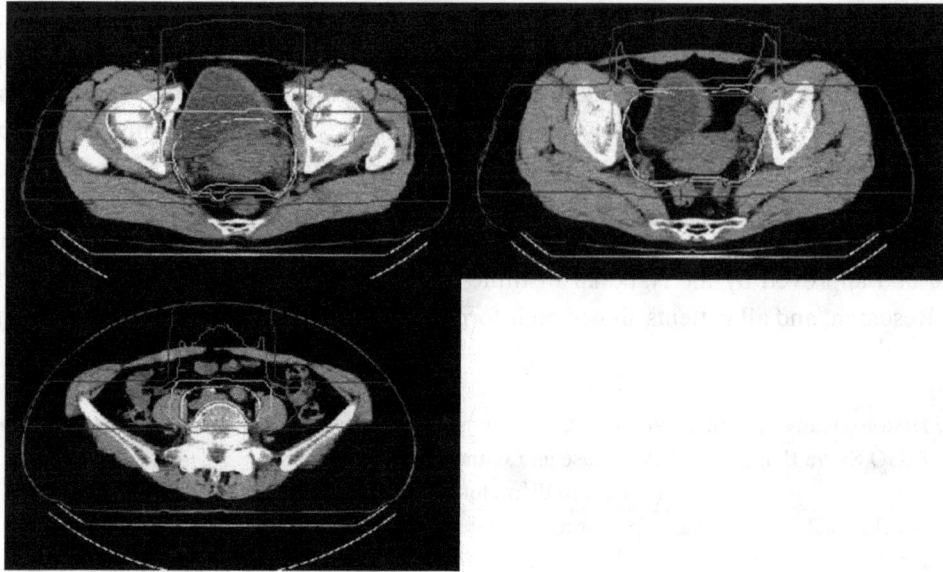

Figure 1: CTV-1 whole pelvic irradiation

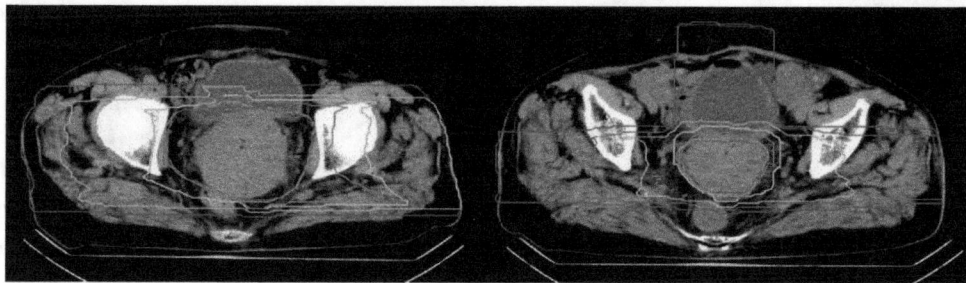

Figure 2: CTV2 and CTV3

The treatment schedule for locally advanced squamous cell carcinoma of the uterus, PTV-1, PTV-2 and PTV-3 were irradiated with 13, 5 and 2 fractions, respectively. First 3 clinical trials (Protocol 9403, 9702 and 9902) are dose escalation trials, and forth clinical trial (Protocol 0508) includes extended-field irradiation. In Protocol 9902, based on DVH analysis of Protocols 9403 and 9702, the doses to PTV-1 and PTV-2 were fixed at 39.0 GyE for 13 fractions and 15.0 GyE for 5 fractions (3.0 GyE per fraction), respectively. With regard to local boost, a dose-escalation study was planned with an initial dose of 10 GyE for 2 fractions to PTV-3. The dose to all GI tracts was strictly limited to < 60 GyE to prevent major late toxicities. The initial dose was determined based on the results of Protocols 9403 and 9702, in which 18% of patients developed major late GI complications, and dose escalation to 18 GyE for 2 fractions was performed after careful observation of late toxicity according to discussions of the Working Group of the Gynecological Tumor on a semi-annual basis. Total dose to the cervical tumor was 64.0 – 72.0 GyE for 20 fractions (Figure 3). In Protocol 0508, CTV-1 is CTV of whole pelvic irradiation with para-aortic lymph node area. The doses to PTV-1, PTV-2 and PTV-3 in 0508 were fixed at 39.0 GyE for 13 fractions, 15.0 GyE for 5 fractions and 18 GyE for 2 fractions, respectively (Figure 3).

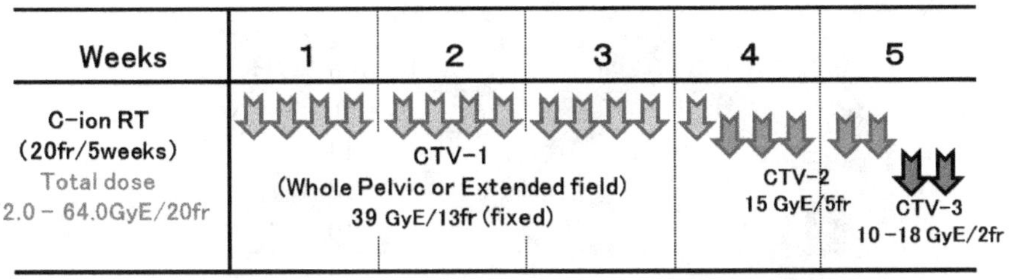

Figure 3: Treatment schedule of protocol 0508 and 9902

The treatment schedule for locally advanced adenocarcinoma of the uterus (Protocol 9704), PTV-1, PTV-2 and PTV-3 were irradiated with 12, 4 and 4 fractions, respectively. This clinical trial was dose escalation trials. Based on the results of a previous study (Protocol 9403), the dose to PTV-1 was fixed at 36.0 GyE for 12 fractions (3.0 GyE per fraction) in this protocol. With regard to local boost, a dose-escalation study was planned with an initial dose of 26.4 GyE for 8 fractions, then gradually increasing up to 38.4 GyE for 8 fractions by 2.4 or 3.6 GyE increments. Dose escalation was performed after careful observation of acute normal tissue responses according to discussion twice per year of the Working Group of the Gynecological Tumor. Total dose to the cervical tumor was 62.4 – 74.4 GyE over 20 fractions (Figure 4).

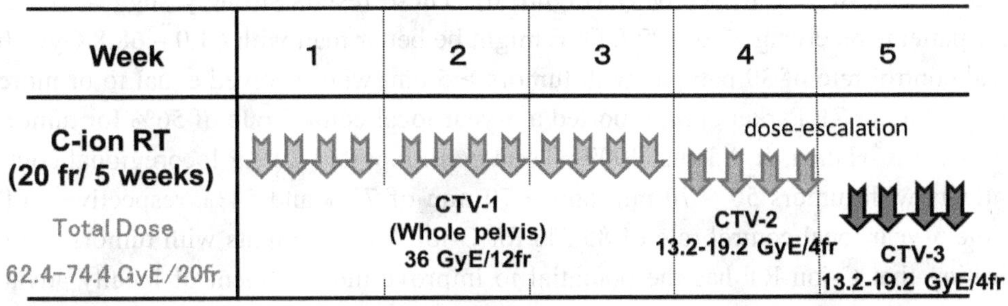

Figure 4: Treatment schedule of protocol 9704

4 Results of C-ion RT

4.1 Locally Advanced Squamous Cell Carcinoma of the Uterus (9702, 9902 and 0508)

Between December 1997 and January 2011, 62 patients for Protocols 9702, 9902 and 0508 were treated with C-ion RT. Protocols 9702 and 9902 were dose escalation studies and protocol 0508 was included in the prophylactic extended-field radiotherapy of pelvic and para-aortic lymph nodes. Patients with histories of prior chemotherapy or pelvic radiotherapy were excluded from the studies. Patient characteristics are summarized in Table 2. Histologically, all patients had squamous cell carcinoma. The numbers of patients with stage IIB, IIIB, and IVA disease were 14, 38, and 10, respectively. All patients with stage IVA had bladder invasion but no rectal invasion. All patients had bulky tumors 4.0 – 12.0 cm in maximum diameter, median diameter 6.4 cm. Thirty-eight of the 62 patients had pelvic lymph node metastases. Staging laparotomy was not performed, and no histologic confirmation of CT-positive pelvic or para-aortic lymph nodes was obtained. No patient underwent lymph node resection. Twenty-three patients re-

No. of patients	62
Follow-up, range (median)(mo)	8 – 168 (29)
Age, range (mean) (y)	31 – 80 (59)
Stage IIB	14
IIIB	38
IVA	10
Lymph node status Negative	24
Positive	38
Tumor size (cm) range (median)	4.0 – 12.0 (6.4)
< 5.0	10
5.0-6.9	30
≥ 7.0	22

Table 2: Patient characteristics of Protocol 9702,9902 and 0508

ceived 64.0 – 68.8 GyE, and 39 patients had 72.0 – 72.8 GyE. Overall treatment time (OTT) ranged from 32 to 48 days, with a median of 36 days. The median follow-up duration was 29 months.

The 5-year overall survival rate and local control rate were 74.1% and 53.4%, respectively (Figure 5). The 5-year local control rates in patients with 64.0 – 68.8 GyE (23 cases) and 72.0 – 72.8 GyE (39 cases) were 60.9% and 82.1%, respectively (Figure 6). These results strongly suggested that the local control rate for patients receiving 72.0 – 72.8 GyE might be better than with 64.0 – 68.8 GyE. In addition, the 5-year local control rate of 30 patients with tumors > 5 cm, who received equal to or more than 72.0 GyE, was 85.3% (Figure 7). Parker *et al.* reported a 5-year local control rate of 56% for tumors > 50 mm (Parker, Gallop-Evans, Hanna, & Adams, 2009). Toita *et al.* reported 2-year locoregional control rates of CCRT for patients with tumors 50 – 70 mm and > 70 mm of 72% and 54%, respectively (Toita *et al.*, 2012). Thus, the 5-year local control rate of 85.3% for C-ion RT in patients with tumors > 5 cm was favorable, indicating that C-ion RT has the potential to improve the treatment of locally advanced bulky cervical cancer. However, the 5-year overall survival rate in patients receiving 72.0 – 72.8 GyE was only 61.2% (Figure 5), and 12 of the 39 patients showed distant metastases. Despite the better local tumor control for C-ion RT compared with CCRT, distant metastases frequently occurred, and the 5-year overall survival rate was still unsatisfactory. The high rate of distant metastasis can be ascribed to the advanced stage of the tumors, which includes bulky tumors and a high rate of pelvic lymph node metastasis. To improve the survival rate as well as the local control rate, the use of chemotherapy in combination with C-ion RT should be further explored. Thus, we are now conducting a new clinical trial of C-ion RT with concurrent chemotherapy for locally advanced squamous cell carcinoma of the uterus.

4.2   Locally Advanced Adenocarcinoma of the Uterus (9704)

Between April 1998 and February 2010, 55 patients with locally advanced adenocarcinoma of the uterine cervix (Protocol 9704) were treated with C-ion RT. Patient characteristics are summarized in Table 3. The numbers of patients with stage IIB, IIIB, and IVA disease were 20, 33, and 2, respectively. All patients with stage IVA had bladder invasion but no rectal invasion. Tumor size was 3.0 – 11.8 cm in maximum diameter, median diameter 5.5 cm, and that of stage IIIB and IVA cases was 3.5 – 9.2 cm (median 5.8 cm). Histologically, 45 of 55 patients had adenocarcinoma and 13 patients had adenosquamous cell carcinoma. Twenty-four of the 55 patients had pelvic lymph node metastases. Seven of 55 patients re-

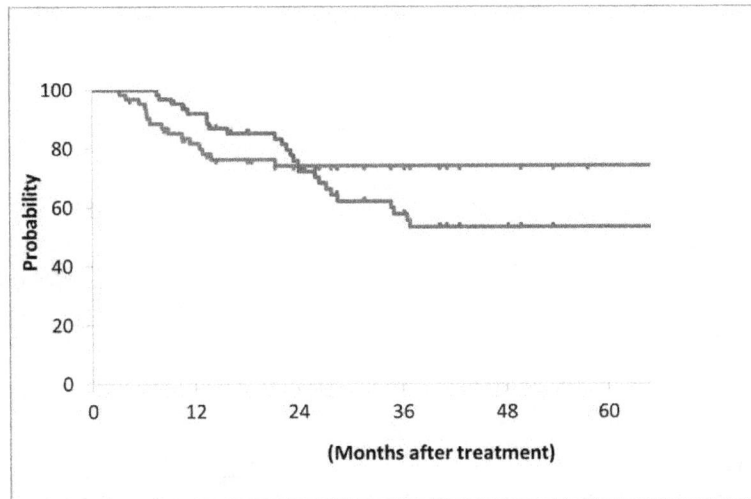

Figure 5: Overall survival and local control curves in Protocol 9702, 9902, 0508 (Squamous cell carcinoma): Red line is overall survival curve; blue line is local control curve.

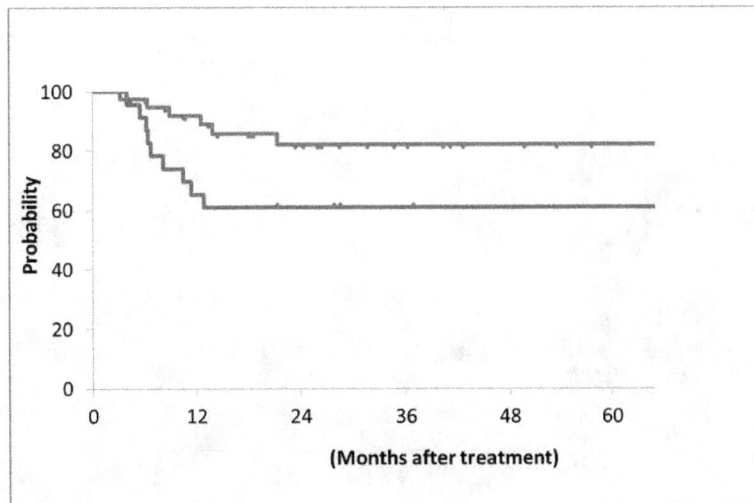

Figure 6: Local control curves in patients with 64.0 – 68.8 GyE (n=23) (red line) and 72.0 – 72.8 GyE (n=39) (blue line).

ceived 62.4 – 64.8 GyE, 10 patients had 68.0 GyE, 21 patients had 71.2 GyE and 17 patients had 74.4 GyE. OTT ranged from 32 to 40 days, with a median of 35 days. Median follow-up duration was 38 months (range, 7 to 141 months).

The 5-year local control rate, local control rate including salvage surgery, and overall survival rate in all cases were 54.5%, 68.2% and 38.1%, respectively (Figure 8). In stage IIIB and IVA cases, the rates were 57.9%, 69.2% and 42.4%, respectively (Figure 9). Several studies have reported treatment outcomes of adenocarcinoma of the uterine cervix treated with RT or CCRT. Niibe et al. reported a 5-year local control rate of 36% for stage IIIB by RT alone or CCRT (Niibe et al., 2010). Grigsby et al. reported

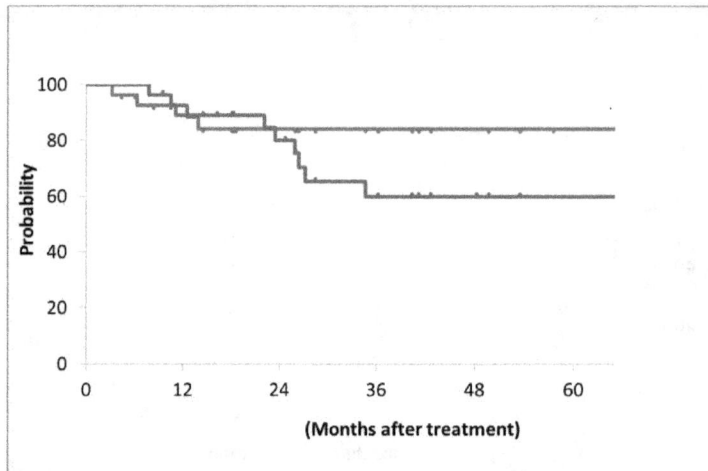

Figure 7: Local control (blue line) and overall survival (red line) curves in patients with 72.0 – 72.8 GyE and tumors > 5 cm.

No. of patients	62
Follow-up, range (median) (mo)	7-141 (38)
Age (median)	28 - 85 years (59 years)
Histology	
Adenocarcinoma	42
Adenosquamous carcinoma	13
FIGO Stage IIB	20
IIIB	33
IVA	2
Lymph node N1	24
N0	31
Dose (C-ion RT) 62.4 GyE / 20 fr	3
64.8 GyE / 20 fr	4
68.0 GyE / 20 fr	10
71.2 GyE / 20 fr	21

Table 3: Patient characteristics of Protocol 9704

33% for stage III adenocarcinoma of the uterine cervix by RT alone (Grigsby *et al.*, 1988). Huang *et al.* reported 58% for stage III and 48% for stage IB-IIA bulky (> 4 cm) by RT alone or CCRT (Huang *et al.*, 2011). In the present study, the 5-year overall local control rate for stage IIIB or IVA was 57.9% even though the median tumor size of our cases was 5.8 cm (3.5-9.2 cm). Although the number of patients in this study was small, the local control rate was relatively better than in the conventional studies.

On the other hand, the overall survival rate was less than satisfactory in this study (2-year: 65.5%, 5-year: 38.1%), even though there was a relatively favorable local control rate for bulky tumors. Several researchers showed that locally advanced adenocarcinoma of the uterine cervix had poor progno-sis, with 5-year survival rates being only 25-29% (Eifel, Morris, Oswald, Wharton, & Delclos, 1990; Grigsby *et al.*, 1988; Huang *et al.*, 2011; Niibe *et al.*, 2010). They suggested that the reasons were poor

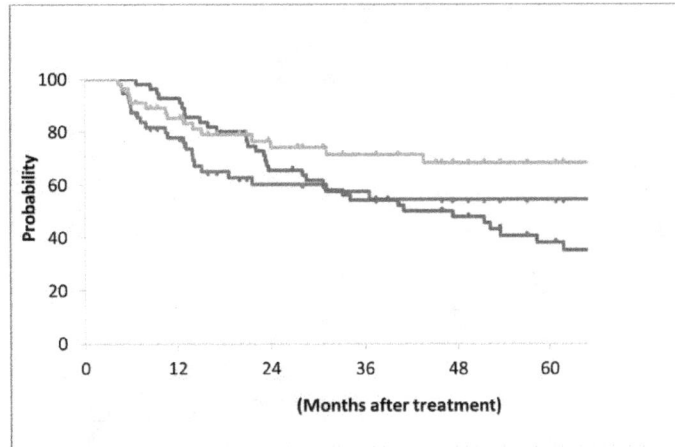

Figure 8: Local control rate, local control rate including salvage surgery and overall survival rate in Protocol 9704(Cervical adenocarcinoma): Red line is overall survival curve, blue line is local control curve, and green line is local control curve including salvage surgery.

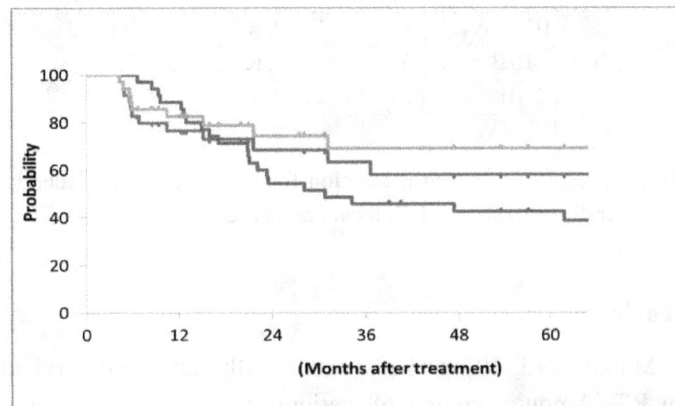

Figure 9: Local control rate, local control rate including salvage surgery and overall survival rate in stage IIIB-IVA: Red line is overall survival curve, blue line is local control curve, and green line is local control curve including salvage surgery.

local control and greater distant metastases. Huang et al. reported a 5-year distant metastasis rate of 46% for stage III patients after RT alone or CCRT (Huang *et al.*, 2011), and Eifel *et al.* reported that 45% of patients with stage IIB or III showed distant metastases after RT (Eifel *et al.*, 1990). In the present study, 2-year and 5-year cumulative distant metastasis rates were 49.4% and 64.8%, respectively (Figure 10). These rates were higher than those in the other studies because our patients did not receive concurrent chemotherapy, tumor size was larger than in the other studies, and the overall survival rate was higher than in the other studies. Thus, to improve the distant metastasis and local control rates, the use of chemotherapy in combination with C-ion RT should receive further consideration.

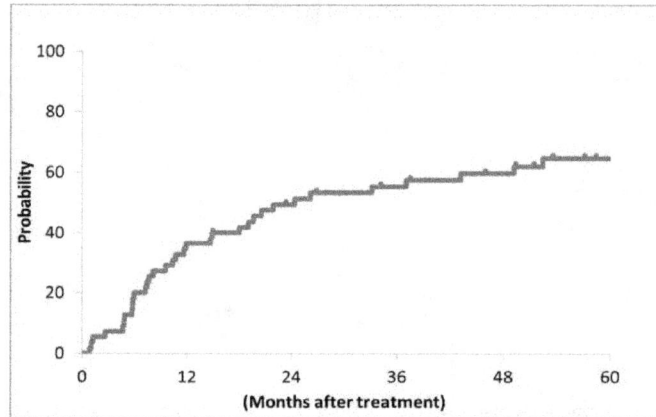

Figure 10: Cumulative distant metastasis rate

Author (year)	Stage	No.	Treatment	(2y) 5y OS (%)	5y LC (%)
Grigsby PW (1988)	III	12	RT	25	33
Eifel PJ (1990)	III	61	RT	(33) 26	46
Lee JS (2002)	III-IVA	36	RT / CRT	(13) 0	
Niibe Y (2010)	IIIB	61	RT / CRT	22	36
Huang Y-T (2011)	III	28	RT / CRT	29	58
NIRS (Protocol 9704)	IIIB-IVA	38	C-ion RT	(54) 42	58

Table 4: Treatment results of photon irradiation for locally advanced adenocarcinoma of the cervix. OS: overall survival rate, LC: local control rate

4.3   Acute and Late Toxicities

Between June 1995 and March 2013, 197 patients with locally advanced cervical cancer in 7 protocols were treated with C-ion RT. Among the first 68 patients treated between 1995 and 2001, 8 patients (11.8%) developed major (Grade 4) GI complications. All patients were surgically salvaged and remained free of intestinal problems. According to these results, the treatment technique was revised after 2002. The dose to the GI tracts was limited to < 60 GyE according to DVH analysis (Kato *et al.*, 2006), and this limitation had higher priority than the prescription to CTV-3 as final boost irradiation. In addition, vaginal packing for the space between tumor of uterine cervix and rectum has been placed at the time of C-ion RT (Figure 11). Since 2002, there has been no grade 3 or higher major GI complication in 129 patients.

Acute toxicity was graded according to the National Cancer Institute - Common Toxicity Criteria version 3.0. Of 117 patients for of Protocols 9702, 9704, 9902 and 0508, all of the observed acute and late toxicities are listed in Table 5 and 6. Although 51 patients (43.6%) developed acute GI toxicity (G1-G2) and 26 patients (22.2%) had acute GU toxicity (G1-G2), all patients completed the scheduled therapy. No patient developed Grade 3 or higher acute toxicity.

Late toxicity was graded according to the Radiation Therapy Oncology Group/European Organization for Research and Treatment of Cancer late radiation morbidity scoring scheme. Thirty patients (25.6 %) had mild or intermediate bleeding of the rectum or sigmoid colon. Two patients (1.7%) had Grade 4 rectal complications that were surgically salvaged, and one patient (0.9%) had severe rectal

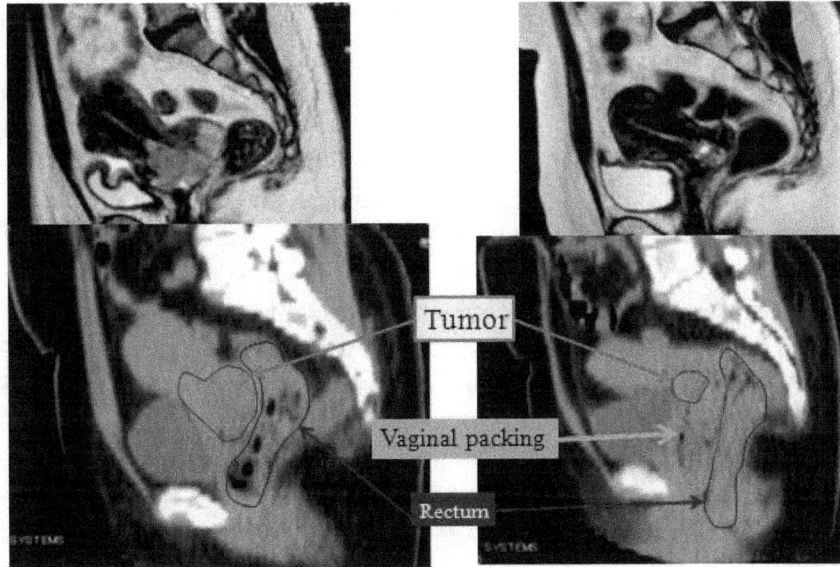

Figure 11: Vaginal packing for the space between tumor of uterine cervix and rectum.

	No.	(CTCAE ver 3.0)				
		Grade 0	Grade 1	Grade 2	Grade 3	Grade 4-5
GI tract	117	66	43	8	0	0
GU tract	117	91	24	2	0	0

Table 5: Acute toxicities of Protocol 9702,9704,9902and 0508

	No.	(RTOG / EORTC)				
		Grade 0	Grade 1	Grade 2	Grade 3	Grade 4
GI tract	117	84	24	6	1	2
GU tract	117	94	12	11	0	0

Table 6: Late toxicities of Protocol 9702,9704,9902and 0508

bleeding. These cases were treated before revision of the treatment technique. Twenty-three patients (19.7%) had Grade 1 or 2 late GU toxicities, and none developed Grade 3 or higher toxicity.

4.4   Overall Treatment Time (OTT)

Carbon-ion RT for several carcinomas has achieved shorter OTT. It is well known that OTT is an important factor of RT for several cancers including cervical cancer. Several studies reported that prolongation of OTT of RT for uterine cervical cancer had a significant impact on treatment outcome because of biological factors such as cell repopulation and increased proliferation (Girinsky *et al.*, 1993; Perez, Grigsby, Castro-Vita, & Lockett, 1996). Thus, they suggested that RT for patients with uterine cervical cancer should be delivered in the shortest possible overall time. In addition, shorter OTT obviously offers a better quality of life for the patients. OTT ranged from 45 to 60 days in most clinical trials for uterine cervical cancer by CCRT. On the other hand, median OTT for C-ion RT in these trials was only 35 or 36 days. Even though C-ion RT was delivered in a shorter OTT, there were no higher incidences of acute or late complications than those for CCRT. This indicates that C-ion RT achieved shorter OTT in a safe manner.

5   Conclusion

Carbon-ion RT has been established as a safe short-term treatment for locally advanced uterine cervical cancer. Although the patient population in these trials was small, it was shown that C-ion RT has the potential to improve the treatment for locally advanced bulky squamous cell carcinoma or adenocarcinoma of the uterine cervix, with the results supporting the view that investigations should be continued to confirm the therapeutic efficacy. In addition, we are now conducting a new clinical trial of C-ion RT with concurrent chemotherapy.

Acknowledgement

The authors thank the members of The Working Group of the Gynecological Tumor for their constructive discussion and precious advice.

References

Ando, K., Koike, S., Nojima, K., Chen, Y. J., Ohira, C., Ando, S., . . . Kanai, T. (1998). Mouse skin reactions following fractionated irradiation with carbon ions. Int J Radiat Biol, 74(1), 129-138.

Chemoradiotherapy for Cervical Cancer Meta-Analysis, C. (2008). Reducing uncertainties about the effects of chemoradiotherapy for cervical cancer: a systematic review and meta-analysis of individual patient data from 18 randomized trials. J Clin Oncol, 26(35), 5802-5812. doi: 10.1200/JCO.2008.16.4368

Eifel, P. J., Morris, M., Oswald, M. J., Wharton, J. T., & Delclos, L. (1990). Adenocarcinoma of the uterine cervix. Prognosis and patterns of failure in 367 cases. Cancer, 65(11), 2507-2514.

Eifel, P. J., Winter, K., Morris, M., Levenback, C., Grigsby, P. W., Cooper, J., . . . Mutch, D. G. (2004). Pelvic irradiation with concurrent chemotherapy versus pelvic and para-aortic irradiation for high-risk cervical cancer: an update of radiation therapy oncology group trial (RTOG) 90-01. J Clin Oncol, 22(5), 872-880. doi: 10.1200/JCO.2004.07.197

Girinsky, T., Rey, A., Roche, B., Haie, C., Gerbaulet, A., Randrianarivello, H., & Chassagne, D. (1993). Overall treatment time in advanced cervical carcinomas: a critical parameter in treatment outcome. Int J Radiat Oncol Biol Phys, 27(5), 1051-1056.

Green, J. A., Kirwan, J. M., Tierney, J. F., Symonds, P., Fresco, L., Collingwood, M., & Williams, C. J. (2001). Survival and recurrence after concomitant chemotherapy and radiotherapy for cancer of the uterine cervix: a systematic review and meta-analysis. Lancet, 358(9284), 781-786. doi: 10.1016/S0140-6736(01)05965-7

Grigsby, P. W., Perez, C. A., Kuske, R. R., Camel, H. M., Kao, M. S., Galakatos, A. E., & Hederman, M. A. (1988). Adenocarcinoma of the uterine cervix: lack of evidence for a poor prognosis. Radiother Oncol, 12(4), 289-296.

Huang, Y. T., Wang, C. C., Tsai, C. S., Lai, C. H., Chang, T. C., Chou, H. H., . . . Hong, J. H. (2011). Long-term outcome and prognostic factors for adenocarcinoma/adenosquamous carcinoma of cervix after definitive radiotherapy. Int J Radiat Oncol Biol Phys, 80(2), 429-436. doi: 10.1016/j.ijrobp.2010.02.009

Kagei, K., Tokuuye, K., Okumura, T., Ohara, K., Shioyama, Y., Sugahara, S., & Akine, Y. (2003). Long-term results of proton beam therapy for carcinoma of the uterine cervix. Int J Radiat Oncol Biol Phys, 55(5), 1265-1271.

Kanai, T., Endo, M., Minohara, S., Miyahara, N., Koyama-ito, H., Tomura, H., . . . Kawachi, K. (1999). Biophysical characteristics of HIMAC clinical irradiation system for heavy-ion radiation therapy. Int J Radiat Oncol Biol Phys, 44(1), 201-210.

Kato, S., Ohno, T., Tsujii, H., Nakano, T., Mizoe, J. E., Kamada, T., . . . Working Group of the Gynecological, T. (2006). Dose escalation study of carbon ion radiotherapy for locally advanced carcinoma of the uterine cervix. Int J Radiat Oncol Biol Phys, 65(2), 388-397. doi: 10.1016/j.ijrobp.2005.12.050

Nagai, Y., Toita, T., Wakayama, A., Nakamoto, T., Ooyama, T., Tokura, A., . . . Aoki, Y. (2012). Concurrent chemoradiotherapy with paclitaxel and cisplatin for adenocarcinoma of the cervix. Anticancer Res, 32(4), 1475-1479.

Nakano, T., Suzuki, M., Abe, A., Suzuki, Y., Morita, S., Mizoe, J., . . . Tsujii, H. (1999). The phase I/II clinical study of carbon ion therapy for cancer of the uterine cervix. Cancer J Sci Am, 5(6), 362-369.

Niibe, Y., Kenjo, M., Onishi, H., Ogawa, Y., Kazumoto, T., Ogino, I., . . . Hayakawa, K. (2010). High-dose-rate intracavitary brachytherapy combined with external beam radiotherapy for stage IIIb adenocarcinoma of the uterine cervix in Japan: a multi-institutional study of Japanese Society of Therapeutic Radiology and Oncology 2006-2007 (study of JASTRO 2006-2007). Jpn J Clin Oncol, 40(8), 795-799. doi: 10.1093/jjco/hyq053

Parker, K., Gallop-Evans, E., Hanna, L., & Adams, M. (2009). Five years' experience treating locally advanced cervical cancer with concurrent chemoradiotherapy and high-dose-rate brachytherapy: results from a single institution. Int J Radiat Oncol Biol Phys, 74(1), 140-146. doi: 10.1016/j.ijrobp.2008.06.1920

Perez, C. A., Grigsby, P. W., Castro-Vita, H., & Lockett, M. A. (1996). Carcinoma of the uterine cervix. II. Lack of impact of prolongation of overall treatment time on morbidity of radiation therapy. Int J Radiat Oncol Biol Phys, 34(1), 3-11.

Rose, P. G., Ali, S., Watkins, E., Thigpen, J. T., Deppe, G., Clarke-Pearson, D. L., . . . Gynecologic Oncology, G. (2007). Long-term follow-up of a randomized trial comparing concurrent single agent cisplatin, cisplatin-based combination chemotherapy, or hydroxyurea during pelvic irradiation for locally advanced cervical cancer: a Gynecologic Oncology Group Study. J Clin Oncol, 25(19), 2804-2810. doi: 10.1200/JCO.2006.09.4532

Toita, T., Kitagawa, R., Hamano, T., Umayahara, K., Hirashima, Y., Aoki, Y., . . . Cervical Cancer Committee of Japanese Gynecologic Oncology, G. (2012). Phase II study of concurrent chemoradiotherapy with high-dose-rate intracavitary brachytherapy in patients with locally advanced uterine cervical cancer: efficacy and toxicity of a low cumulative radiation dose schedule. Gynecol Oncol, 126(2), 211-216. doi: 10.1016/j.ygyno.2012.04.036

Tsujii, H., & Kamada, T. (2012). A review of update clinical results of carbon ion radiotherapy. Jpn J Clin Oncol, 42(8), 670-685. doi: 10.1093/jjco/hys104

Chrysin in PI3K/AKT and Other Apoptosis Signalling Pathways, and its Effect on HeLa Cells

Khoo Boon Yin
Institute For Research In Molecular Medicine (INFORMM)
Universiti Sains Malaysia, Malaysia

1   Introduction

Over 4,000 flavonoids have been identified as a broad class of plant secondary metabolites (Kuntz *et al.*, 1999; Samarghandian *et al.*, 2011). Flavonoids originate naturally in plants are synthesised from amino acid phenylalanine by the phenylpropanoid metabolic pathways, such as shikimate and arogenate pathways (Harborne & Turner, 1984; Soumajit & Ramesh, 2010). Flavonoids display brilliant colours in the flowering parts of plants (Clifford & Cuppett, 2000). These compounds exhibit protective effects against microorganisms, UV light and spread of diseases; and are dietary polyphenols essential to both human and animal health (Khoo *et al.*, 2010; Manika *et al.*, 2012). Flavonoids cannot be synthesised by humans or animals. In contrast, plants have to manufacture what the plants need, not merely to grow, but to defend, protect and heal from stress that would help humans or animals under similar circumstances. Flavonoids are classified into at least 10 main chemical groups. Those are flavanones, flavones, isoflavonoids, flavanols, anthocyanins and flavonols (Table 1) (Cook & Samman, 1996; Bravo, 1988; Aherne & Obrien, 2002; Lakhanpal & Rai, 2007). Flavonoids are ubiquitously present in the green plants and human diet, including in vegetables, fruits, honey, nuts, seeds, coffee, tea and wine (Ho *et al.*, 1992; Kuntz *et al.*, 1999), but the subclasses of flavonoid do not seem to be uniformly distributed (Neuhouser *et al.*, 2009). In addition, flavonoids content is influenced by surrounding factors, such as season, sunlight, climate, food preparation and processing. The average daily flavonoid intakes seem to vary greatly between countries where the lowest intakes (2.6 mg/d) are in Finland and the highest intakes (68.2 mg/d) are in Japan (Nijveldt *et al.*, 2001). Nonetheless, it is extremely difficult to estimate the daily human intake of flavonoids, especially the lack of standardized analytical methods (Scalbert & Williamson, 2000). Similar to daily intake, it is also quite complex to assess and quantify the bioavailability of flavonoids due to the significantly difference between metabolized flavonoids and native compounds present in blood (Russo *et al.*, 2007). It is important to note that flavonoids are biologically active compounds, which contain multiple potent biological effects, including anti-allergic, anti-thrombotic, anti-inflammatory, anti-oxidant, anti-viral and anti-cancer activities (Samarghandian *et al.*, 2011). The flavonoids modulate also the function of sex hormones and the hormones' receptors. Certain flavonoids, such as isoflavone genistein, are estrogenic (Wang *et al.*, 1996; Zand *et al.*, 2000), whereas others, such as chrysin, can interfere with steroid synthesis and metabolism. Although flavonoids are often called phytoestrogens, only a limited number are estrogen receptor agonists, indeed. In contrast, many flavonoids are known to interfere to a greater or lesser extent with various P450 enzymes, including those in steroidogenesis. Epidemiological studies have shown that the consumption of flavonoids is associated with a low risk of cancer (Block *et al.*, 1992). The cancer chemopreventive properties of flavonoids have become an important topic of investigation. Flavonoids are safe to use and are associated with low toxicity, making these compounds (constituents) potential chemopreventive agents against several types of human cancer, in general. Moreover, the abilities of the compounds to inhibit the cell cycle, cell proliferation and oxidative stress; to activate detoxification enzymes and apoptosis induction; to influence signal transduction pathway, as well as to enhance the immune system, making the compounds ideal candidates for cancer chemoprevention (Yao *et al.*, 2004; Birt *et al.*, 1999). Therefore, flavonoids have gained importance in the pharmaceutical field. The flavonoids are widely available as nutritional supplements, which could be extensively used as primary sources of complementary and alternative health care products or economic in-house regimens for cancer patients. It is still controversial whether all natural flavonoids are beneficial for the prevention and treatment of human cancers. The biological actions of flavonoids depend on the structure and the

Groups	Compounds	Food Sources
Flavonols	Quercetin, Kaempferol, Myricetin, Isorhamnetin, Querctagetin	Yellow onion, Curly kale, Leek, Cherry, Tomato, Broccoli, Apple, Green & Black tea, Black grapes, Blueberry, Olives, Lettuce, Parsley
Flavones	Tangeretin, Heptamethoxyflavone, Nobiletin, Sinensetin, Quercetogetin, **Chrysin**, Apegenin, Luteolin, Disometin, Tricetin	Parsley, Celery, Capsicum pepper, Apple skins, Berries,
Flavanones	Naringenin, Eriodictyol, Hesperetin, Dihydroquercetin, Dihydrofisetin, Dihydrobinetin	Orange juice, Grapefruit juice, Lemon juice
Flavanols	Silibinin, Silymarin, Taxifolin, Pinobanksin	Cocoa, Cocoa beverages, Chocolates
Catechins (Proanthocyanidins)	(+) Catechin, Gallocatechin, (-) Epicatechin, Epigallocatechin, Epicatechin 3-gallate, Epigallocatechin 3-gallate	Chocolate, Beans, Apricot, Cherry, Grapes, Peach, Red wine, Cider, Green & Black tea, Blackberry
Isoflanones	Daidzein, Genistein, Glycitein	Soy cheese, Soy flour, Soy bean, Tofu
Anthocyanins	Cyanidin, Delphinidin, Malvidin, Pelargonidin, Peonidin, Petunidin	Blueberry, Blackcurrant, Black grapes, Cherry, Rhubarb, Plum, Strawberry, Red wine, Red cabbage

Table 1: Classification of flavonoids. The flavonoid in bold is under our current study. This table is derived from the article by Lakhanpal & Rai, 2007.

structural properties may be crucial for the actions of the compounds (Jin *et al.*, 2007 & Yang *et al.*, 2006).

2   Chrysin

Chrysin (5,7-dihydroxyflavone) is the natural and biologically active flavones group of flavonoids. It is the focus of this review (Nijveldt *et al.*, 2001; Awad *et al.*, 2003; Zheng *et al.*, 2003; Ernst, 2006; Huang *et al.*, 2006; Scheck *et al.*, 2006; Cole *et al.*, 2008; Kale *et al.*, 2008; Parajuli *et al.*, 2009) (Figure 1). Chrysin can be extracted from plants, such as passion flower (Beaumont *et al.*, 2008), silver linden, honey and propolis of some geranium species (Samarghandian *et al.*, 2011). It has been reported that chrysin can also be found in a species of mushroom, *Pleurotus ostreatus* (Anandhi *et al.*, 2013). In addition to be food flavourant and pigment, chrysin has been identified as food constituent that plays important biological roles in nitrogen fixation and chemical defences (Khoo *et al.*, 2010). The chemical structure of chrysin shares the common flavone structure, which composed of fused A and C rings, and a phenyl B ring attached to position 2 of the C ring, with hydroxyl groups at position 5 and 7 of ring A (Figure 1). Chrysin has been shown to be an analogue of galangin, baicalein, apigenin, kaempferol, luteolin and quercetin. However, its anti-cancer properties have seldom been studied in details compare with other flavonoids. Preliminarily, chrysin is observed to have lowered cytotoxic activity *in vitro* in certain human cancer cells, compared with other flavonoids. However, the potential apoptotic effect of chrysin has been reported in human cervical cancer cells, leukemic cells, esophageal squamous carcinoma cells, malignant glioma cells, breast carcinoma cells, prostate cancer cells, Non-Small Cell Lung Cancer (NSCLC) cells and

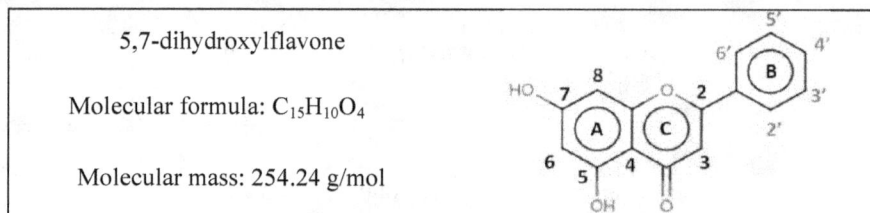

Figure 1: General information and chemical structure of chrysin.

colon cancer cells (Khoo *et al.*, 2010). Activation of apoptosis is the key molecular mechanism responsible for the anti-cancer activities of most of the flavonoids currently being studied, including chrysin.

In fact, chrysin exhibited promising cytotoxic effects with an EC_{50} value of 100 µM in a variety of human cancer cell lines, including breast cancer cell lines (MCF-7 and MDA-MB-231), malignant glioma cell lines (U87-MG and U-251), colon cancer cell lines (Lovo, DLD-1) and prostate cancer cell line (PC3) (Chang *et al.*, 2008; Khoo *et al.*, 2010; Androutsopoulos *et al.*, 2011). Furthermore, treatment of human melanoma cells (A375) with chrysin at lowers concentration; 40 µM showed a drastic decreasing in the levels of anti-apoptotic proteins, such as $Bcl-x_L$ (a Bcl-2 family protein) and survivin (Manika *et al.*, 2012). Interestingly, an increase in the level of effector caspase (caspase-3) was also observed in the study. Thus, these observations suggested that the chrysin had a potential role in causing caspase-dependent apoptosis. Besides, a recent study proved that the chrysin not only induced apoptosis in cancer cells by activation of caspases, but it also suppressed some of the well-known anti-apoptotic proteins, such as IAP and c-FLIP; inhibited IKK and NF-κB activities and influenced the PI3K/AKT signalling pathway (Sawicka *et al.* 2012). All of the studies done are significantly elucidated that chrysin induces apoptosis *via* dose- and time-dependent manners. However, a systematic study of the apoptotic activity of chrysin in the aforementioned human cancer cell lines has yet to be fully elucidated. Further studies are necessary not only to understand the exact mechanism of chrysin-induced apoptosis in cancer cells, but to facilitate the studies demonstrate that the chrysin exhibits a broad range of pharmacological effects ranging from anti-inflammatory properties to anti-oxidation and anti-cancer properties by induction of apoptosis in a diverse range of human and rat cells (Zheng *et al.*, 2003; Kale *et al.*, 2008; Khoo *et al.*, 2010; Teh *et al.*, 2010).

Chrysin is also reported as a potent inhibitor of aromatase which is responsible for blocking the conversion of androgen to estrogens (Sanderson *et al.*, 2004; Khoo *et al.*, 2010). Estrogens are known as cell proliferators and their metabolites, such as catechols, are carcinogens. A local expression of aromatase is suggested to be closely connected with tumour initiation, promotion and progression (Chen, 1998). Therefore, chrysin seems to be a promising way for treatment towards steroid hormone-dependent cancers (breast and prostate), as well as preventing menopausal symptoms by blocking the aromatase activities (Nga & Walle, 2007). However, its blockade should not interfere with the production of other steroids (Hodek *et al.*, 2002). The situation may be different when high intake of chrysin is made, whereby it may result accumulation of flavonoid in tissue that are sufficiently high to inhibit aromatase activity. The sharp decreases of aromatase activity in females may also lead to disruption of the menstrual cycle (Brodice *et al.*, 1989) and loss of bone density (Turner *et al.*, 1994). As for men, decrease estrogen systhesis may also result in deleterious effects on bone homeostasis (Vanderschueren *et al.*, 1998) and disruption of spermatogenesis (Carreau *et al.*, 2003). Although, aforementioned of flavonoids plays a role in modulating the function of sex hormones and their receptors. However, the function of chrysin as a putative inhibitor for aromatase is poorly elucidated. Most of the studies reported that chrysin was used to raise or stimulated testosterone concentration (Kellis *et al.*, 1984; von Brandenstein *et al.*, 2008) that increased it marketing values by health food stores and is used by many body builders (Nga & Walle, 2007). The oral bioavailability of chrysin was lacking circumstantial clinical evidence in the past years. Nonetheless, recent studies suggested that extensive metabolism by adsorption cells was the factor that caused the oral bioavailability of chrysin was much too low for any biological activity in humans (Galijatovic *et al.*, 1999; Walle *et al.*, 1999; Walle *et al.*, 2001).

Chrysin has also been demonstrated to inhibit the activation of human immunodeficiency virus in models of latent infection (Critchfield *et al.*, 1996; Khoo *et al.*, 2010). Most of these studies focused on the inhibitory activity of reverse transcriptase, or RNA-directed DNA polymerase, but there were other studies on chrysin acted as anti-integrase and anti-protease activities were also described (Nijveldt *et al.*, 2001). However, all of these effects require further clinical validation and verification. An exhaustive line of research shows that chrysin demonstrates anxiolytic properties, which inhibit surgical and non-surgical suppression of Natural Killer (NK) cells activity (Beaumont *et al.*, 2008). NK cells are crucial for defence against infectious diseases and cancers. Several factors have been shown to suppress NK cells activity, including stress, anxiety, surgical procedures and certain anesthetics (Locke *et al.*, 1984; Melamed *et al.*, 2003; Ben-Eliyahu *et al.*, 1999), and hence, surgical suppression of NK cells activity accompanied by prolonged stress may promote metastatic spread of cancers. Therefore, anxiety control and pain management must be an essential element of care and is often accomplished through the use of pharmaceutical agents. This inhibition by chrysin may lead to the suppression of cancer cells metastasis (Beaumont *et al.*, 2008). However, the recent study elucidates the anxiolytic effect of chrysin is blocked by the administration of flumazenil, suggesting that chrysin has a higher possibility to bind to the α-subunit of ϒ-aminobutyric acid (GABA) receptor (Dhawan *et al.*, 2002), and hence, further studies are required to elucidate the effects of chrysin on NK cells activity fully under surgical and non-surgical conditions.

3   *In vitro* activities of chrysin

3.1   Chrysin suppresses HIF-1α/VEGF and angiogenesis

As mentioned in the introduction, chrysin is a natural flavonoid and has been shown recently to have anti-cancer effects on various cancer cells. However, the molecular mechanisms underlying chrysin on cancer inhibition are not well studied. In this section, investigation showed that chrysin suppresses *in vitro* expression of Hypoxia-inducible Factor-1 alpha (HIF-1α) in tumour cells and inhibits *in vivo* expression of tumour cell-induced angiogenesis through multiple HIF/VEGF pathways, a crucial step in metastasis (Fu *et al.*, 2007; Samarghandian *et al.*, 2011).

In a nutshell, Hypoxia-inducible Factor-1 (HIF-1) is a transcription factor with a heterodimeric structure composed of oxygen regulated α and ubiquitously expressed β subunits. HIF-1α is constitutively expressed during hypoxia, but rapidly degraded by the ubiquitin-proteasome pathway in normoxia (Salceda & Caro, 1997; Kallio *et al.*, 1999; Fu *et al.*, 2007). The prolyl hydroxylation of HIF-1α at the Oxygen-dependent Degradation Domain (ODD) is critical in the regulation of HIF-1α steady state (Fu *et al.*, 2007). Under hypoxic condition, the absence of oxygen prevents the prolyl hydroxylase from modifying HIF-1α, allowing HIF-1α to accumulate (Jaakkola *et al.*, 2001, Ivan *et al.*, 2001). Besides, HIF-1α has been demonstrated to heterodimerize with HIF-1β, and this HIF-1 complex acts as a regulator for more than 70 genes involved in cellular response to reduce oxygen level, thus playing a role in adaptation, survival and progression of tumour cells, including Vascular Endothelial Growth Factor (VEGF) (Miranda *et al.*, 2013) (Figure 2). The intricate interplay between HIF-α isomers in cancer is complicated and yet to be fully deciphered, but the role of HIF-1α activity has been correlated with tumourigenicity and angiogenesis. Many anaerobic human cancers cells are observed to overexpress HIF-1α, because it is induced by hypoxia, cytokines, growth factors, hormones, activated oncogenes and inactivated tumour suppressors (Maxwell *et al.*, 1997; Fukuda *et al.*, 2002; Traxler *et al.*, 2004; Fu *et al.*, 2007; Nagle & Zhou, 2006). Hypoxic tumour cells are more resistant to ionizing radiation and chemotherapy than normoxic tumour cells. These cells are also more invasive and metastatic, resistant to apoptosis and genetically unstable (Melillo *et al.*, 2007). Such areas have been found in a wide range of malignancies: cancers of breast, uterine cervix, vulva, head and neck, prostate, rectum, pancreas, lung, brain tumours, soft tissue sarcomas, non-Hodgkin's lymphomas, malignant melanomas, metastatic liver tumours and renal cell cancer (Vaupel *et al.*, 2007).

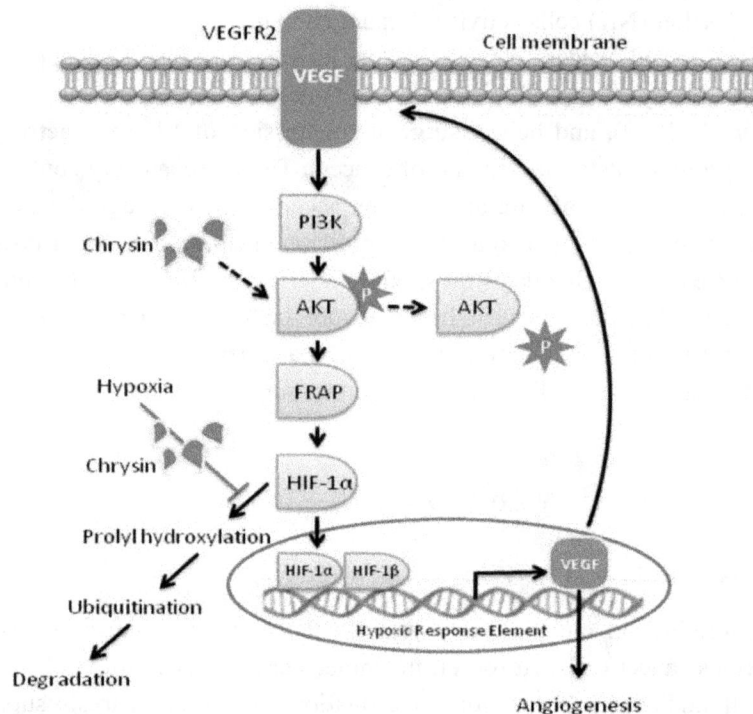

Figure 2: The proposed schematic diagram of the mechanism of HIF-1α and VEGF in angiogenesis. Chrysin is consistently demonstrated to inhibit tumour angiogenesis by targeting multiple HIF-1α/VEGF mechanisms *via* reducing the HIF-1α stability, dephosphorylating the AKT in the mechanism and reducing the interaction of HIF-1α with Hsp90.

VEGF that is involved in tumour angiogenesis is regulated by HIF-1α in the transcriptional level (Ferrara & Davis-Smyth, 1997; Folkman, 2002; Fu *et al.*, 2007). HIF-1α activates the expression of VEGF gene by binding to the Hypoxia Response Element (HRE) in VEGF promoter (Fang *et al.*, 2005).

In addition to the induction of HIF-1α, other microenvironmental factors are also shown to influence VEGF expression; among them are glucose depletion, glutamine deprivation and acidic extracellular pH (Vaupel *et al.*, 2007). Angiogenesis is critical in tumourigenesis because *de novo* blood vessel formation must occur to maintain oxygen and nutrient exchange between the tumour periphery and the hypoxic core and metastasis (Folkman 2007). Tumour angiogenesis is stimulated by angiogenic growth factors, such as VEGF, basic Fibroblast Growth Factor (bFGF), Transforming Growth Factor (TGF) and Interleukin-8 (IL-8). VEGF and its receptors have been described as the fundamental regulators of angiogenesis and play an important role in tumour progression (Fang *et al.*, 2005). Therefore, an anti-angiogenic therapy that targets HIF-1α/VEGF system by reducing the HIF-1α level proportionally reducing the expression of VEGF mRNA is a promising strategy for the treatment of human cancers.

The correlation between chrysin and HIF-1α in hypoxia and angiogenesis has been demonstrated and showed that chrysin reduces HIF-1α stability by increasing the prolyl hydroxylation of Oxygen-dependent Domains (ODDs), resulting in an increase in the ubiquitination and proteasome degradation of HIF-1α (Fu *et al.*, 2007) (Figure 2). However, the mechanism of chrysin affecting ODDs remains unknown. A separate study demonstrated that chrysin had the ability also to reduce HIF-1α stability by inhibiting the interaction between HIF-1α and Heat Shock Protein 90 (Hsp90), a chaperone protein (Minet *et al.*, 1999; Isaacs *et al.*, 2002; Katschinski *et al.*, 2002; Nagle & Zhou, 2006). In the studies, the authors suggested that Hsp90 bound to the HIF-1α PAS domains stabilized HIF-1α protein from degradation.

The expression of HIF-1α is regulated not only through protein degradation. It has been reported that growth factors, cytokines and other signalling molecules stimulated also the HIF-1α expression through Phosphatidylinositol 3-kinase (PI3K) (Blancher *et al.*, 2001; Laughner *et al.*, 2001; Stiehl *et al.*, 2002) and target of rapamycin signalling pathways (Treins *et al.*, 2002). Briefly, PI3K/AKT signalling pathway plays an important role in the expression of HIF-1α (Jiang *et al.*, 2001; Blancher *et al.*, 2001). PI3K is a key player in PI3K/AKT signalling pathway, and it is a heterodimeric enzyme composed of 110 kDa catalytic subunit and an 85 kDa regulatory subunit (Carpenter *et al.*, 1990). The best-known downstream target of PI3K is the Serine Threonine Kinase (AKT), which transmits survival signals from growth factors (Chan *et al.*, 1999; Duronio *et al.*, 1998). PI3K/AKT signalling cascade is essential for VEGF expression through HIF-1α response to growth factor stimulation and oncogene activation (Zunde

et al., 2000; Blancher *et al.*, 2001; Zhong *et al.*, 2000; Jiang *et al.*, 2001; Fukuda *et al.*, 2002). Conclusively, the role of PI3K/AKT signalling pathway in cancer and angiogenesis is firmly established. Lately, chrysin was found and observed to act as an inhibitor of AKT phosphorylation, and overexpression of active AKT reversed the chrysin-inhibited HIF-1α expression (Fu *et al.*, 2007). Indirectly, this suggests chrysin may inhibit HIF-1α/VEGF-regulated angiogenesis *via* the AKT signalling pathway (Figure 2). It was also reported that flavonoids or related compounds, such as apigenin (Fang *et al.*, 2005; Osada *et al.*, 2004), resveratrol (Cao *et al.*, 2004), and epigallocatechin-3-gallate (Zhang *et al.*, 2006), inhibited the expression of HIF-1α not only through PI3K/AKT pathway, but multiple signalling pathways. This novel finding provides new insight for chrysin as a potent and versatile inhibitor of angiogenesis and tumorigenesis.

3.2   Chrysin downregulates NFκB and its target genes

The anti-cancer potential of chrysin has been further addressed and enhanced by assessing the sensitisation effect of chrysin on Tumour Necrosis Factor-alpha (TNFα)-mediated apoptosis and its related molecular mechanisms (Li *et al.*, 2010; Samarghandian *et al.*, 2011). This sensitisation effect of chrysin is closely associated with its inhibitory effect on Nuclear Factor kappa B (NFκB) activation, which reduces the expression of NFκB target genes, such as c-FLIP-L that blocking caspase-8 activity (Samarghandian *et al.*, 2011) (Figure 3). Generally, NFκB is a transcription factor involved in multiple cellular processes, including apoptosis. Therefore, it is also a target gene for chemopreventive properties of phytochemicals (Li *et al.*, 2010; Samarghandian *et al.*, 2011). Periodically, NFκB appears as a complex of NFκB:IκB in cytoplasm. The binding of IκB to NFκB prevents NFκB protein to translocate into the nucleus, and hence maintains inactive NFκB in cytoplasm (Hayden & Ghosh, 2004). However, the dynamic balance between cytosolic and nuclear localizations of NFκB is altered upon IκB degradation, resulting in translocation of the activated NFκB into the nucleus where the dimer binds to specific sequences in the promoter or enhancer regions of target genes, such as iNOS, TNFα, IL-1, IL-8, COX-2, CAMs and c-FLIC-L (Ingaramo *et al.*, 2013).

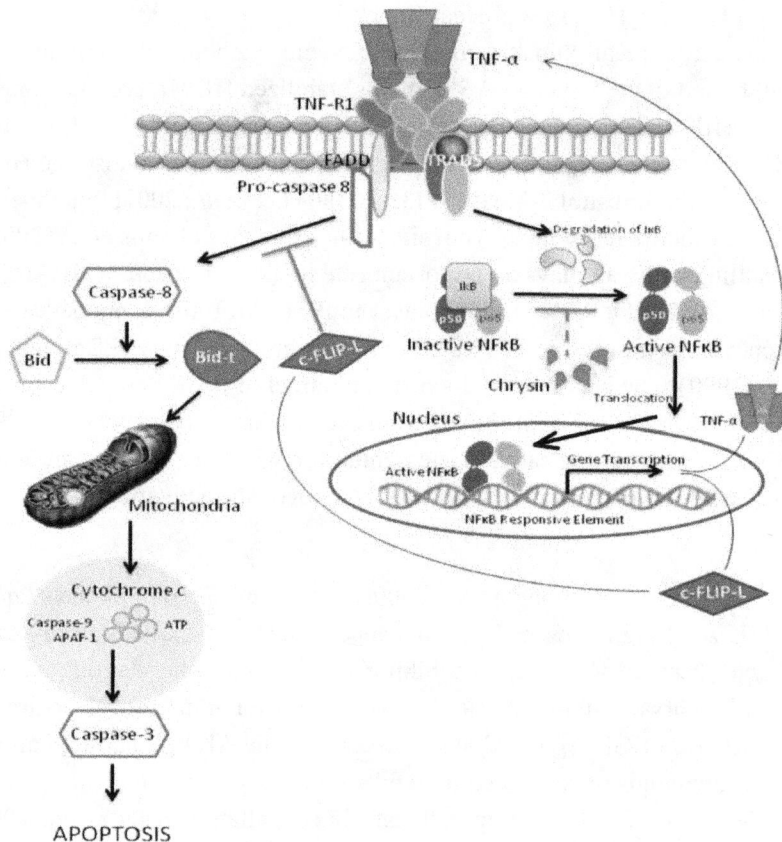

Figure 3: The proposed schematic diagram of the mechanism of NFκB activation induced by TNFα signalling pathway. Chrysin downregulates NFκB and its target genes whereby enhances the activation of caspase-8 in the apoptotic mechanism.

The sensitisation effect of chrysin on TNFα-induced cell death is achieved through downregulation of NFκB, whereby it reduces of NFκB target gene; cFLIP-L which followed by enhancement of caspase-8 activation. Caspase-8 is the initial caspase in the death receptor signalling pathway that typically induces apoptosis post-ligand treatment. Furthermore, chrysin also shows potential in inducing MAPKp38 and activating NFκB/p65 in cell-cycle arrest and apoptosis (Samarghandian *et al.*, 2011; von Brandenstein *et al.*, 2008).

3.3   Chrysin inactivates PI3K/AKT signalling pathway in apoptosis

Generally, the important effects of chrysin in cellular processes can be concluded to be (1) the inhibition of HIF-1α/VEGF-regulated angiogenesis *via* the AKT signalling pathway and (2) the sensitisation of TNFα-induced cell death *via* downregulation of NFκB and activation of caspase-8. In addition, (3) chrysin induces also apoptosis *via* activation of caspase-3, which involves the inactivation of AKT signalling pathway and downregulation of the X-linked Inhibitor of Apoptosis Protein (XIAP) (Samarghandian *et al.*, 2011). This phenomenon is observed on leukemic cell line (U937) in a previous study that provides the first evidence of a more detailed molecular mechanism on how chrysin induces apoptosis *via* AKT dephosphorylation in the PI3K signalling pathway. The AKT signalling pathway attracts much attention because of its role in cell survival and the ability to evade cell death pathways in cancer progression. In an overview, the AKT signalling pathway, begins from PI3K to Phosphoinositide-dependent Kinase-1 (PDK1) and end with AKT, mediates apoptosis in human cancer cells. The activation of AKT *via* phosphorylation prevents apoptosis (Roberts, 2000), whereas dephosphorylation initiates apoptosis. Phosphorylation of AKT phosphorylates Bcl-2-associated Death protein (BAD) and a non-active form of caspase-9, which are the hosts of the cell-signalling proteins. The signalling cascade continues when phosphorylated BAD binds to cytosolic 14-3-3 proteins, resulting in a failure of the protein to heterodimerise with Bcl-2 at the mitochondrial membrane (Kelekar *et al.*, 1997). Dephosphorylation of BAD releases itself from cytosolic 14-3-3 proteins, which subsequently form heterodimers with Bcl-2 family proteins and migrate into the mitochondrial membrane. This is where the heterodimers induce the release of cytochrome *c* by altering the membrane pores (Pelengaris *et al.*, 2002; Debatin, 2004). Free cytochrome *c* in the cytoplasm combines with Apoptotic Protease Activating Factor-1 (APAF-1) and caspase-9 to form a complex called apoptosome with the presence of ATP in order to activate the caspase-9 (Debatin, 2004). Subsequently, caspase-9 initiates the downstream executor caspase-3. The activation of caspase-3 follows by degradative events trigger apoptosis (Yoshida *et al.*, 2003; Debatin, 2004). The role of BAD in this molecular mechanism has been investigated. However, the involvement of Bcl-2 Homologous Antagonist/Killer protein (BAK) in this mechanism has not been elucidated in any study previously. It is hypothesized that BAK may have different capacity than BAX to induce apoptosis in cancer cells. Besides, chrysin has also been reported to have the ability to abolish Stem Cell Factor (SCF)/c-Kit signalling by inhibiting the PI3K/AKT pathway (Lee *et al.*, 2007). Monasterio *et al.* (2004) reported that flavonoids, including chrysin, induced apoptosis *via* a mechanism that required the activation of caspase-3 and caspase-8, indicating that chrysin-induced apoptosis could operate *via* a ligand receptor-dependent cell death mechanism. This study suggested also a relationship between AKT and NFκB signalling pathway in the cells. Thus, the study elucidates the relationship between AKT and NFκB with respect to the effects of chrysin in human cancer cells is warranted.

4   Chrysin inhibits proliferation and induces apoptosis in HeLa

4.1   Cervical cancer in Malaysia

Malaysia is a rapidly developing South-East Asian country with an intermediate Gross Domestic Product (GDP) per capita and a significant burden of cervical cancer (Othman & Rebolj, 2009). According to Power Over Cervical Cancer (POCC) in a campaign initiated by the National Cancer Society Malaysia (NCSM), cervical cancer is the third most common cancer among Malaysian females following breast and colorectal cancers. Among the ethnic groups in Malaysia, Indians ranked the highest incidence rate in 2007 at 10.3 per 100,000 persons, followed by Chinese and Malays at 9.5 and 5.3 per 100,000 persons, respectively. On the other hand, the National Cancer Registry (NCR) revealed that the highest number of cancer cases in the country is breast cancer (18.1%), followed by colon cancer (12.3%), lung cancer (10.2%), nasopharynx cancer (5.2%) and cervical cancer (4.6%). On a larger scale, woman dies of cervical cancer every two minutes worldwide. As in other countries in Southeast Asia, the burden of cervical cancer in Malaysia is moderately high. The costs of nationwide spent for cytology-based screening approaches, such as Pap testing that effective in preventing cervical cancer are limited in the region. Moreover, the use of alternative screening modalities, such as visual inspection of the cervix aided by acetic acid (VIA) with or without magnification, is plainly for inspection only. Although prophylactic Human Papillomavirus (HPV) vaccination for the prevention of infection and related disease is considered as an additional cervical cancer control strategy, the service is not accessible to all women in the country. In addition, more efforts should be dedicated to the policy-making context; improve awareness and increase knowledge about cervical cancer using mass media, electronic media, posters and pamphlets to maintain a healthy lifestyle in the community.

Leading a healthy lifestyle has been a way to reduce the risk and the cause of cervical cancer in Malaysia. These efforts include campaigns of consumption more fruits and vegetables, exercising, quitting smoking, taking vitamins, minerals, food supplements and healthcare products. Consuming more fruits and vegetables that contain high levels of flavonoids e.g. chrysin can prevent cervical cancer. Naturally occurring chrysin products are found in the passion flowers *Passiflora caerulea* and *Passiflora incarnata*, honeycomb, the mushroom *Pleurotus ostreatus*, chamomile, *Oroxylum indicum* and Indian trumpet flower. Malaysia has an abundance of traditional medicinal plants and fruits that can be produced for the above-mentioned purposes (Anandhi *et al.*, 2013). As such, complementary and alternative medicine and healthcare products of chrysin should be developed from local traditional medicinal plants and fruits as the primary source of healthcare products or economical in-house regimens for cancer patients in this region.

4.2   *In vitro* cervical cancer study

Chrysin has been observed to reduce the cytotoxic activity in many human cancer cells. Moreover, the potential apoptotic effect of chrysin has been reported in human cervical cancer, leukemia, esophageal squamous carcinoma, malignant glioma, breast carcinoma, prostate cancer, NSCLC and colorectal cancers (Khoo *et al.*, 2010). Although chrysin has showed to sensitize various human cancer cells to apoptosis substantially (Li *et al.*, 2010), detailed studies of the apoptotic activity of chrysin in cancer cells remain to be elucidated. Furthermore, the apoptotic effect exhibited by chrysin in cervical cancer cells has not extensively being reviewed with respect to leukemia previously (Table 2). Therefore, chrysin remains its values to be studied for the treatment of human cervical cancer.

Immortal cancer cell lines are used as a useful tool, to facilitate the *in vitro* screening of novel cytotoxic compounds in human cancer research. Additionally, cell culture facilitates also the study of mechanisms and actions of novel compounds and the structure-activity relationship of the compounds, as well as others *in vitro* study, for the development of novel anti-cancer agents (Middleton *et al.*, 1994; Lopez-Lazaro *et al.*, 2002). The HeLa cell line is the best known and most widely used human cervical cancer cell line. Indeed, it was the first successful immortal cell line used for the study of human cancers (Masters *et al.*, 2002). Briefly, the HeLa cell line was derived from an adenocarcinoma on the cervix of a 31-year-old black woman, according to the American Type Culture Collection (ATCC). The cells are epithelial, adherent, contain human papillomavirus and react as a suitable transfection host that can be used to

Cancer Type	Reference	Effect and Molecular Mechanism
Cervical cancer	Zhang *et al.* (2004)	Chrysin (IC_{50}=14.2 μM) inhibited proliferation and induced apoptosis in HeLa cells, though the effects were not as potent as those of its synthetic derivative compounds.
	von Brandenstein *et al.* (2008)	Chrysin (30 μM) potentially induced p38 and NFkappaB/p65 activation in HeLa cells.
	Lird-prapamongkol *et al.* (2013)	Chrysin (20-60 μM) sensitized HeLa cells to TRAIL-induced apoptosis by inhibiting STAT3 and downregulating Mcl-1.
Leukemia	Monasterio *et al.* (2004)	Chrysin (IC_{50} = 16 μM) showed to be the most potent flavonoid to reduce cell viability and induced apoptotic DNA fragmentation in U937 cells.
	Woo *et al.* (2004), Woo *et al.* (2005)	Chrysin induced apoptosis in Bcl-2 overexpressing U937 leukemia cells, was associated with activation of caspase-3 and PLC-γ1 degradation. The induction of apoptosis was accompanied by down-regulation of XIAP and inactivation of AKT.
	Lee *et al.* (2007)	Chrysin had the ability to abolish SCF/c-Kit signaling by inhibiting the PI3K pathway in myeloid leukemia cells (MO7e).
	Ramos *et al.* (2008)	Chrysin, alone or in combination with other compounds, decreased AKT phosphorylation and potentially caused mitochondrial dysfunction in THP-1 and HL-60 leukemia cells.

Table 2: The apoptotic effects of chrysin in leukemia and cervical cancer *in vitro* (Khoo *et al.*, 2010).

screen for *Escherichia coli* strains with invasive potential. HeLa cells are indispensable to cancer research, indeed. Therefore, many pharmacological studies and biological evaluations have been carried out using this cell line. For example, several natural and synthetic flavonoids, such as chrysin, are used to determine whether these compounds can inhibit the growth of HeLa cells by inhibiting cell cycle, cell proliferation, oxidative stress, and to induce detoxification enzymes, apoptosis or activate the immune system. Although many efforts have been dedicated to the screening of the preliminary effects of chrysin using HeLa cells, the exact molecular mechanisms and effects exhibited by chrysin in HeLa cells are not fully understood yet.

One contemporary study showed that the chrysin possibly induced p38 to activate NFκB/p65 in HeLa cells, leading to the apoptosis of the cells (von Brandenstein *et al.*, 2008). Similarly, a few studies also showed that treatment of HeLa cells with 30 μM chrysin for 24 hours induced a significant improvement of NFκB/p65 ranges in the cells, as demonstrated by EMSA. The signals could be suppressed by a specific p38 or p65 inhibitor, indicating that p38 or p65 could be helpful therapeutic target of chrysin in managing gene expression in HeLa cells. More studies are required to determine whether this phenomenon can occur in different manners in HeLa cells, in which NFκB remains the target of research to uncover the mechanisms of apoptosis induced by chrysin in HeLa cells.

4.3   Improving the effects of chrysin in cervical cancer

The biological properties and potential anti-cancer effects of chrysin in human cervical carcinoma (HeLa) can be improved by synthesising dietyl chrysin-7-yl phosphate (CPE: $C_{19}H_{19}O_7P$) and the tetraethyl bis-phosphoric ester of chrysin (CP: $C_{23}H_{28}O_{10}P_2$) through a simplified Antheron Todd reaction (Zhang *et al.*, 2004). The chemical structures indicate the formation of CPE and CP can be achieved by replacing the hydroxyl groups at positions 5 and/or 7 of the A ring in chrysin with phosphate groups (Figure 4). Mass spectroscopy analysis revealed that CPE formed a non-covalent compound with lysozyme, and hence, phosphate esters of chrysin enhanced the interaction of phosphorylated (modified) chrysin with proteins compared to the interaction induced by non-phosphorylated chrysin. The phosphorylated chrysin was concluded to be more effective in inhibiting cancer cell growth and inducing apoptosis in HeLa cells, compared to the original one. This phenomenon can be observed in cultured HeLa cells treated with chrysin, CP and CPE at a concentration of 10 μM for 24 hours, 48 hours and 72 hours. The replacement of both hydroxyl groups at positions 5 and 7 of the A ring in chrysin with phosphate groups proved more effective of the phosphorylated chrysin in inhibiting the growth of cancer cells and inducing apoptosis in HeLa cells more efficiently, compared to the original one. At the same time, this result showed that the cell viability declined in a time-dependent fashion. All chrysin, CPE and CP showed inhibition potency upon proliferation and apoptosis induction in the following order; CP (IC50 = 9.8 μM) > CPE (IC50 = 10.3 μM) > chrysin (IC50 = 14.2 μM) in HeLa cells, using methyl green-pyronin staining and Terminal Deoxynucleotidyl Transferase-mediated dUTP Nick End Labeling (TUNEL) assay, confirming the aforementioned hypothesis. In addition, chrysin, CPE and CP were shown to reduce cell viability by induction of apoptosis and downregulation of the Proliferating Cell Nuclear Antigen (PCNA) in the cells assessed by PCNA immunohistochemistry. Therefore, chrysin and phosphorylated chrysin are suggested as potential potent anti-cancer agents for the treatment of human cervical carcinoma.

5   Perspectives

In conclusion, chrysin inhibits proliferation, induces apoptosis and reduce angiogenesis in most tested cancer cells, including cervical cancer cells. Studies of the mechanisms and actions of the phytochemical reveal that chrysin likely operates by suppressing HIF-1α/VEGF, downregulating NFκB and inactivating PI3K/AKT signalling pathways. However, the inter-relationship of these mechanisms in chrysin-induced apoptosis remains unclear, even though they are known to act *via* the caspase activation cascade. Other

Bcl-2 family proteins, such as BAK1 and BAK2, might enhance the effect of chrysin-induced apoptosis in HeLa cells. Our current research supports this preliminary hypothesis. However, more studies are warranted. The biological activities of chrysin may be improved by modification of the original structure of chrysin or combination therapy. In addition to structure modification or combination therapy, it is necessary to have chrysin that would not cause general cytotoxicity-related side effects. Although most studies support the conclusion that chrysin induces apoptosis in various tumour cell lines, studies published to date are often haphazardly performed and occasionally contradictory. Hence, more significant research

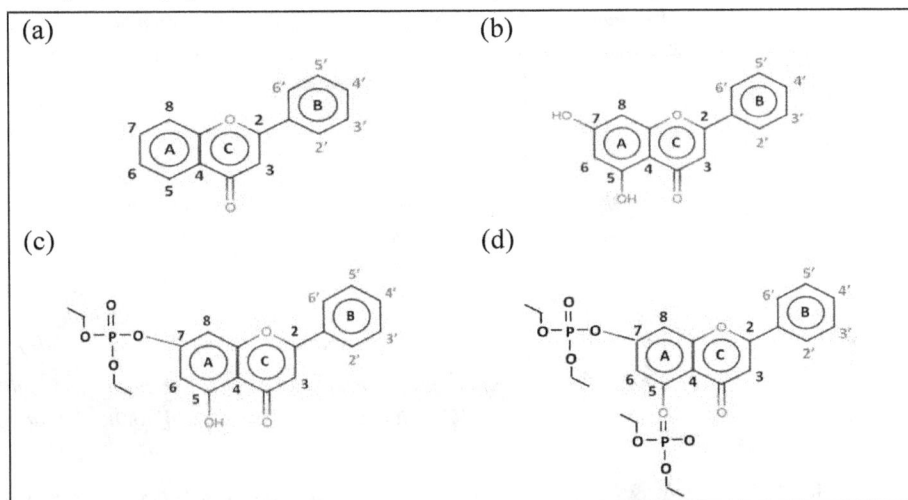

Figure 4: (a) Common chemical structure of flavones, (b) chemical structure of chrysin, (c) chemical structure of dietyl chrysin-7-yl phosphate (CPE) and (d) chemical structure of tetraethyl bis-phosphoric ester of chrysin (CP).

that combine well-designed bioassays and unique sources of chemical diversity are required to understand the exact mechanisms and actions of apoptosis induced by chrysin in human cancers. Results of these studies may help to develop ways of improving the effectiveness of chrysin in the treatment of human cancers.

Acknowledgements

This book chapter was funded by a Research University Grant Scheme (Grant number 1001/CIPPM/811208) from Universiti Sains Malaysia. The first author is grateful for the support of Ernst-von-Leyden Scholarship, from Berliner Krebsgesellschaft E.V. (BKG) and Dr. Ranjeet Bhagwan Singh Medical Research Trust Fund during her postdoctoral training. The author thanks also Mr. Benjamin Khoo Wu-Yang for his technical assistance in preparing this book chapter.

References

Aherne, A. S. & Obrien, N. M. (2002). Dietary flavonols: Chemistry, food content and metabolism. Nutrition, 18(1), 75-81.

Anandhi, R., Annadurai, T., Anitha, T. S., Muralidharan, A. R., Najmunnisha, K., Nachiappan, V., Thomas, P. A. & Geraldine, P. (2013). Antihypercholesterolemic and antioxidative effects of an extract of the oyster mushroom, Pleurotus ostratus, and its major constituent, chrysin, in Triton WR-1339-induced hypercholesterolemic rats. Journal of Physiology and Biochemistry, 69(2), 313-323.

Androutsopoulos, V. P., Papakyriakou, A., Vourloumis, D. & Spandidos, D. A. (2011). Comparative CYP1A1 and CYP1B1 substrate and inhibitor profile of dietary flavonoids. Bioorganic & Medicinal Chemistry, 19(9), 2842-2849.

Awad, R., Arnason, J. T., Trudeau, V., Bergeron, C., Budzinski, J. W., Foster, B. C. & Merali, Z. (2003). Phytochemical and biological analysis of skullcap (Scutellaria lateriflora L.): A medicinal plant with anxiolytic properties. Phytomedicine, 10(8), 640-649.

Beaumont, D. M., Mark, T. M. Jr., Hills, R., Dixon, P., Veit, B. & Normalynn, G. (2008). The effect of chrysin, a Passiflora incarnata extract, on natural killer cell activity in male Sprague-Dawley Rats undergoing abdominal surgery. AAANA Journal, 76(2), 113-117.

Ben-Eliyahu, S., Page, G. G., Yirmiya, R. & Shakhar, G. (1999). Evidence that stress and surgical interventions promote tumour development by suppressing natural killer cell activity. International Journal of Cancer, 80(6), 880-888.

Birt, D. F., Shull, J. D. & Yaktine, A. (1999). Chemoprevention of cancer. In Modern Nutrition in Health and Diesease Baltimore (eds Shils ME, Olson JE, Shike M, Ross & AC). Lippincott, Williams and Wilkins, Philadelphia, 9, 1283-1295.

Blancher, C., Moore, J. W., Robertson, N. & Harris, A. L. (2001). Effects of ras and von Hippel-Lindau (VHL) gene mutations on hypoxia-inducible factor (HIF)-1alpha, HIF-2alpha, and vascular endothelial growth factor expression and their regulation by the phosphatidylinositol 3'-kinase/Akt signaling pathway. Cancer Research, 61(19), 7349-7355.

Block, G., Patterson, B. & Subar, A. (1992). Fruit, vegetable and cancer prevention: A review of the epidemiological evidence. Nutrition and Cancer, 18(1), 1-29.

Bravo, L. (1988). Polyphenols: Chemistry, dietary sources, metabolism, and nutritional significance. Nutrition Reviews, 56(11), 317-333.

Brodie, A. M., Hammond, J. O., Ghosh, M., Meyer, K. & Albrecht, E. D. (1989). Effect of treatment with aromatase inhibitor 4-hydroxandrostenedione on the nonhuman primate menstrual cycle. Cancer Research, 49(17), 4780-4784.

Cao, Z., Fang, J., Xia, C., Shi, X. & Jiang, B. H. (2004). Trans-3,4,5'-Trihydroxystibene inhibits hypoxia-inducible factor 1alpha and vascular endothelial growth factor expression in human ovarian cancer cells. Clinical Cancer Research, 10(15), 5253-5263.

Carpenter, C. L., Duckworth, B. C. Auger, K. R., Cohen, B., Schaffhausen, B. S. & Catley, L. C. (1990). Purification and characterization of phosphoinositide 3-kinase from rat liver. Journal of Biological Chemistry, 265(32), 19704-19711.

Carreau, S., Lambard, S., Delelande, C., Denis-Galeraud, I., Bilinska, B. & Bourguiba, S. (2003). Aromatase expression and role of estrogens in male gonad: A review. Reproductive Biology and Endocrinology, 1, 35.

Chan, T. O., Rittenhouse, S. E. & Tsichlis, P. N. (1999). AKT/PKB and other D3 phosphoinositide-dependent phosphorylation. Annual Review of Biochemistry, 68, 965-1014.

Chang, H., Mi, M., Ling, W., Zhu, J., Zhang, Q., Wei, N., Zhou, Y., Tang, Y. & Yuan, J. (2008). Structurally related cytotoxic effects of flavonoids on human cancer cells in vitro. Archives of Pharmacal Research, 31(9), 1137-1144.

Chen S. (1998). Aromatase and breast cancer. Frontiers in Bioscience, 3, 922-933.

Clifford, A. H. & Cuppett, S. L. (2000). Anthocyanins - nature, occurrence and dietary burden. Journal of the Science of Food and Agriculture, 80(7), 1063-1072.

Cole, I. B., Cao, J., Alan, A. R., Saxena, P. K. & Murch, S. J. (2008). Comparisons of Scutellaria baicalensis, Scutellaria lateriflora and Scutellaria racemosa: Genome size, anti-oxidant potential and phytochemistry. Planta Medica, 74(4), 474-481.

Cook, N. C. & Samman, S. (1996). Flavonoids-chemistry, metabolism, cardioprotective effects, and dietary sources. The Journal of Nutritional Biochemistry, 7(2), 66–76.

Critchfield, J. W., Butera, S. T. & Folks, T. M. (1996). Inhibition of HIV activation in latently infected cells by flavonoid compounds. AIDS Research and Human Retroviruses, 12(1), 39-46.

Debatin, K. M. (2004). Apoptosis pathways in cancer and cancer therapy. Cancer Immunology, Immunotherapy, 53(3), 153-159.

Dhawan, K., Kumar, S. & Sharma, A. (2002). Suppression of alcohol-cessation-oriented hyper-anxiety by the benzoflavone moiety of Passiflora incarnate linneaus in mice. Journal of Ethnopharmacology, 81(2), 239-244.

Duronio, V., Scheid, M. P. & Ettinger, S. (1998). Downstrem signalling events regulated by phosphatidylinositol 3-kinase activity. Cellular Signalling, 10(4), 233-239.

Ernst, E. (2006). Herbal remedies for anxiety - a systematic review of controlled clinical trials. Phytomedicine, 13(3), 205-208.

Fang, J., Xia, C., Cao, Z. X., Zheng, J. Z., Reed, E. & Jiang, B. H. (2005). Apigenin inhibits VEGF and HIF-1 expression via PI3K/AKT/p70S6K1 and HDM2/p53 pathways. The FASEB Journal, 19(3), 342-353.

Ferrara, N. & Davis-Smyth, T. (1997). The biology of vascular endothelial growth factor. Endocrine Reviews, 18(1), 4-25.

Folkman, J. (2007). Angiogenesis: an organizing principle for drug discovery? Nature Reviews Drug Discovery, 6, 273-286.

Folkman, J. (2002). Role of angiogenesis in tumor growth and metastasis. Seminars in Oncology, 29(6), 15-18.

Fu, B., Xue, J., Li, Z., Shi, X., Jiang, B. H. & Fang, J. (2007). Chrysin inhibits expression of hypoxia-inducible factor-1alpha through reducing hypoxia-inducible factor-1alpha stability and inhibiting its protein synthesis. Molecular Cancer Therapeutics, 6(1), 220-226.

Fukuda, R., Hirota, K., Fan, F., Jung, Y. D., Ellis, L. M. & Semenza, G. L. (2002). Insulin-like growth factor 1 induces hypoxia-inducible factor 1-mediated vascular endothelial growth factor expression, which is dependent on MAP kinase and phosphatidylinositol 3-kinase signaling in colon cancer cells. The Journal of Biological Chemistry, 277(41), 38205-38211.

Galijatovic, A., Otake, Y., Walle, U. K. & Walle, T. (1999). Extensive metabolism of the flavonoid chrysin by human Caco-2 and Hep G2 cells. Xenobiotica, 29(12), 1241-1256.

Gambelunghe, C., Rossi, R., Sommavilla, M., Ferranti, C., Rossi, R., Ciculli, C., Gizzi, S., Micheletti, A. & Rufini, S. (2003). Effects of chrysin on urinary testosterone levels in human males. Journal of Medicinal Food, 6(4), 387-390.

Harborne, J. B. & Turner, B. L. (1984). Plant Chemosystematics. London: Academic Press.

Hayden, M. S. & Ghosh S. (2004). Signalling to NF-kappaB. Genes & Development, 18, 2195-2224.

Ho, C. T., Lee, C. Y. & Huang, M. T. (1992). Phenolic compounds in food and their effects on health I. Analysis, Occurrence & Chemistry. Austin, TX: American Chemical Society.

Hodek, P., Trefil, P. & Stiborova, M. (2002). Flavonoids-potent and versatile biologically active compounds interacting with cytochromes P450. Chemico-Biological Interactions, 139(1), 1-21.

Huang, W. H., Lee, A. R. & Yang, C. H. (2006). Anti-oxidative and anti-inflammatory activities of polyhydroxyflavonoids of Scutellaria baicalensis GEORGI. Bioscience, Biotechnology, and Biochemistry, 70(10), 2371-2380.

Ingaramo, P. I., Francés, D. E., Ronco, M. T. & Carnovale, C. E. (2013). Diabetes and its hepatic complication, hot topics in endocrine and endocrine-related diseases, Dr. Monica Fedele (Ed.), ISBN: 978-953-51-1080-4, InTech.

Isaacs, J. S., Jung, Y. J., Mimnaugh, E. G., Martinez, A., Cuttitta, F. & Neckers, L. M. (2002). Hsp90 regulates a von Hippel Lindau-independent hypoxia-inducible factor-1 alpha-degradative pathway. The Journal of Biological Chemistry, 277(33), 29936-29944.

Ivan, M., Kondo, K., Yang, H., Kim, W., Valiando, J., Ohh, M., Salic, A., Asara, J. M., Lane, W. S. & Kaelin, W. G. Jr. (2001). HIF-alpha targeted for VHL-mediated destruction by proline hydroxylation: implications for O_2 sensing. Science, 292 (5516), 464-468.

Jaakkola, P., Mole, D. R., Tian, Y. M., Wilson, M. I., Gielbert, J., Gaskell, S. J., von Kriegsheim, A., Hebestreit, H. F., Mukherji, M., Schofield, C. J., Maxwell, P. H., Pugh, C. W. & Ratcliffe, P. J. (2001). Targeting of HIF-alpha to the von Hippel-Lindau ubiquitylation complex by O_2-regulated prolyl hydroxylation. Science, 292 (5516), 468-472.

Jiang, B. H., Jiang, G., Zheng, J. Z., Jiang, B. H., Jiang, G., Zheng, J. Z., Lu, Z., Hunter, T. & Vogt, P. K. (2001). Phosphatidylinositol 3-kinase signaling controls levels of hypoxia-inducible factor 1. Cell Growth and Differentiation, 12(7), 363-369.

Jin, F., Jin, X. Y., Jin, Y, L., Sohn, D. W., Kim, S. A., Sohn, D.H., Kim, Y. C. & Kim, H. S., (2007). Structural requirements of 2',4',6'-tris(methoxymethoxy) chalcone derivatives for antiinflammatory activity: the importance of a 2'-hydroxy moiety. Archives of Pharmacal Research, 30(11), 1359-1367.

Kale, A., Gawande, S. & Kotwal, S. (2008). Cancer phytotherapeutics: Role for flavonoids at the cellular level. Phytotherapy Research, 22(5), 567-577.

Katschinski, D. M., Le, L., Heinrich, D., Wagner, K. F., Hofer, T., Schindler, S. G. & Wenger, R. H. (2002). Heat induction of the unphosphorylated form of hypoxia-inducible factor-1alpha is dependent on heat shock protein-90 activity. The Journal of Biological Chemistry, 277(11), 9262-9267.

Kelekar, A., Chang, B. S., Harlan, J. E., Fesik, S. W. & Thompson, C. B. (1997). Bad is a BH3 domain-containing protein that forms an inactivating dimer with Bcl-XL. Molecular and Cellular Biology, 17(12), 7040-7046.

Kellis, J. T. Jr. & Vickery, L. E. (1984). Inhibition of human estrogen synthetase (aromatase) by flavones. Science, 225(4666), 1032-1034.

Khoo, B. Y., Chua, S. L. & Balaram, P. (2010). Apoptotic effects of chrysin in human cancer cell lines. International Journal of Molecular Sciences, 11(5), 2188-2199.

Kuntz, S., Wenzel, U. & Daniel, H. (1999). Comparative analysis of the effects of flavonoids on proliferation, cytotoxicity and apoptosis in human colon cancer cell lines. European Journal of Nutrition, 38(3), 133-142.

Lakhanpal, P. & Rai, D. M. (2007) Quercetin: A versatile flavonoid. Internet Journal of Medical Update, (2)2, 22-37.

Laugher, E., Taghavi, P., Chiles, K., Mahon, P. C. & Semenza, G. L. (2001). HER2 (neu) signalling increases the rate of hypoxia-inducible factor 1alpha (HIF-1aplha) synthesis: novel mechanism for HIF-1-mediated vascular endothelial growth factor expression. Molecular and Cellular Biology, 21(12), 3995-4004.

Lee, S. J., Yoon, J. H. & Song, K. S. (2007). Chrysin inhibited stem cell factor (SCF)/c-Kit complex-induced cell proliferation in human myeloid leukemia cells. Biochemical Pharmacology, 74(2), 215-225.

Li, X., Huang, Q., Ong, C. N., Yang, X. F. & Shen, H. M. (2010). Chrysin sensitizes tumor necrosis factor-alpha-induced apoptosis in human tumor cells via suppression of nuclear factor-kappaB. Cancer Letters, 293(1), 109-116.

Lirdprapamongkol, K., Sakurai, H., Abdelhamed, S., Yokoyama, S., Athikomkulchai, S., Viriyaroj, A., Awale, S., Ruchirawat, S., Svasti, J. & Saiki, I. (2013). Chrysin overcomes TRAIL resistance of cancer cells through Mcl-1 downregulation by inhibiting STAT3 phosphorylation. International Journal of Oncology, 43(1), 329-337.

Locke, S. E., Kraus, L., Leserman, J., Hurst, M. W., Heisel, J. S. & William, R. M. (1984). Life change stress, psychiatric symptoms and natural killer cell activity. Psychosomatic Medicine, 46(5), 441-453.

Lopez-Lazaro, M., Gavez, M., Cordero, M. & Ayuso, M. (2002). Cytotoxicity of flavonoids on cancer cell lines. Structure-activity relationship. Atta-ur-Rahman (Ed.) Studies in Natural Products Chemistry. Elsevier Science B. V., 27, 891-932.

Pal-Bhadra, M., Ramaiah, M. J., Reddy, T. L., Krishnan, A., Pushpavalli, S., Babu, K. S., Tiwari, A. K., Rao, J. M., Yadav, J. S. & Bhadra, U. (2012). Plant HDAC inhibitor chrysin arrst cell growth and induce p21^{WAF1} by altering chromatin of STAT response element in A375 cells. BMC Cancer, 12, 180.

Maxwell, P. H., Dachs, G. U., Gleadle, J. M., Nicholls, L. G., Harris, A. L., Stratford, I. J., Hankinson, O., Pugh, C. W. & Ratcliffe, P. J. (1997). Hypoxia-inducible factor-1 modulates gene expression in solid tumors and influences both angiogenesis and tumor growth. Proceedings of the National Academy of Sciences U.S.A., 94(15), 8104-8109.

Melamed, R., Bar-Yosef, S., Shakhar, G., Shakhar, K. & Ben-Eliyahu, S. (2003). Suppresion of natural killer activity and promotion of tumour metastasis by ketamine, thiopental and halothane, but not by propool: mediating mechanisms and prophylactic measures. Anesthesia and Analgesia, 97(5), 1331-1339.

Melillo, G. (2007). Targeting hypoxia cell signalling for cancer therapy. Cancer and Metastasis Reviews, 26(2), 341-352.

Middleton, E. & Kandaswami, C. (1994). The flavonoids: Advances in research since 1986, In Harborne, J. B. Ed.; Chapman and Hall: London, 619-652.

Minet, E., Mottet, D., Michel, G., Roland, I., Raes, M., Remacle, J. & Michiels, C. (1999). Hypoxia-induced activation of HIF-1: role of HIF-1alpha-Hsp90 interaction. FEBS Letters, 460(2), 251-256.

Miranda, E., Nordgren, I. K., Male, A. L., Lawrence, C. E., Hoakwie, F., Cuda, F., Court, W., Fox, K. R., Townsend, P. A., Packham, G. K., Eccles, S. A. & Tavassoli, A. (2013). A cyclic peptide inhibitor of HIF-1 heterodimerization that inhibits hypoxia signalling in cancer cells. Journal of the American Chemical Society, 135(28), 10418-10425.

Monasterio, A., Urdaci, M. C., Pinchuk, I. V., Lopez-Moratalla, N. & Martinez-Irujo, J. J. (2004). Flavonoids induce apoptosis in human leukemia U937 cells through caspase- and caspase-calpain-dependent pathways. Nutrition and Cancer, 50(1), 90-100.

Nagle, D. G. & Zhou, Y. D. (2006). Natural product-based inhibitors of hypoxia-inducible factor-1 (HIF-1). Current Drug Targets, 7(3), 355-369.

Neuhouser, M. L. (2009). Dietary flavonoids and cancer risk: Evidence from human population studies. Nutrition and Cancer, 50(1), 1-7.

Nga, T. & Walle, T. (2007). Aromatase inhibition by bioavailable methylated flavones. The Journal of Steroid Biochemistry and Molecular Biology, 107(1-2), 127-129.

Nijveldt, R. J., van Nood, E., van Hoorn, D. E, Boelens, P. G., van Norren, K. & van Leeuwen, P. A. (2001). Flavonoids: A review of probable mechanisms of action and potential applications. The American Journal of Clinical Nutrition, 74(4), 418-425.

Osada, M., Imaoka, S. & Funae, Y. (2004). Apigenin suppresses the expression of VEGF, an important factor for angiogenesis, in endothelial cells via degradation of HIF-1alpha protein. FEBS Letters, 575(1-3), 59-63.

Othman, N. H. & Rebolj, M. (2009). Challenges to cervical screening in a developing country: The case of Malaysia. Asian Pacific Journal of Cancer Prevention, 10(5), 747-752.

Parajuli, P., Joshee, N., Rimando, A. M., Mittal, S. & Yadav, A. K. (2009). In vitro anti-tumor mechanisms of various Scutellaria extracts and constituent flavonoids. Planta Medica, 75(1), 41-48.

Pelengaris, S., Khan, M. & Evan, G. (2002). c-MYC: More than just a matter of life and death. Nature Reviews Cancer, 2(10), 764-776.

Ramos, A. M. & Aller, P. (2008). Quercetin decreases intracellular GSH content and potentiates the apoptotic action of the anti-leukemic drug arsenic trioxide in human leukemia cell lines. Biochemical Pharmacology, 75(10), 1912-1923.

Roberts, R. (2000). Apoptosis in toxicology. Taylor & Francis: London, UK, 22-40, 214-232.

Russo, G. L. (2007). Ins and outs of dietary phytochemicals in cancer chemoprevention. Biochemical Pharmacology, 74(4), 533-544.

Saarinen, N., Joshi, S. C., Ahotupa, M., Li, X., Ammala, J., Makela, S. & Santti, R. (2001). No evidence for the in vivo activity of aromatase-inhibiting flavonoids. The Journal of Steroid Biochemistry and Molecular Biology, 78(3), 231-239.

Salceda, S. & Caro, J. (1997). Hypoxia-inducible factor 1alpha (HIF-1alpha) protein is rapidly degraded by the ubiquitin-proteasome system under normoxic conditions. Its stabilization by hypoxia depends on redoxinduced changes. The Journal of Biological Chemistry, 272 (36), 22642-22647.

Samarghandian, S., Afshari, J. T. & Davoodi, S. (2011). Chrysin reduces proliferation and induces apoptosis in the human prostate cancer cell line pc-3. Clinics, 66(6), 1073-1079.

Sanderson, J. T., Hordijk, J., Denison, M. S., Springsteel, M. F., Nantz, M. H. & van den Berg, M. (2004). Induction and inhibition of aromatase (CYP19) activity by natural and synthetic flavonoid compounds in H295R human adrenocortical carcinoma cells. Toxicological Sciences, 82(1), 70-79.

Sawicka, D., Car, H., Borawska, M. H. & Niklinski, J. (2012). The anticancer activity of propolis. Folia Histochemica Et Cytobiologica, 1(50), 25-37.

Scalbert, A. & Williamson, G. (2000). Dietary intake and bioavailability of polyphenols. Journal of Nutrition, 130, 2073-2085.

Scheck, A. C., Perry, K., Hank, N. C. & Clark, W. D. (2006). Anti-cancer activity of extracts derived fromthe mature roots of Scutellaria baicalensis on human malignant brain tumor cells. BMC Complementary and Alternative Medicine, 6, 27-35.

Soumajit, M. & Ramesh, S. (2010). Potential of the bioflavonoids in the prevention/treatment of ocular disorders. Journal of Pharmacy and Pharmacology, 62(8), 951-965.

Stiehl, D. P., Jelkman, W., Wenger, R. H. & Hellwig-Burgel, T. (2002). Normoxic induction of the hypoxia-inducible factor 1-alpha by insulin and interleukin-1-beta involvers the phophatidylinositol 3-kinase pathway. FEBB Letters, 512(1-3), 157-162.

Teh, B. K., Anizah, R., Thaneswary, Y., Maimumah, A. & Khoo, B. Y. (2010). Potential effects of Chrysin on MDA-MB-231 cells. International Journal of Molecular Sciences, 11(3), 1057-1069.

Traxler, P., Allegrini, P. R., Brandt, R., Brueggen, J., Cozens, R., Fabbro, D., Grosios, K., Lane, H. A., McSheehy, P., Mestan, J., Meyer, T., Tang, C., Wartmann, M., Wood, J. & Caravatti, G. (2004). AEE788: a dual family epidermal growth factor receptor/ErbB2 and vascular endothelial growth factor receptor tyrosine kinase inhibitor with antitumor and antiangiogenic activity. Cancer Research, 64(14), 4931-4941.

Treins, C., Giorgetti-Peraldi, S., Murdaca, J., Semenza, G. L. & Van Obberghen, E. (2002). Insulin stimulates hypoxia-inducible factor 1 through a phosphatidylinositol 3-kinase/target of rapamycin-dependent signalling pathway. The Journal of Biological Chemistry, 277(31), 27975-27981.

Turner, R. T., Riggs, B. L. & Spelsberg, T. C. (1994). Skeletal effects of estrogen. Endocrine Reviews, 15(3), 275-300.

Vabderschueren, D., Boonen, S. & Bouillon, R. (1998). Action of androgens versus estrogens in male skeletal homeostasis. Bone, 23, 391-394.

Vaupel, P. & Mayer, A. (2007). Hypoxia in cancer: significance and impact on clinical outcome. Cancer and Metastasis Reviews, 26(2), 225-239.

von Brandenstein, M. G., Ngum Abety, A., Depping, R., Roth, T., Koehler, M., Dienes, H. P. & Fries, J. W. (2008). A p38-p65 transcription complex induced by endothelin-1 mediates signal transduction in cancer cells. Biochimica et Biophysica Acta, 1783(9), 1613-1622.

Walle, T., Otake, Y., Brubaker, J. A., Walle, U. K. & Halushka, P. V. (2001). Disposition and metabolism of the flavonoid chrysin in normal volunteers. Journal of Clinical Pharmacology, 51(2), 143-146.

Walle, U. K., Galijatovic, A. & Walle, T. (1999). Transport of the flavonoid chrysin and its conjugated metabolites by the human intestinal cell line Caco-2. Biochemical Pharmacology, 58(3), 431-438.

Wang, T. T., Sathyamoorthy, N. & Phang, J. M. (1996). Molecular effects of genistein on estrogen receptor mediated pathways. Carcinogenesis, 17(2), 271-275.

Woo, K. J., Jeong, Y. J., Park, J. W. & Kwon, T. K. (2004). Chrysin-induced apoptosis is mediated through caspase activation and Akt inactivation in U937 leukemia cells. Biochemical and Biophysical Research Communications, 325(4), 1215-1222.

Woo, K. J., Yoo, Y. H., Park, J. W. & Kwon, T. K. (2005). Bcl-2 attenuates anti-cancer agents-induced apoptosis by sustained activation of Akt/protein kinase B in U937 cells. Apoptosis, 10(6), 1333-1343.

Yang, H. M., Shin, H. R., Cho, S. H., Song, G. Y., Lee, I. J., Kim, M. K., Lee, S. H., Ryu, J. C., Kim, Y. & Jung, S.H., (2006). The role of the hydrophobic group on ring A of chalcones in the inhibition of interleukin-5. Archives of Pharmacal Research, 29(11), 969-976.

Yao, L. H., Jiang, Y. M., Shi, J., Tomas-Barberan, F. A., Datta, N., Singanusong, R. & Chen, S. S. (2004). Flavonoids in food and their health benefits. Plan Food for Human Nutrition, 59(3), 113-122.

Yoshida, K., Hirose, Y., Tanaka, T., Yamada, Y., Kuno, T., Kohno, H., Katayama, M., Qiao, Z., Sakata, K., Sugie, S., Shibata, T. & Mori, H. (2003). Inhibitory effects of troglitazone, a peroxisome proliferator-activated receptor gamma ligand, in rat tongue carcinogenesis initiated with 4-nitroquinoline 1-oxide. Cancer Science, 94(4), 365-371.

Zand, R. S., Jenkins, D. J. & Diamandis, E. P. (2000). Steroid hormone activity of flavonoids and related compounds. Breast Cancer Research and Treatment, 62(1), 35-49.

Zhang, Q., Tang, X., Lu, Q., Zhang, Z., Rao, J. & Le, A. D. (2006). Green tea extract and (-)-epigallocatechin-3-gallate inhibit hypoxia- and serum-induced HIF-1alpha protein accumulation and VEGF expression in human cervical carcinoma and hepatoma cells. Molecular Cancer Therapeutics, 5(5), 1227-1238.

Zhang, T., Chen, X., Qu, L., Wu, J., Cui, R. & Zhao, Y. (2004). Chrysin and its phosphate ester inhibit cell proliferation and induce apoptosis in Hela cells. Bioorganic & Medicinal Chemistry, 12(23), 6097-6105.

Zheng, X., Meng, W. D., Xu, Y. Y., Cao, J. G. & Qing, F. L. (2003). Synthesis and anticancer effect of chrysin derivatives. Bioorganic & Medicinal Chemistry Letters, 13(5), 881-884.

Zhong, H., Chiles, K., Feldser, D., Laughner, E., Hanrahan, C., Georgescu, M. M., Simons, J. W. & Semenza, G. L. (2000). Modulation of hypoxia-inducible factor 1alpha expression by the epidermal growth factor/ phosphatidylinositol 3-kinase/ PTEN/AKT/FRAP pathway in human prostate cancer cells: implications for tumor angiogenesis and therapeutics. Cancer Research, 60(6), 1541-1545.

Zundel, W., Schindler, C., Hass-Kogan, D., Koong, A., Karper, F., Chen, E., Gottschalk, A. R., Ryan, H. E., Johnson, R. S., Jefferson, A. B., Stokoe, D. & Giaccia, A. J. (2000). Loss of PTEN facilitates HIF-1mediated gene expression. Genes & Development, 14(4), 391-396.

Human Papillomavirus Vaccination in BC: The Case for Physician Advocates

Sana Shahram

Interdisciplinary Graduate Studies
University of British Columbia, USA

1   Statement of the Problem

In 2005, the incidence rate of cervical cancer in British Columbia was 6.7 per 100,000 women and the mortality rate was 2.0 per 100,000 women (British Columbia Cancer Agency, 2005). These rates are representative of the observed national decrease in incidence and mortality of cervical cancer between 1996 and 2004 of 2.3% and 3.3% per year respectively (Canadian Cancer Society, 2009). These decreases have largely been attributed to the widespread regular use of Papanicolaou (Pap) test screening whereby malignant as well as pre-malignant lesions can be detected early and treated (Canadian Cancer Society, 2009); it is estimated that much larger decreases in cervical cancer will be observed if optimal uptake of the vaccine against Human Papillomavirus (HPV) is achieved.

Currently in British Columbia, there is a publically-funded school-based HPV immunization program for girls in grades 6 and 9. Given the minor status of these girls, their parents not only serve as their primary source for guidance and support regarding immunization issues (Zimet, 2005), but are also required to provide the consent for the immunization itself, and so it follows that parental attitudes towards the vaccine play a crucial role in HPV vaccine uptake (Ogilvie et al., 2007). Last year, the school-based program's first year in British Columbia, the program successfully immunized approximately 64% of eligible girls in the program, a result that is in agreement with the results from a recent national survey which estimated parental intention to immunize their daughters against HPV in British Columbia at 63% (Ogilvie et al., 2007). Given this vaccine's huge potential impact on the incidence of HPV infection and/or cervical cancer, and by extension the morbidity and mortality associated with them, it is an important public health priority to achieve maximum uptake of this important vaccine.

Research has shown that one of parents' most trusted sources of information regarding their own and their children's health is a health care professional, specifically their family physician (Dempsey, Zimet, Davis, & Koutsky, 2006). Additionally, it has been shown that there is a lack of perceived severity and susceptibility associated with HPV infection among parents, and that this coupled with a lack of trusted and unbiased information regarding the safety of the vaccine are main factors in a parent's reluctance to have his or her daughter immunized in the school based program (Ogilvie et al., 2007). Accordingly, this project hopes to identify potential opportunities to involve physicians in the promotion of the HPV vaccine in BC, following the logic that parents will be most likely to accept the promotion strategy's messages if they are being delivered and/or supported by physicians.

Although the survey itself is not based on a health communication theory, the rationale behind the need for this particular survey lends itself to the Health Belief Model (Glanz, Lewis, & Rimer, 1990). In explanation, the health belief model stipulates that in order for behavior change to occur, in this case for a mother (the more likely decision maker regarding daughters' health issues, and the typical focus of research regarding parental vaccination decision-making) to consent to having her daughter vaccinated, the mother must perceive her daughter to be susceptible to HPV infection, and believe that the implications of this infection are severe. Similarly, the mother must also believe that the benefits of this behavior are high (i.e. will effectively protect her daughter from HPV infection), and that the barriers to the behavior are low. These changes in perception can only be accomplished through changes in attitudes, beliefs and knowledge associated with the HPV infection and vaccination among parents. These substantial changes in parents' perspectives will be difficult to accomplish, and will only be helped if the changes are supported by a trusted source like a family physician.

Given these conditions, the behavioural focus of the resulting communications campaign will be to have parents, specifically mothers, of girls between the ages of 10-13 consent to HPV immunization in the school-based program. There has been much research into mothers' attitudes towards immunization in general, as well as towards HPV immunization specifically. Factors that have been identified as contributing to acceptance of HPV immunization among these women include the benefit to society (Constantine & Jerman, 2007), the desire to protect her children from harm (Gonik, 2006), concern about the disease characteristics (Mays, Sturm, & Zimet, 2004), and physician recommendations (Ogilvie *et al.*, 2007). Barriers to accepting the HPV vaccine were identified as low perception of severity of and susceptibility to HPV infection of their children (Zimet, 2005), concerns over vaccine safety and efficacy (Constantine & Jerman, 2007), concerns about the influence of immunization on sexual behaviour (Ogilvie *et al.*, 2007), and her desire to wait until her daughter is older to receive the immunization (Marlow, Waller, & Wardle, 2007).

Overall, most studies have found that approximately 75% of mothers intend to have their daughters immunized in the school-based program, while only 6% claimed they would not accept the vaccine under any circumstances (Marlow, Waller, & Wardle, 2007). A significant proportion (19%), however, claimed that they were unsure about the immunization (Marlow, Waller, & Wardle, 2007). The competing behaviour among these mothers, then, is to not sign the consent form on account of feeling unable to make the right decision regarding HPV immunization for their daughters. A successful campaign will focus on eliminating this uncertainty by increasing the perceived benefits of immunizing their daughters against HPV for the mothers through highlighting the health benefits for their daughters, while decreasing the barriers to the behaviour, through education surrounding vaccine efficacy and misconceptions about its effects on sexual behavior. These messages will be increasingly effective when they are delivered by physicians, since they are already strong influencers of the behavior on an individual basis. Similarly, decreasing the benefits of not consenting to the immunization for the mothers will involve demonstrating the risk of infection to their daughters through the establishment of severity and susceptibility of HPV infection, while creating conceptual barriers to not consenting by establishing this behaviour as a lost opportunity to protect their daughters from cervical cancer in the future. Again, these messages will be especially poignant coming from a physician, since mothers already view physicians as people who are charged with protecting their daughter's health.

Research has shown that the success of an HPV vaccine promotion campaign will depend on changing mothers' beliefs and attitudes as well as increasing their knowledge about HPV and the vaccine. (Kahn, 2007). Numerous studies have demonstrated that there is low knowledge among most people surrounding HPV infection and its association with genital warts and cervical cancer (Gonik, 2006). Although HPV is the most widespread sexually transmitted disease in Canada, and most sexually active people will be exposed to HPV infection within their lifetime, perceived susceptibility to HPV of daughters, remains low among mothers. (Ogilvie *et al.*, 2007). Some of this lack of susceptibility may be due to a lack of knowledge about HPV infection itself and how widespread it actually is among adolescents (Kahn, 2007). Similarly, there is a demonstrated lack of understanding among mothers about the potential severity of HPV infection, and many surveyed mothers were completely unaware of the link between HPV infection and cervical cancer (Friedman & Shepeard, 2007). This link must be firmly established through information and education, so that mothers begin to view the HPV vaccine as a vaccine against cancer, rather than a vaccine against a sexually transmitted infection (Friedman & Shepeard, 2007).

In addition to knowledge needs surrounding HPV infection itself, there have been demonstrated knowledge gaps for mothers around the HPV vaccine. There is a need to further educate mothers about the safety and efficacy of the vaccine in an effort to quell their concerns about potential side-effects to immunization (Mays, Sturm, & Zimet, 2004). In the same vein, many of the undecided mothers claim that they would be willing to immunize their daughters at a later age, which demonstrates a lack of understanding of the prophylactic nature of the vaccine (Marlow, Waller, & Wardle, 2007). As such, education materials aimed at these mothers will have to include a good justification for why the vaccine is recommended at a particular age if they are going to be successful in convincing the mothers to consent to HPV immunization through the provincial grade 6 programs (Marlow, Waller, & Wardle, 2007). Although there is a demonstrated need for more information about HPV and HPV immunization for parents, research has shown that simply educating mothers is not sufficient, and it is necessary to consider their beliefs and attitudes since these may be more influential than knowledge on the parental decision-making process (Dempsey, Zimet, Davis, & Koutsky, 2006).

One of the main barriers to mothers consenting to immunizing their daughters against HPV is the belief that their child is not, or should not be, susceptible to infection by a virus that is sexually transmitted (Mays, Sturm, & Zimet, 2004). This belief manifests itself in a number of ways from mothers either believing that their child will wait until marriage to have sex and therefore is not at risk of infection, to the belief that deciding to immunize their daughter implicitly or explicitly acknowledges that they believe that their daughter is at risk for an STI, or that they are in some way condoning their daughters sexual activity (Mays, Sturm, & Zimet, 2004). In fact, since it has been shown that vaccine acceptance, unlike vaccine rejection, is not linked to a mother's perceived sexual behaviour of their daughter, it is important to shift a mother's belief about HPV immunization towards protection from cervical cancer, and remove its association with sexual activity (Mays, Sturm, & Zimet, 2004). Similarly, mothers must believe that preventing HPV infection in their daughters is not necessarily within their control, and that immunization is the best and most reliable protection from infection; indeed, many mothers reasoned in favour of the vaccine due to the provision of added protection against unpredictable and uncontrollable circumstances (Mays, Sturm, & Zimet, 2004). Therefore, it is important for mothers to understand and believe that HPV immunization is safe, effective and important to protecting their daughters from cervical cancer, in order to carry out the campaign's behavioural objective of consenting to having them immunized during the school-based program in Grade 6.

Given the complexity of the issues that need to be addressed when attempting to persuade mothers to consent to having their daughters vaccinated in the school-based program against HPV, it is essential to add physicians to the promotion effort in order to establish a sense of trust and validity among the target population. It is for this reason that this survey is being conducted, in an effort to design an effective communications campaign that utilizes physicians to affect behaviour change among mothers within the health belief model framework.

Specifically for this project, the BC Center for Disease Control (BCCDC) has pre-determined that the desired target group for this survey and communications strategy will be General Practitioner Oncologists (GPOs), or a general practitioner who provides oncology care in a primary care setting. The rationale for this is two-fold: first, these physicians are particularly well suited to serving as HPV vaccine advocates since as General Practitioners they are parents' likely source for information about the vaccine; and second, as doctors who treat cervical cancer, their intimate knowledge about the morbidity and mortality associated with the disease makes them particularly passionate about the vaccine, and the prevention of the disease. Indeed, this group of physicians has already demonstrated support for the HPV vaccine through their participation in education events throughout the province, and through their biannual newsletter.

1.1   Surveying Physicians

Research has shown that physicians have lower response rates to questionnaires than do other health care professionals. According to one study, while the average response rate following the first mailing of questionnaires to other health professionals is 62%, that average response rate drops down to 54% among physicians (Bhandari, *et al.*, 2003). Despite this fact, however, research continues to show that surveying physicians is one of the most effective ways to elicit their opinions on issues affecting practice, the delivery of clinical preventive services, as well as the implementation of public health interventions (Kellerman & Herold, 2001). Given this fact, it is important to understand how to increase physician response rates, in order to protect the validity and generalizability of this study's results.

The low response rate among physicians is surprising, when considering that mail surveys of highly educated, professional persons (like physicians) should theoretically elicit higher response rates than those of less educated respondents (Kellerman & Herold, 2001). Some possible explanations for this discrepancy may be that some professionals may resist surveys or questions that stereotype or generalize issues, are restrictive in answers, do not make sense to them, or take too much time out of an already overburdened schedule (Kellerman & Herold, 2001). In a systematic review of all of the literature on methodological strategies to increasing physician response rates to surveys, several key strategies were identified (Kellerman & Herold, 2001). Strategies shown to increase response rates were the use of first-class postage, the use of shorter (i.e. one to two pages) surveys, personalized packaging of the mail-outs, and monetary incentives (Kellerman & Herold, 2001). Indeed, research consistently showed that monetary incentives, regardless of the amount, were consistently associated with increased response rates, as was the timing of such incentives, pre-payment being preferable to post-payment (Kellerman & Herold, 2001). Specifically, one study found that when incentives were used the odds of response were more than doubled when money was the incentive and were almost doubled when incentives were not conditional on response (Edwards, *et al.*, 2002). Other strategies to increase response rates include making questionnaires and letters more personal, follow up contact, providing non-respondents with a second copy of the questionnaire, and designing questionnaires to be of more interest to participants (Edwards, *et al.*, 2002). Lastly, questionnaires originating from universities were more likely to be returned than questionnaires from other sources (Edwards, *et al.*, 2002).

Strategies that were shown to have negligible effects on increasing the response rate were: Pre-notification of survey participants, the use of non-monetary incentives or a phone call as follow-up, or the use of phone calls or personal interviews as survey methods versus mailed surveys (Kellerman & Herold, 2001). Another issue that has been examined is the role of non-response bias in physician surveys. Studies on this topic have found that there was little difference in demographic variables among respondents and non-respondents when surveying physicians (Kellerman & Herold, 2001). This can be explained by the fact that physicians as a group are more homogenous regarding knowledge, training, attitudes, and behaviour than the general population, and variations that do exist among physicians may not be associated with willingness to respond or survey content as in the general population (Kellerman & Herold, 2001). This finding has two implications in surveying physicians: One, considering the consistently positive effect of monetary incentives, limited resources may be best directed towards a sufficient monetary incentive in the first mailing, rather than to follow-up mailings (Kellerman & Herold, 2001); and, second, during the interpretation of data gathered from physician surveys with low response rates, non-response bias may not be as crucial as in surveys for the general population (Kellerman & Herold, 2001).

Finally, since the mailed questionnaire is recommended when the respondent needs greater control over time, pace, and sequence or response, when privacy of response is important, and when the sample is a highly literate population (Edwards, *et al.*, 2002), this option serves as the best method for surveying physicians. Similarly, as advances have been made with web-based surveys, this offers a good alternative to the mailed survey (Braithwaite, Emery, de Lusignan, & Sutton, 2003), albeit with acknowledged shortcomings. The main consideration with web-based surveys is that respondents are not usually representative of the general population, even within a certain health care specialty (Braithwaite, Emery, de Lusignan, & Sutton, 2003). For this reason, if an electronic survey is to be used, there must be an alternative hard copy survey that can be completed by those who prefer to do so, to eliminate any potential biases (Braithwaite, Emery, de Lusignan, & Sutton, 2003).

2   Description of the Field Organization

The BC Centre for Disease Control (BCCDC) provides provincial and national leadership in public health through surveillance, detection, treatment, and prevention of infectious diseases and also provides consultation services. The Centre provides both direct diagnostic and treatment services for people with diseases of public health importance and analytical and policy support to all levels of government and health authorities. BCCDC investigates and evaluates the occurrence of communicable diseases in BC and is the provincial reporting centre for reportable cases and categories of communicable diseases. In addition, the Centre creates opportunities for scientists, health professionals, University and other partners to contribute their knowledge and experience in resolving the outstanding health challenges facing British Columbians.

The BCCDC is an agency of the Provincial Health Services Authority (PHSA), which is one of six health authorities – the other five health authorities serve geographic regions of BC. PHSA's primary role is to ensure that BC residents have access to a coordinated network of high-quality specialized health care services.

This project will be completed in close cooperation with the Department of Communications at the BCCDC, as well as the Department of Epidemiology Services, specifically its Division of Immunizations. The project preceptor is the Director of Communications, while most of the other support for the project comes from within the Division of Immunizations. This division has been involved in many projects surrounding the HPV vaccine and has specific funding for HPV vaccine research and promotion, and this project hopes to add to that stream of knowledge. While this specific project is being undertaken, the department of STI/HIV services is also conducting a larger, more general survey of all general practitioner physicians to determine their knowledge, attitudes and beliefs surrounding the HPV vaccine. The staff at the BCCDC is very experienced in conducting surveys in general, as well as surveys of physicians, and their expertise in this area will be invaluable to this project. The BCCDC is affiliated with the University of British Columbia (UBC) for research. As such, all research done at the BCCDC must be approved by UBC's independent ethics review board, before it can be conducted.

3   Scope of Work and Methods

This project is intended to increase the potential public health impact of the HPV vaccine by increasing the vaccine's uptake in British Columbia's provincially funded school-based grades 6 and 9 immunization programs. The BCCDC hopes to accomplish this increase through a strategic communications campaign that utilizes General Practitioner Oncologists (GPOs) as spokespeople, since they have been shown to be one of the main influencers of the target behavior. This project intends to inform this campaign by conducting a survey to assess GPOs' current practices, attitudes and beliefs towards the HPV vaccine, as well as potential opportunities to involve GPOs in HPV vaccine promotion, in order to develop informed and evidence-based communications recommendations to achieve maximum vaccine uptake in British Columbia.

3.1   Methods

From October 20th to November 16th, 2009 a survey was conducted regarding HPV vaccine promotion in a provincial sample of General Practitioner Oncologists in British Columbia. This study was reviewed by the University of British Columbia's Behavioural Research Ethics Board and was approved as minimal risk research.

3.1.1   Population

The target population of the survey were General Practitioners in Oncology in British Columbia. Since the BCCDC did not have access to contact information for all GPOs in BC, and also did not have the GPOs' consent for being contacted to conduct research, the British Columbia Cancer Agency (BCCA) where these physician's are trained was contacted. The BCCA had contact information, as well as the permission to contact all of the GPO's in BC. It was therefore determined from a logistical perspective that the best option was to collaborate with the BCCA to conduct a survey of 44 GPOs who currently work within the community. (Currently there are 77 total members of the General Practitioner in Oncology Network in BC, although only 44 of these GPOs work within the community, which for our research purposes are the relevant physicians).

3.1.2   Survey Design

The survey instrument was designed with the focus of identifying specific activities that the GPOs would be willing to participate in, as well as to ask them for the permission to contact them in the future to actually participate in the stated activities. Additionally, it was important to determine the physicians' current knowledge about the HPV vaccination program, as well which resources, if any, they were currently using to promote HPV vaccination. Lastly, it was also important to determine if the physicians themselves felt that they needed more resources or information to effectively promote the HPV vaccination.

The survey was also designed according to proven strategies to increase response rates among physicians. For this reason, two introduction letters were written, one from a respected physician at the BCCDC and the other from a respected physician at the BCCA, to not only show support for the study among the GPOs colleagues, but also to explain the importance of the study to the GPOs in a way that personalized the research for the physician, a proven strategy for increasing response rates. In addition, the survey was designed to be short (only 15 questions long), and allowed the physician's the option to write-in responses whenever appropriate, so as not to turn them off by providing limiting responses. The survey was also made to fit on two pages, since research has shown that surveys that are longer than 2 pages have lower response rates. Lastly, a $20 gift certificate to Starbucks Coffee was included with the survey, as a pre-paid, condition free incentive for completing the survey.

The survey was pilot-tested and reviewed by a physician at the BCCDC in order to determine the survey's clarity and accuracy. The physician's suggestions were incorporated to the final copy of the survey.

3.1.3   Survey Administration

Each physician was mailed a package which included an introduction letter from the BCCDC and from the BCCA respectively, a hard copy of the survey with a consent statement and instructions, a postage-paid pre-labeled return envelope and a $20 gift certificate for Starbucks Coffee. The instructions specified that the physician had the option to complete the hard-copy of the survey and return it via mail or fax, or that he or she could access an online version of the survey hosted by Survey Monkey and complete the survey online.

Two email reminders were sent to all of the GPOs, encouraging them to complete the survey, and also provided a hyperlink in the email to the online survey. Responses from all channels were accepted until November 16th, 2009.

4   Results

4.1   Survey Response and Characteristics of Respondents

Of the 44 General Practitioner Oncologists that were contacted to participate in the survey, two mailed packages were returned to sender due to incorrect mailing addresses. Of the 42 surveys that were delivered, 24 GPOs (57%) returned completed surveys, with 83% of respondents responding by mail and only 17% of respondents opting to complete the survey online (Table 1). As presented in Table 2, the majority of survey respondents were between the age of 45 to 54 years old, worked in a community with a population less than 30,000 people, had been in practice for over 15 years, and were mostly of White/Caucasian ethnic and/or racial background. Male and females were approximately evenly represented. There is no demographic data available for survey non-respondents.

4.2   Knowledge and attitudes towards HPV vaccine

Responses to survey questions regarding knowledge and attitudes towards HPV vaccine are shown in Table 3. As suspected in this group, there was a high level of awareness of the provincially-funded HPV program in BC, and approximately 67% of respondents have received some form of Continuing Medical Education training about the HPV vaccine. Similarly, 75% of respondents claimed to recommend the HPV vaccine to eligible girls all the time; Two respondents left the question blank, but wrote into the comments that the question was not applicable since they did not see this demographic in their practices. Three respondents claimed to recommend the vaccine sometimes, with one respondent commenting simply that "some parents worry." The remaining comments discussed that it was often parents, not the girls, requesting advice/information, and that there is a need for more materials targeted at parents. Only one respondent claimed to never recommend the vaccine, and commented that there is currently no proof that the vaccine actually decreases the risk of cervical cancer.

Surveys Returned	24	
Response Rate (n=42)	57%	
Survey Method	**Number of Respondents**	**Percentage (n=24)**
Returned by Mail	20	83%
Returned Online	4	17%

Table 1: Survey Response Rate.

Characteristic	Number of Respondents	Percentage (n=24)
Age		
35-44 years old	7	29.2%
45-54 years old	12	50.0%
55-64 years old	5	20.8%
Total	24	100.0%
Gender		
Male	10	41.7%
Female	13	54.2%
Prefer not to disclose	1	4.2%
Total	24	100.0%
Years in practice		
6 to 10 years	6	25.0%
11 to 15 years	4	16.7%
More than 15 years	14	58.3%
Total	24	100.0%
Population Size of Community		
Less than 5,000	2	8.3%
5,000 - 10,000	5	20.8%
10,001 - 30,000	8	33.3%
30,001 - 50,000	2	8.3%
50,0001 - 100,000	5	20.8%
More than 100,000	2	8.3%
Total	24	100.0%
Ethnic/Racial Background		
White	22	91.7%
Black	1	4.2%
Prefer not to disclose	1	4.2%
Total	24	100.0%

Table 2: Survey Respondents' Characteristics.

	Number of Respondents	Percentage (n=24)
Have you ever received any continuing medical education training about the HPV vaccine?		
Do not remember	4	16.7%
No	4	16.7%
Yes	16	66.7%
Total	24	100%
How aware are you of the current provincially-funded school-based grades 6 & 9 HPV immunization program for BC girls?		
Very aware	15	62.5%
Somewhat aware	9	37.5%
Not aware	0	0.0%
Total	24	100%
Do you currently recommend the HPV vaccine to your eligible girls for the grades 6 & 9 program?		
Yes, all the time	18	75.0%
Yes, sometimes	3	12.5%
No, never	1	4.2%
No response	2	8.3%
Total	24	100.0%

Table 3: Respondents' current knowledge and practices regarding HPV vaccination.

4.3   Resources, Information and Relationships

Table 4 and Figures 1 and 2 show a breakdown of the resources these physicians are using to counsel their patients about the HPV vaccine, their information needs regarding the HPV vaccine, as well as the current working relationships they have with other health care professionals in their community. Notably, 41.7% of respondents claimed that they required more information about statistics regarding HPV infection and vaccination. Most of the respondents also claimed to have working relationships with family physicians in private practice (91.7%) and pharmacists in the community (83.3%), while only 2 respondents claimed to have working relationships with a School Nurse in the community. The three most common resources respondents used for HPV vaccine counseling were the Canadian Immunization Guide, the information from the vaccine manufacturer and information from health units.

4.4   Physicians as public supporters of the HPV vaccine

As shown in Table 4, 41.7% of respondents agreed to share their contact information as well as the activities that they were willing to participate in as public supporters of the HPV vaccine with their local health authorities. Of the two that did not respond, one commented that he or she was not actually a community physician, and several of the physicians who declined to share their contact information wrote in reasons such as that they were uncomfortable with public speaking, or that they would be away from their practice for a year. Table 5 and Figure 3 also show the activities that respondents are willing to participate in as public supporters of the HPV vaccine, with organizing Continuing Medical Education (CME) on HPV as the activity most are willing to participate in at 37.5% of respondents, followed by conducting CMEs and making local presentations at 33.3% each, respectively. Several comments were also written in suggesting that this participation was contingent on training and/or support to carry out the tasks.

	Number of Respondents	Percentage (n=24)
What are the resources you currently use to counsel patients about HPV and HPV vaccine? Select all that apply.		
ImmunizeBC website	5	20.8%
Canadian Paediatric Society Manual	1	4.2%
Canadian Immunization Guide	9	37.5%
Vaccine manufacturer's materials	8	33.3%
Information from Health Units	8	33.3%
Society of Obstetricians and Gynaecologists of Canada	5	20.8%
None of the Above	4	16.7%
Other	5	20.8%
Do you require more information about HPV Vaccine:		
Safety	5	20.8%
Immunogenicity	2	8.3%
Duration of coverage	5	20.8%
Statistics such as HPV infection, cervical cancer, or genital warts rates	10	41.7%
Adverse Events	7	29.2%
No, I do not require more information	11	45.8%
Do you currently have a working relationship with any of the following healthcare professionals in your community?		
School Nurse	2	8.3%
Health Units	15	62.5%
Medical Health Officer	5	20.8%
Family Physician in private practice	22	91.7%
Specialist in private practice	11	45.8%
Pharmacist	20	83.3%
Other	1	4.2%

Table 4: Respondents' HPV Vaccine Resource Usage and Needs.

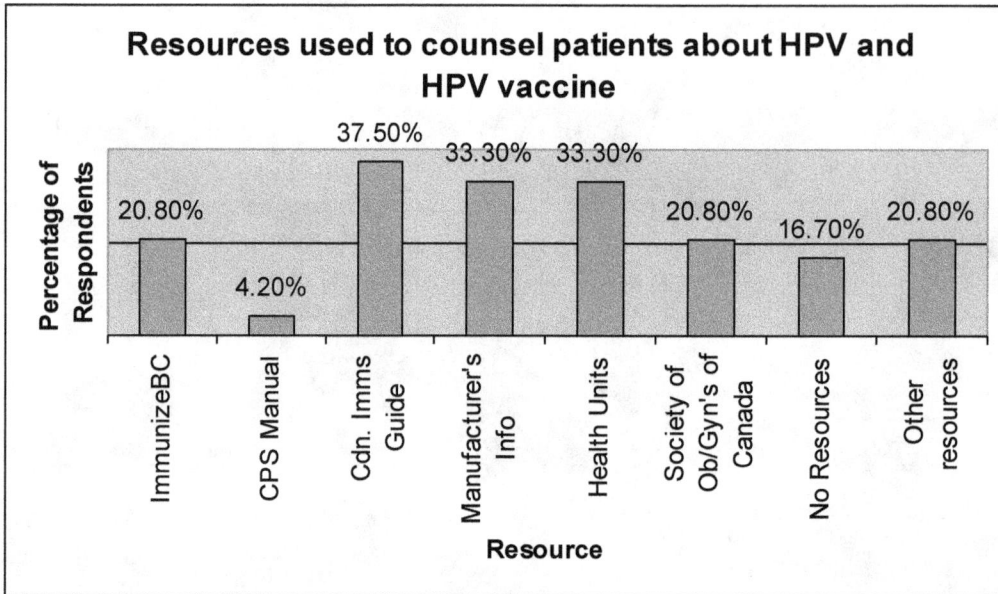

Figure 1: Resource usage for HPV vaccine counseling.

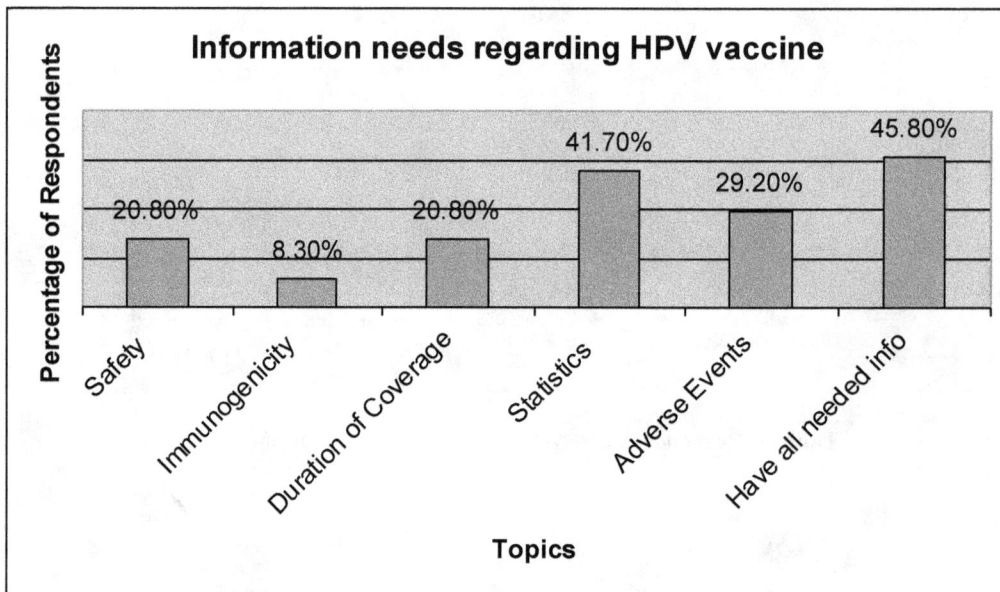

Figure 2: Information needs for HPV vaccine counselling.

	Number of respondents	Percentage of respondents (n=24)
Do you agree to share your contact information, as well as specified activities, with your local health authority?		
Yes, please	10	41.7%
No, thank you	12	50.0%
No Response	2	8.3%
Total	24	100.0%
As a public Supporter of HPV would you be willing to:		
Be available as an expert relating to HPV issues for media inquiries in my community	6	25.0%
Make presentations at local schools to parents and staff, parent advisory groups, or at local town hall meetings	8	33.3%
Help conduct Continuing Medical Education on HPV in my community/for my colleagues	8	33.3%
Help organize Continuing Medical Education on HPV in my community/for my colleagues	9	37.5%
Write a letter to local newspapers supporting the HPV vaccine and/or school based program	7	29.2%
Other	2	8.3%

Table 5: Respondents' activity within the community.

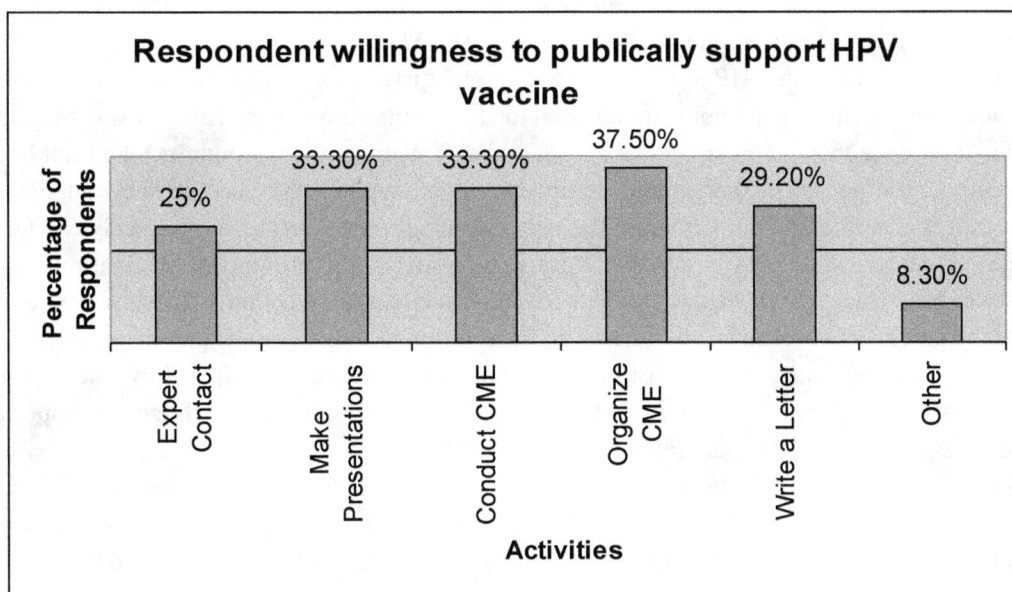

Figure 3: Public supporters of HPV vaccine activities.

5   Discussion

The survey response rate of 57% was similar to the average response rate of physicians to surveys, which according to most studies conducted is 54%. An interesting observation is that 83% of respondents chose to return a hard-copy of the survey by mail, rather than completing the survey online. One factor which may have played a role is that the original mailing contained a copy of the survey, as well as a pre-addressed postage paid envelope, which may have made this option more appealing than having to take an extra step to access the online survey. The physicians did receive two email reminders which contained electronic links to the online survey which attempted to make this option an easier choice, however if most of the physicians did not feel completely proficient with computers and/or the internet, this may have had no effect. Over 70% of the respondents were above the age of 45 and therefore they may have felt more comfortable using the more traditional mail survey method. Also, approximately 62% of respondents lived in communities with populations under 30,000 which may have had an impact on internet access or reliance of the respondents. Lastly, research has shown that physicians as a group tend to shy away from limiting multiple choice answers, and the online version of the survey may have been more restricting in this case; Indeed, on the online version of the survey, you could only write in additional information in designated places, while many of the physicians wrote in qualifying statements next to their responses in the mailed surveys, while others also wrote in explanations when they left a question blank. For this reason, the mail survey may have been the survey method of choice since it provided the physician with more control over his or her answers, and also allowed for a pseudo conversation between the people administering the survey, and the people completing the survey.

As suspected, this group of physicians was highly supportive of the HPV vaccine. There was however one physician who noted his or her opposition to the vaccine, which is an indication that there is still perhaps a need for more education of health care professionals about the vaccine. That being said, 66.7% of respondents had received some continuing medical education training about the HPV vaccine, and this was a likely factor in the high proportion (87.5%) of respondents who either always or sometimes recommended the HPV vaccine to eligible girls. Most of those who only sometimes recommended the vaccine, or did not respond, provided an explanation as to why this was the case (such as that they didn't see this demographic, or that they didn't work in the community), and implied that if these exceptions did not exist, they would be always recommending the vaccine. This support is very important as it is clear that the physician buy-in exists, although it has yet to be effectively capitalized on. In the same vein, only 62.5% of physicians were very aware of the provincial vaccination program in British Columbia, which also speaks to a need for increased communication between the public health sector and the professional realm since these physicians are often a first contact point for parents trying to decide to vaccinate their daughters. It is impossible for physicians to support or buy into a program if they are not aware of it, or are not provided the opportunity, and this serves as a huge lost opportunity to maximize the success of an important public health program.

Although 91.7% and 83.3% of respondents claimed to have working relationships with other family physicians and pharmacists in their community, respectively, only 62% claimed to have a working relationship with their health unit. This suggests that the health units and private practices in these communities are not integrated, and that there is not as much communication between these units as there should be. Achieving physician support and buy-in of public health programs will only serve to increase their success, while physicians will be better able to care and provide for their patients' health when they are aware of all of the programs that are offered. Indeed, a move to a more integrated and holistic health care system will be mutually beneficial to all health care professionals involved, as well as to the health of all British Columbians.

One notable observation in terms of the resources physicians are using is that only 20.8% of physicians claim to use the BCCDC's website "ImmunizeBC" as a resource to counsel patients about HPV and HPV vaccine. When asked, however, what other resources they would like to counsel patients, a few of the physicians wrote that they would like a website. This suggests that there is likely not enough awareness of this website, or possibly that the website does not meet the needs of these respondents, and this finding merits some further evaluation to optimize the website. Further to this, 41.7% of respondents noted that they would like more information on statistics about HPV infection rates, cervical cancer rates or genital warts rates. In fact, there was at least some need for more information in every suggested category, and considering these respondents are physicians and should be experts on the topic, it is important to meet these information needs immediately. Other resources that the respondents wrote in that they would like included an informational video, and more materials such as brochures and pamphlets with comprehensive information that was targeted at parents. This information is useful since it demonstrates that most respondents would like to further inform their patients about the vaccine, but that they require appropriate support and resources to accomplish this task. Further research could focus on what resources in particular would be the most effective and efficient, with input from these important stakeholders.

The overarching goal of this study was to identify specific opportunities to involve general practitioner oncologists in the promotion of the HPV vaccine. Almost half of the respondents agreed to have their contact information, as well as the activities that they were willing to participate in to promote the vaccine, with their local health unit. This is an important outcome not only functionally for the health units who will now have a contact list for physicians that they can contact as resources for publically supporting the vaccine, but also structurally for the field of public health which has typically been thought of as separate or at times even counter to the practices of private physicians. This study has demonstrated that physicians are willing to and have a desire to be involved with public health programs, and has identified specific ways in which they are willing to achieve this involvement. In this case, these particular physicians were identified to be surveyed, since by virtue of their specialty they were considered to already have a vested interest in the HPV vaccination program, and were therefore important stakeholders in the program. Future public health programs would likely also benefit by identifying potential health care professional stakeholders prior to the roll-out of a program, in an effort to achieve buy-in and support from the people who will likely have great influence on the program's success. Indeed it is likely that if GPOs had been more involved in the planning or roll-out of the publically funded school-based HPV vaccination program, the program may have been met with more support initially. Regardless, now that these public supporters have been identified, it will be imperative to act on their offered support to ensure the maximum uptake of this vaccine to help decrease the morbidity and mortality associated with HPV infection, genital warts and cervical cancer.

This study was subject to several limitations. Due to the small sample size, there were some limitations to the analysis of the data. If further research is done with larger sample sizes, it will be possible to test for association between certain demographic factors and HPV vaccine attitudes, practices and knowledge. Additionally, this survey was conducted on a specific specialty of physicians, and further research will have to be done to determine the generalizability of the results. General practitioners will also have important roles in the success of the HPV vaccination program, and so their views will also be important to assess. Although the response rate was satisfactory for this survey, it is not known whether non-respondents had different views about HPV vaccination than did survey respondents.

5.1   Specific Recommendations

How to Involve General Practitioner Oncologists in an HPV Vaccine Promotions Strategy

1. **Centralize**
    - Establish initial contact with the volunteered physicians within one month
    - Centralize the HPV promotions campaign at the BCCDC to ensure efficiency

2. **Educate**
    - Create a CME course on HPV, and organize events throughout the province

3. **Propagate**
    - Create a public relations plan for province-wide media coverage of physician written support letters and public presenations

4. **Train**
    - Provide training and support to the volunteered physicians so that they are on message for the promotions campaign

5. **Expand**
    - Solicit volunteered physicians for names of other interested physicians, as well as set up sign-up opportunities at CME events

6. **Unify**
    - Create one comprehensive, low-health literacy, research-driven, parent-targeted booklet about HPV and the vaccination program to distribute to physician's offices and to health units

7. **Optimize**
    - Assess how to optimize the ImmunizeBC website

8. **Communicate**
    - Establish a BCCDC monthly newsletter to physicians to inform them about current public health research, programs, and insights into the social aspects of health

5.2   Recommendations Rationale

Ten physicians have offered their personal contact information to be contacted to act as public supporters of the HPV vaccine, and it could be quite discouraging if this offer for help was not accepted and pursued in a timely manner. It is therefore important that a communications strategy be formed to include these physicians in HPV vaccine promotion, not only to continue on the path of outreach to include physicians as stakeholders in the vaccination program, but also to allow observation and evaluation of the impact of physician-promoted public health programs to inform future endeavours of this nature.

Since the health units are all run fairly independently, logistically and strategically speaking it would be best to centralize the execution of an HPV promotion strategy involving these physicians in an agency like the BC Centre for Disease Control. A centralized campaign will allow for an organized and appropriately allotted use of these physicians, as well as allow for a stream-lined and research-supported placement of these physicians given that there are only ten of them. If the campaign is centralized at the BCCDC, the first step to organizing a promotion strategy will be to personally contact these ten physicians to establish an initial dialogue, and to acknowledge their offer of support. This engagement will ensure that these physicians feel appreciated and involved, which will maintain their interests as stakeholders in the program.

Given the activities that the physicians have indicated that they are willing to participate in, the BCCDC will have to evaluate how and if it will facilitate each of these activities. For example, over one third of respondents indicated that they are willing to either organize or conduct Continuing Medical Education (CME) training within their communities, and since the results show that there are still some gaps in knowledge among these physicians regarding the school-based HPV vaccination program itself, as well as HPV infection and vaccination information and statistics, facilitating these sessions will be an important step in HPV promotion. Of the physicians who have provided their contact information, the ones who have indicated that they are willing to participate in organizing or conducting CME training are important contacts for moving forward with this initiative.

Research has shown that there is a need for a professional and unbiased information source presence regarding HPV infection and vaccination in the media. For this reason, the physicians who have indicated that they are willing to write letters to local newspapers or to be available as experts for media inquiries are invaluable assets to an HPV promotion strategy. In addition to providing an important component of a successful campaign to change parental behaviours, in this case to encourage them to consent to the school-based HPV vaccination program, these physicians can participate in these activities across the province; Although only a few of the physician contacts have agreed to participate in these specific activities, the activities lend themselves to being easily disbursed across the province. For example, a physician in Terrace BC can write a letter to a local newspaper, but that letter can also be distributed to newspapers province-wide. Or, the BCCDC can pro-actively provide contact information to media outlets of the physicians who have agreed to act as experts, who can obviously be contacted by any media sources within the province by either phone or email. As several of the physicians themselves indicated, however, it will be important for the BCCDC to provide these so-called "HPV vaccine representatives" with the proper training and support to ensure that they remain on message and synchronized with the promotion strategies as a whole.

The BCCDC currently has two powerpoint presentations targeted at parents and teachers respectively about the HPV vaccine and the school-based program, originally intended to be used by public health nurses during school presentations. These presentations can also be adapted to be presented by the physicians who have agreed to make presentations within their communities. Again, training should be provided to support these physicians, as well as to prepare them for questions from specific audiences. Again, given the limited amount of physicians willing to participate in this activity, it will be important for the BCCDC to strategize (in consultation with the appropriate health units) where the best places and times are for making these presentations. Also, consideration should be given to possibly obtaining media coverage of the events to further the reach of the presentation, and the public endorsement of the physician of the vaccination program in order to fully capitalize on limited resources.

Lastly, this survey may not be representative of how many family practitioner oncologists are willing to participate in the suggested activities. Although the response rate of 57% was typical for physician surveys, this does not automatically mean that the remaining 43% are unsupportive of the vaccine, or unwilling to act as public supporters. There may have been time constraints which kept them from completing the survey, they may have not received it, or they may have been away from their office. With this in mind, it may be fruitful to ask the physician's currently on the contact list if they are aware of any other physicians who might be willing to participate in a promotion strategy, and if they would be willing to share their contact information. This will provide an opening to begin a dialogue with more Family Practitioner Oncologists. Additionally, if and when CME trainings are held, it will be important to provide attendees of these events with the opportunity to sign up as public supporters, should they want to do that.

In terms of resources for counselling patients about HPV, several physicians indicated that there was a need for comprehensive materials such as a brochure, that were targeted at parents. One physician suggested that a BC Cancer Agency endorsed information booklet would also be helpful. The information that most physicians wanted in these materials was mostly related to statistics about HPV infection, cervical cancer and genital warts, as well as more information surrounding vaccine safety and adverse events. (Although more research should be done to confirm that this information will be useful to parents, the physician's seemed to suggest that this information would be helpful to them when counselling parents.) In order to support physicians in promoting the HPV vaccination program, they must have the appropriate materials. It is therefore essential for the BCCDC and/or the BCCA create a comprehensive publication that can act as the authority on all things HPV related, that is available for physicians and/or public health nurses to give to parents. This document should be research-driven in terms of messaging and in terms of addressing the top concerns of undecided parents, and it should be written for low-literacy audiences such that it is accessible to all BC residents. Relating to current resources, one notable observation was that only 20.8% said that they used the BCCDC's ImmunizeBC website, while two physicians actually commented that they would like a website with resources. Depending on the BCCDC's priorities, it may be worthwhile to assess whether this is a result of low awareness of the website, or rather that it does not cater to this particular group in terms of content. Either way, the website does contain helpful information and it would be beneficial to increase its usage.

As a general observation, it appears that there may be a disconnect between physicians in private practice and public health professionals. In fact, one physician, rather than completing the survey, provided a lesson in the social aspects of this issue. This lesson illustrated that physicians in private practice may not be familiar with the type of work and research that is done at the BCCDC, and this can be detrimental to any public health program. Ultimately, both groups are striving for the same goal of keeping British Columbians healthy, and it therefore makes perfect sense that there should be a shift to convergence between these disciplines. Furthermore, awareness of public health programs and research among physicians will only help this convergence, while generally bringing the physicians in as partners and stakeholders in public health programs, ultimately making them more successful. In terms of this issue, I highly recommend that the BCCDC, in partnership with the health units, create a regular form of communication with the physicians of British Columbia. One way to do this would be to establish a monthly newsletter that details current public health programs and initiatives, as well as provides in-depth coverage of some of the social aspects of disease and health. This step alone will go a long way in creating a more harmonious health system in British Columbia. This idea can also be taken further to become more interactive, using social media, forums, and mixers in the future.

This study has illustrated that there are opportunities to involve physicians in the promotion of a public health program, and specifically in this case, that family physician oncologists are willing to act as public supporters for the HPV vaccine and school-based program. With the support of these trusted voices among parents, the HPV vaccine program will hopefully achieve optimal uptake, and BC girls will be protected from cervical cancer.

5.3   General Considerations for an HPV Promotions Campaign

Involving physician's as public supporters of the HPV vaccine will serve as one component of a successful HPV promotion strategy. Ultimately, however, the campaign's success will be dependent on its basis on research-driven messaging and delivery. Specifically, when designing a comprehensive publication for physicians to distribute to mothers about HPV infection and vaccination, based on current research surrounding HPV, there are four key communication strategies that must be employed to increase their acceptance and uptake of the HPV vaccine.

The first strategy is empowerment (Friedman & Shepeard, 2007). This can be accomplished by educating mothers on the natural history, transmission and prevention of HPV while also emphasizing available options for preventing and treating its potential consequences. Secondly, it is critical to promote accurate portrayals of HPV risk without creating undue anxiety or complacency (Friedman & Shepeard, 2007). This delicate balance must be established so that the ubiquitous nature of HPV does not lead to exaggerated fears of cancer, but still challenges the current public perception that HPV infection is mostly harmless, a perception which can inadvertently promote complacent attitudes towards immunization. Thirdly, there is a need to distinguish HPV infection from other sexually transmitted infections (Friedman & Shepeard, 2007). This strategy has two justifications: the first is that the global movement to de-stigmatize STIs may lead people to miss-identify HPV infection as something that can easily be tested for and treated through antibiotics, despite the fact that HPV's natural history is not necessarily amenable to this process; Secondly, it is important to stress that most people who have been sexually active will have been exposed to HPV, in an effort to disassociate the infection from the notion of promiscuity or stigma. Lastly, current limitations and gaps in HPV science should be disclosed to the public (Friedman & Shepeard, 2007). This strategy is essential to earning the public's trust by showing transparency through sharing of what is and is not known about HPV, so as to maintain credibility as the science continues to evolve. All of these strategies should be kept in mind when designing the promotion materials for the HPV vaccine.

Before a booklet for parents is finalized, it will be important to run focus groups with the target audience, in this case mothers, to determine if the booklet has any shortcomings and whether or not it is accomplishing the desired outcome. This will ensure that the resource is effective and beneficial to promoting HPV vaccine uptake among mothers. Also, since most of the mothers will be thinking about this topic when completing the consent form, it may be beneficial to also send out this booklet with the consent forms, which will allow mothers to access the important information immediately. Consideration however should be given to perhaps providing supplementary information regarding all of the vaccines on the consent form so as not to contribute to the fears of mothers by flagging the HPV vaccine as a vaccine of special interest.

Promotion of HPV immunization must happen through several strategies. In terms of advertising, there is a decided need for demonstrated support of HPV immunization that is not linked to the corporate beneficiaries of the vaccine (Ogilvie et al., 2007). Extensive advertising by the vaccine's manufacturers may have lead to reservations among the public towards the vaccine's true value, and unbiased and trusted advertisements are necessary to assert and defend the government's position in favour of HPV immunization. Also, due to the media's unprecedented focus on the HPV vaccine, it is crucial that the promotion of the vaccine also focus on publicity. It is important to increase the media's coverage of the government's support for the program, as well as to use the media to clear up any misconceptions about the HPV vaccine. And, since physicians and health care providers are repeatedly mentioned as trusted sources of information, forming partnerships with these people and providing them with the resources and encouragement to promote the HPV vaccine on an individual basis, as well as through providing expert opinions or public endorsements of the immunization program will only add to any promotion strategy.

Consumers have identified the following acceptable vehicles and settings for delivering information regarding HPV infection and immunization: the internet, their health care provider, gynaecologists, clinics, schools, magazines, local television news, and national television advertisements (Friedman & Shepeard, 2007). Participants stressed the need for factual information to be delivered in a serious tone in clear, simple language (Friedman & Shepeard, 2007). Paid advertisements should be targeted to TV programs that mothers of daughters aged 10-13 are likely to watch, radio stations that they are likely to listen to, and print materials should be placed in areas of high visibility to these particular women. These three channels are necessary since the vaccine manufacturers have used these means, and it is important to supplement their ads with reliable and unbiased information. The publicity can be targeted at local and provincial news outlets (TV, radio and print) as well as through school newsletters and word of mouth through physicians, family and friends. Consumers have also suggested the use of an average person's testimony about his or her experience with HPV immunization as a reliable message source (Friedman & Shepeard, 2007), so another promotion strategy will be to have school information sessions where mothers can explain why they chose to have their daughter immunized. This face-to-face interaction could provide another crucial interaction with the target audience to further promote providing consent for HPV immunization.

Since the HPV vaccine is provided in British Columbia for free, a price strategy must focus on the more intangible costs and benefits of providing consent for HPV immunization. One cost that undecided mothers may face when deciding to give consent is the time and effort it will take to seek more information about the HPV vaccine. By providing these mothers with a booklet about HPV infection and immunization that accompanies the consent form, they no longer need to make extra effort to learn more. Even with this information however, mothers may still feel overwhelmed or not qualified to make this decision for their daughters and these concerns have associated emotional costs. By focusing the promotion campaign around physicians as public supporters of the vaccine, the anxiety associated with this decision will be minimized. In regards to the issues surrounding the sexual implications of the vaccine, mothers may experience conflicting messages as to how best to protect their daughters. Focusing on the HPV vaccine's role in protecting against a severe and life threatening disease such as cervical cancer will be paramount to outweighing these moral costs with tangible health benefits for the women's daughters. Lastly, it is important to highlight the convenience of the school-based program, and remind the mothers that if they do not consent now, but choose to have their daughter immunized later, not only may she be less protected, but the mother will have to make the extra time and effort to take her to a public health nurse for immunization. This will involve making a strong argument as to why girls need to be immunized now, rather than later.

All aspects of an HPV promotion strategy should be focused around the clear message that the HPV vaccine is an important, safe and effective way to protect girls against cervical cancer. And, of course, all aspects of the promotion strategy should be continuously evaluated throughout the course of the campaign, as well as following the campaign.

6 Conclusion

This study has shown that involving physicians in the promotion of public health programs and initiatives is a viable option. Given the authority that physicians have with the public on health care decisions, achieving physician support of public health programs will help to increase the success and impact of these programs, and is therefore an important consideration when designing any promotion or communications campaign in support of the public's health. Specifically in this study, several opportunities have been identified to involve General Practitioner Oncologists in British Columbia in the promotion of the publically funded, school-based HPV immunization program. Future public health programs should aim to identify specific groups of physicians who are likely stakeholders in the program early in the development phases to help ensure and promote public acceptance. There should also be efforts made to establish a dialogue between the public health field and the private practice physicians in BC, as mutual understanding and appreciation of each other's roles will allow for more convergence between the two streams of health care. Future research could focus on the most effective ways to involve physicians in the promotion of public health programs, as well as evaluate the impact of physician support on the success of public health programs.

Appendix

1. Have you received any continuing medical education training about the HPV vaccine?
- ☐ Do not remember
- ☐ No
- ☐ Yes, please describe: _____

2. How aware are you of the current provincially-funded school-based grades 6 & 9 HPV immunization program for BC girls?
- ☐ Very aware
- ☐ Somewhat aware
- ☐ Not aware

3. Do you currently recommend the HPV vaccine to your eligible girls for the grades 6 & 9 program?
- ☐ Yes, all the time
- ☐ Yes, sometimes
- ☐ No, never

Additional Comments: _____

4. What are the resources you currently use to counsel patients about HPV and HPV vaccine? Select all that apply.
- ☐ ImmunizeBC website
- ☐ Canadian Paediatric Society Manual
- ☐ Canadian Immunization Guide
- ☐ Vaccine manufacturer's materials
- ☐ Information from Health Units
- ☐ Society of Obstetricians and Gynaecologists of Canada
- ☐ None of the above
- ☐ Other, please specify: _____

5. What other resources would you like to help you counsel patients about HPV vaccine?
_____

6. Do you require more information about HPV vaccine: (Select all that apply)
- ☐ Safety
- ☐ Immunogenicity
- ☐ Duration of coverage
- ☐ Statistics, such as HPV infection rates, cervical cancer rates, or genital warts rates
- ☐ Adverse events
- ☐ No, I do not require more information

7. If you are willing to act as a public supporter for HPV vaccine, would you be willing to: (Select all that apply)
- ☐ Be available as an expert relating to HPV issues for media inquiries in my community.
- ☐ Make presentations at local schools to parents and staff, parent advisory groups, or at local town hall meetings.
- ☐ Help conduct Continuing Medical Education on HPV in my community/for my colleagues
- ☐ Help organize Continuing Medical Education on HPV in my community/for my colleagues
- ☐ Write a letter to local newspapers supporting the HPV vaccine and/or the school-based program
- ☐ Other, please explain other ways you would like to act as a public supporter for HPV vaccine in your community:
_____

8. Do you currently have a working relationship with any of the following health care professionals in your community? (Select all that apply)

☐ School Nurse

☐ Health Units

☐ Medical Health Officers

☐ Family Physicians in private practice

☐ Specialist Physicians in private practice

☐ Pharmacists

☐ I have no working relationships

☐ Other, please specify:

9. May we share your contact information, as well as the activities you are willing to participate in, with your local health authority?

☐ Yes, please

☐ No, thank you

10. If you answered 'Yes, please' to question 9, please provide your contact information:

Name: _____

Address: _____

_____

City/Town: _____

Email Address: _____

Phone Number: _____

DEMOGRAPHICS:

1. What is your age?

☐ 25-34 years old

☐ 35-44 years old

☐ 45-54 years old

☐ 55-64 years old

☐ 65 or over

☐ Prefer not to disclose

2. Do you identify yourself as:

☐ Male

☐ Female

☐ Prefer not to disclose

3. How many years have you been a general practitioner?

☐ 1 to 5 years

☐ 6 to 10 years

☐ 11 to 15 years

☐ More than 15 years

4. What is the population size of the community in which you practice/are employed?

☐ Less than 5,000

☐ 5,000 – 10,000

☐ 10,001 – 30,000

☐ 30,001 – 50,000

☐ 50,001 – 100,000

☐ More than 100,000

5. What is your ethnic/racial background? (Select all that apply)

☐ White/Caucasian

☐ Chinese

☐ South Asian (e.g., East Indian, Pakistani, Punjabi, Sri Lankan, etc.)

☐ Black

☐ First Nation/Aboriginal Peoples of North America (e.g., North American Indian, Metis, Inuit/Eskimo)

☐ Arab/West Asian (e.g., Armenian, Egyptian, Iranian, Lebanese, Moroccan, Saudi Arabian, etc.)

☐ Filipino(a)

☐ South East Asian (e.g., Cambodian, Indonesian, Laotian, Vietnamese, Thai, etc.)

☐ Latin American

☐ Japanese

☐ Korean

☐ Prefer not to disclose

☐ Other, please specify: _____

References

Bhandari, M., Devereaux, P. J., Swiontkowski, M. F., Schemitsch, E. H., Shankardass, K., Sprague, S., et al. (2003). A randomized trial of opinion leader endorsement in a survey of orthopaedic surgeons: effect on primary response rates. *Internation Journal of Epidemiology* , 634-636.

Braithwaite, D., Emery, J., de Lusignan, S., & Sutton, S. (2003). Using the internet to conduct surveys of health professionals: a valid alternative? *Family Practice* , 20 (5), 545-551.

British Columbia Cancer Agency. (2005). Statistics by Cancer Type. Retrieved August 14, 2009, from http://www.cancer.ca/canada-wide/about%20cancer/cancer%20statistics/~/media/CCS/Canada%20wide/Files%20List/English%20files%20heading/pdf%20not%20in%20publications%20section/Stats%202009E%20Cdn%20Cancer.ashx

Canadian Cancer Society. (2009). Canadian Cancer Statistics. Retrieved August 16, 2009, from http://www.cancer.ca/canada-wide/about%20cancer/cancer%20statistics/~/media/CCS/Canada%20wide/Files%20List/English%20files%20heading/pdf%20not%20in%20publications%20section/Stats%202009E%20Cdn%20Cancer.ashx

Constantine, N. A., & Jerman, P. (2007). Acceptance of human papillomavirus vaccination among Californian parents of daughters: A representative statewide analysis. Journal of Adolescent Health , 40, 108-115.

Dempsey, A. F., Zimet, G. D., Davis, R. L., & Koutsky, L. (2006). Factors that are associated with parental acceptance of human papillomavirus vaccines: A randomized intervention study of written information about HPV. Pediatrics , 1486-1493.

Edwards, P., Roberts, I., Clarke, M., DiGuiseppi, C., Pratap, S., Wentz, R., et al. (2002). Increasing response rates to postal questionnaires: systematic review. British Medical Journal , 324, 1183-1192.

Friedman, A. L., & Shepeard, H. (2007). Exploring the knowledge, attitudes, beliefs and communication preferences of the general public regarding HPV: Findings from CDC focus group research and implications for practice. Health Education and Behavior , 34, 471-485.

Glanz, K., Lewis, F. M., & Rimer, B. K. (1990). Health behavior and health education: Theory, research, and practice (Vol. xxxi). San Francisco, CA: Jossey-Bass.

Gonik, B. (2006). Strategies for fostering HPV vaccine acceptance. Infectious Diseases in Obstetrics and Gynecology , 1-4.

Kahn, J. A. (2007). Maximizing the potential public health impact of HPV vaccines: A focus on parents. Journal of Adolescent Health , 40, 101-103.

Kellerman, S. E., & Herold, J. (2001). Physician response to surveys: A review of the literature. American Journal of Preventitive Medicine , 61-67.

Marlow, L. A., Waller, J., & Wardle, J. (2007). Parental attitudes to pre-pubertal HPV vaccination. Vaccine , 25, 1945-1952.

Mays, R. M., Sturm, L. A., & Zimet, G. D. (2004). Parental perspectives on vaccinating children against sexually transmitted infections. Social Science and Medicine , 58, 1405-1413.

Ogilvie, G. S., Remple, V. P., Marra, F., McNeil, S. A., Naus, M., Pielak, K. L., et al. (2007). Parental intention to have daughters receive the human papillomavirus. CMAJ , 177 (12), 1506-1512.

Zimet, G. D. (2005). Improving adolescent health: Focus on HPV vaccine acceptance. Journal of Adolescent Health , 37, S17-S23.

Resolving the Controversial Role of METCAM/MUC18 in the Progression of Human Breast Cancer

Guang-Jer Wu
Department of Bioscience Technology, Center of Biomedical Technology
Chung Yuan Christian University, Chung Li, Taiwan
Department of Microbiology and Immunology
Emory University School of Medicine, Atlanta, USA

1   Introduction: METCAM

Human *METCAM* (*huMETCAM*), a *CAM* in the immunoglobulin-like gene superfamily, is an integral membrane glycoprotein. Alternative names for *METCAM* are *MUC18* (Lehmann *et al.*, 1989), *CD146* (Anfosso *et al.*, 2001), *MCAM* (Xie *et al.*, 1997), *MelCAM* (Shih *et al.*, 1994), *A32* (Shih *et al.*, 1994), and *S-endo 1* (Bardin *et al.*, 1996). To avoid confusion with mucins and to reflect its biological functions, we have renamed *MUC18* as *METCAM* (*met*astasis *CAM*), which means an immunoglobulin-like *CAM* that affects or regulates metastasis, (Wu, 2005). The *huMETCAM* has 646 amino acids that include a N-terminal extra-cellular domain of 558 amino acids, which has 28 amino acids characteristics of a signal peptide sequence at its N-terminus, a transmembrane domain of 24 amino acids (amino acid #559-583), and a cytoplasmic domain of 64 amino acids at the C-terminus. *HuMETCAM* has eight putative N-glycosylation sites (*Asn-X-Ser/Thr*), of which six are conserved, and are heavily glycosylated and si-alylated resulting in an apparent molecular weight of 113,000-150,000. The extra-cellular domain of the protein comprises five immunoglobulin-like domains (V-V-C2-C2-C2) (Lehmann *et al.*, 1989; Wu, 2005) and an X domain (Wu, 2005). The cytoplasmic tail contains peptide sequences that will potentially be phosphorylated by protein kinase A (*PKA*), protein kinase C (*PKC*), and casein kinase 2 (*CK 2*) (Leh-mann *et al.*, 1989; Wu et. al., 2001a; Wu, 2005). My lab has also cloned and sequenced the mouse *METCAM* (*moMETCAM*) cDNA, which contains 648 amino acids with a 76.2% identity with *huMETCAM*, suggesting that *moMETCAM* is likely to have biochemical properties and biological functions similar to the human counter part (Yang *et al.*, 2001). The structure of the *huMETCAM* protein is depicted in Fig. 1, suggesting that *METCAM*, similar to most *CAMs*, plays an active role in mediating cell-cell and cell-extracellular interactions, crosstalk with many intracellular signaling pathways, and modulating the social behaviors of cells (Wu, 2005).

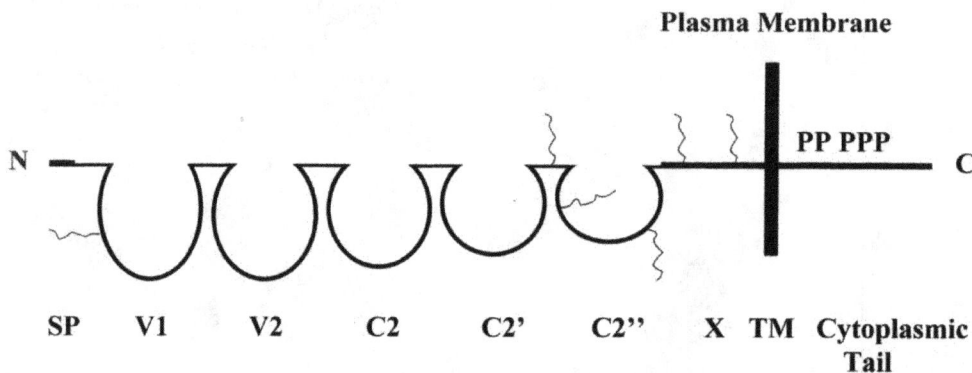

Figure 1: *HuMETCAM* protein structure. SP stands for signal peptide sequence, V1, V2, C2, C2', C2'' for five Ig-like domains (each held by a disulfide bond) and X for one domain (without any disulfide bond) in the extracellular region, and TM for transmembrane domain. P stands for five potential phosphorylation sites (one for *PKA*, three for *PKC*, and one for *CK2*) in the cytoplasmic tail. The six conserved N-glycosylation sites are shown as wiggled lines in the extracellular domains of V1, between C2' and C2'', C2'', and X.

HuMETCAM is expressed in a limited number of normal tissues, such as hair follicular cells, smooth muscle cells, endothelial cells, cerebellum, normal mammary epithelial cells, basal cells of the lung, activated T cells, intermediate trophoblast, (Shih, 1999) and normal nasopharyngeal epithelial cells (Lin et al., 2013). The protein is overly expressed in most (67%) malignant melanoma cells (Lehmann *et al.*, 1989), and in most (more than 80%) pre-malignant prostate epithelial cells (PIN), high-grade prostatic carcinoma cells, and metastatic lesions (Wu *et al.*, 2001b; Wu, 2004). *huMETCAM* is also expressed in other cancers, such as gestational trophoblastic tumors, leiomyosarcoma, angiosarcoma, haemangioma, Kaposi's sarcoma, schwannoma, some lung squamous and small cell carcinomas, some breast cancers, some neuroblastomas (Shih, 1999), and also nasopharyngeal carcinoma (Lin *et al.*, 2014) and ovarian cancer (Aldovini *et al.*, 2006; Wu & Dickerson, 2014).

It is now well documented that cancers from different tissues also express some common genes in addition to tissue specific signatures in different cancer types (Vogelstein & Kinzler, 2004; Christofori, 2006; Gupta & Massague, 2006). One group of them is cell adhesion molecules (*CAMs*). *CAMs* do not merely act as a molecular glue to hold together homotypic cells in a specific tissue or to facilitate interactions of heterotypic cells; *CAMs* also actively govern the social behaviors of cells by affecting the adhesion status of cells and modulating cell signaling (Cavallaro & Christofori, 2005). They control cell motility and invasiveness by mediating the remodeling of cytoskeleton (Cavallaro & Christofori, 2005). They also actively mediate the cell-to-cell and cell-to-extracellular matrix interactions to allow cells to constantly respond to physiological fluctuations and to alter/remodel the surrounding microenvironment for survival (Chambers *et al.*, 2002). They do so by crosstalk with cellular surface growth factor receptors, which interact with growth factors that may be secreted from stromal cells, or released from circulation, and embedded in the extracellular matrix (Chambers *et al.*, 2002; Cavallaro & Christofori, 2005). Thus an altered expression of *CAMs* affects the motility and invasiveness of many tumor cells *in vitro* and metastasis *in vivo* (Chambers *et al.*, 2002; Cavallaro & Christofori, 2005). *CAMs* also play an important role in the favorable soil that provides a proper microenvironment at a suitable period to awaken the dormant metastatic tumor cells to enter into an aggressive growth phase. Actually, the metastatic potential of a tumor cell, as documented in many carcinomas, is the consequence of a complex participation of many over- and under-expressed *CAMs* (Chambers *et al.*, 2002; Cavallaro & Christofori, 2005). Based on the above information, aberrant expression of *METCAM* may also affect the motility and invasiveness of many tumor cells *in vitro* and metastasis *in vivo*. Indeed *METCAM* plays a positive role in the malignant progression of many cancer types, such as melanoma, prostate cancer, and osteosarcomas (Xie *et al.*, 1997; Wu, 2005; Schlagbauer-Wahl *et al.*, 1999; Wu *et al.*, 2008; Wu, 2011). However, it may play an opposite role in the progression of other tumors, such as one mouse melanoma subline, human ovarian cancers, and perhaps haemangiomas and nasopharyngeal carcinomas (Wu, 2012; Wu & Wu, 2012). Shih *et al* first suggested that *huMETCAM* may play a negative role in the progression of breast cancer cell MCF-7 cells (Shih *et al.*, 1997). Later one group also suggested the similar notion for the MDA-MB-231 cells (Ouhtit *et al.*, 2009). In contrast, two other groups suggested the opposite notion that *huMETCAM* may play a positive role in the progression of breast cancer cells (Garcia *et al.*, 2009; Zabouo *et al.*, 2009). To resolve this controversial notion, we re-investigated the role of *huMETCAM* in the progression of four human breast cancer cell lines, which had been previously used by the above four groups. From both *in vitro* and *in vivo* evidence, we strongly suggested that *huMETCAM* plays a positive role in the progression of the four breast cancer cell lines (Zeng *et al.*, 2011; Zeng *et al.*, 2012a). Recently this notion has also been supported by the work done by two other groups (Zeng *et al.*, 2012b; Imbert *et al.*, 2012). In this review we will summarize the work in the followings:

2   METCAM and Breast Cancer Tumorigenesis

HuMETCAM-induced tumorigenesis has been studied in several human breast cancer cell lines. Over-expression of *huMETCAM* may have a negative effect, or a positive effect on tumorigenesis, as shown in the followings:

Shih *et al*. showed in immunohistochemistry that *huMETCAM* was expressed in normal breasts, but only expressed in 18% of breast carcinomas and in 13% of metastatic breast carcinomas (Shih *et al*., 1997). However, this result is misleading because later when breast carcinomas were found to be much more heterogeneous by molecular typing (which were determined by using the gene-expression profile) than by traditional classification (which were determined by using histological and clinical criteria) (Perou *et al*., 2000). As such, breast carcinomas were further divided into at least five different subtypes (Sorlie *et al*., 2001; Charafe-Jauffret *et al*., 2006; Neve *et al*., 2006). *HuMETCAM* was found to be expressed in cell lines and tissues of basal-like and mesenchymal subtypes at levels much higher than that in luminal subtypes, which poorly or very weakly expressed the protein (Garcia *et al*., 2009; Zabouo *et al*. 2009; Imbert *et al*., 2012; Zeng *et al*., 2012b). Thus the reason that *huMETCAM* was only expressed in less than 20% of their specimens is highly likely due to that the luminal subtypes, which had been shown to poorly express *huMETCAM*, were predominantly represented in their collected specimens.

Since *huMETCAM* was not expressed in *MCF-7* cell line, they transfected the *huMETCAM* gene into MCF-7 cells and isolated overly expressed clones for animal studies (Shih *et al*., 1997). They showed that over-expression of *huMETCAM* in *MCF-7* cells suppressed tumor formation of the cells in *SCID* mice, as shown in Fig. 2, suggesting that *huMETCAM* is a possible tumor suppressor in breast cancer (Shih *et al*., 1997).

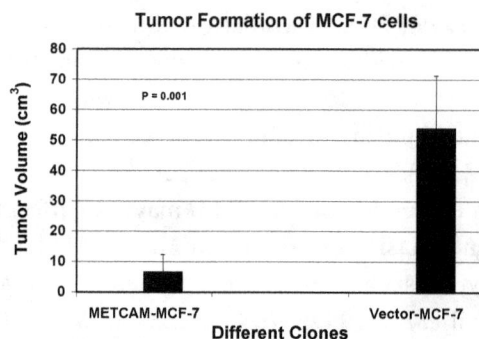

Figure 2: Effect of over-expression of *huMETCAM* on tumor formation of a human breast cancer cell line *MCF-7*. METCAM-MCF-7 was a clone, which expressed a high level of *huMETCAM* after transfection with the cDNA. Vector-MCF-7 was a clone, which did not express any *huMETCAM* after transfection with an empty vector. Cells were injected subcutaneously into female *SCID* mice (Shih *et al*., 1997).

To try to reproduce their results, first we determined the expression of *huMETCAM* in four human breast cancer cell lines, two derived from the luminal subtype (*MCF-7* and *SK-BR3*) and two from the basal-like subtype (*MDA-MB-231* and *MDA-MB-468*), as suggested by the results of recent gene expression profiles of breast cancer cell lines (Charafe-Jauffret *et al*., 2006; Neve *et al*., 2006). As shown in Fig. 3, *huMETCAM* is not expressed in *MCF-7* cells (0%), which is consistent with the observation of Shih *et al.*, ((Shih *et al.*, 1997), weakly expressed in *SK-BR-3* cells (5%), and moderately expressed in the human mammary cancer cell lines, *MDA-MB-231* (a metastatic cell line) (16%), and *MDA-MB-468* (a metastatic cell line) (22%), as shown in Fig. 3.

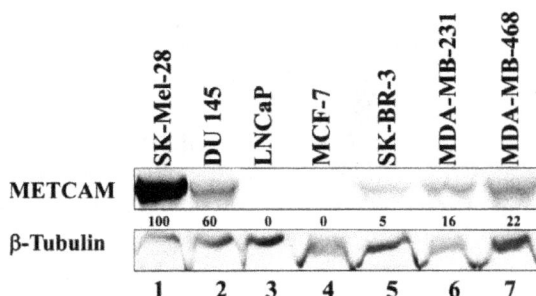

Figure 3: Expression of *huMETCAM* in four human breast cancer cell lines, *MCF-7*, *SK-BR-3*, *MDA-MB-231* and *MDA-MB-468*. *SK-Mel-28*, a human melanoma cell line, which expressed a very high level of *huMETCAM*, was used as a positive control (100%). Two human prostate cancer cell lines, *DU145* and *LNCaP*, which expressed different levels of *huMETCAM* (60% and 0%, respectively) were used as positive and negative controls.

The above results appeared to suggest that *huMETCAM* is not or weakly expressed in cell lines established from luminal subtypes, but it is moderately expressed in cell lines established from basal-like subtype, *MDA-MB-231* and *MDA-MB-468*, consistent with the recent gene expression profiles of many human breast cancer cell lines and different subtypes of clinical breast cancer specimens (Garcia *et al.*, 2009; Zabouo *et al.*, 2009; Zeng *et al.*, 2012b).

Second, we transfected the *huMETCAM* gene into *MCF-7* and *SK-BR-3* cells, isolated overly expressed clones, and used them for *in vitro* tumorigenesis studies (Zeng *et al.*, 2011; Zeng *et al.*, 2012a). We found that over-expression of *huMETCAM* significantly increased the anchorage-independent colony formation of these cell lines in soft agar and a disorganized growth in a 3D basement membrane culture assay, and this augmentation effect was significantly reduced in the presence of the anti-*huMETCAM* antibodies, suggesting that *huMETCAM* increased *in vitro* tumorigenesis of the two luminal-like breast cancer cell lines (Zeng *et al.*, 2011; Zeng *et al.*, 2012a). Since the two basal-like cell lines, *MDA-MB-231* and *MDA-MB-468*, already express *huMETCAM,* we also directly used them for the similar studies in the presence or absence of the anti-*huMETCAM* antibodies. We also found that these two cell lines had a higher ability to form anchorage-independent colonies in soft agar and a higher disorganized growth in a 3D basement membrane culture assay in the absence of than in the presence of the anti-*huMETCAM* antibodies, suggesting also that *huMETCAM* increased *in vitro* tumorigenesis of the two basal-like breast cancer cell lines (Zeng *et al.*, 2011; Zeng *et al.*, 2012a).Thus we concluded that *huMETCAM* expression increased *in vitro* tumorigenesis of the four breast cancer cell lines.

Third, we then used the overly expressed clones of *MCF-7* and *SK-BR-3* cells to reinvestigate the role of *huMETCAM* in *in vivo* tumorigenesis studies in animal models and found that over-expression of *huMETCAM* promoted the tumorigenesis of two human breast cancer cell lines, *MCF7* and *SK-BR-3*, in immunodeficient mouse models (Zeng *et al.*, 2011; Zeng *et al.*, 2012a), as shown in Fig. 4, effect of *huMETCAM* expression on tumorigenesis of *MCF-7* in female *SCID* mice (Zeng *et al.*, 2011) and in Fig. 5, that of *SK-BR-3* in female athymic nude mice (Zeng *et al.*, 2012a).

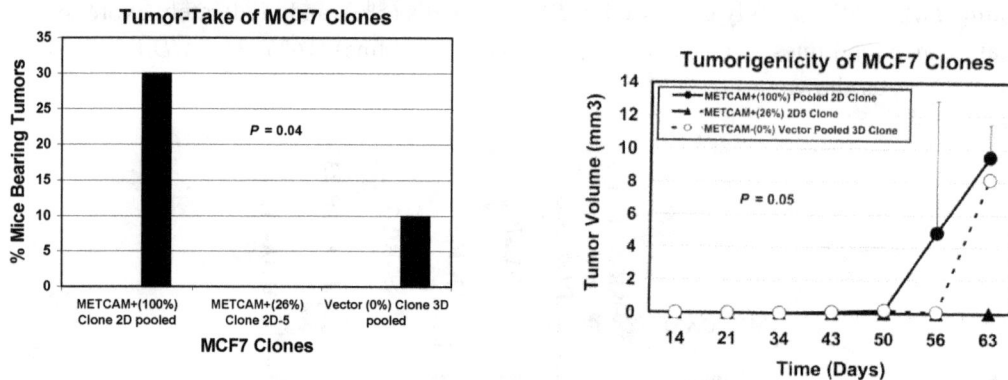

Figure 4: Effect of over-expression of *huMETCAM* on tumor-take (left panel) and tumorigenicity (right panel) of a human breast cancer cell line *MCF-7 in female SCID mice*. METCAM+ clone 2D pooled was a pooled clone, which expressed 100% of *huMETCAM*, and METCAM+ clone 2D-5, which expressed 26% of *huMETCAM*, after transfection with the *huMETCAM* cDNA. Vector clone 3D pooled was a pooled clone, which did not express any *huMETCAM*, after transfection with an empty vector. Cells were injected subcutaneously into female SCID mice (Zeng *et al.*, 2011).

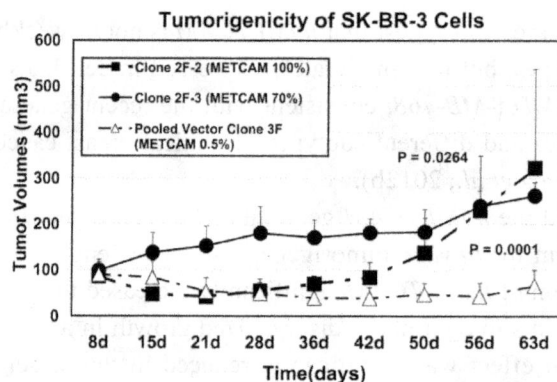

Figure 5: Effect of over-expression of *huMETCAM* on tumor formation of a human breast cancer cell line *SK-BR-3* in female nude mice (Zeng *et al.*, 2012a). Clone 2F-2 and clone 2F-3 expressed 100% and 70% of *METCAM*, respectively. Pooled vector clone 3F expressed only about 0.5% of *METCAM*, as a vector control.

Taken together, the suppression role of *huMETCAM* in tumorigenesis of human breast cancer cells originally observed by Shih *et al.*, is not supported by the above evidence (Zeng *et al.*, 2011; Zeng *et al.*, 2012a) and also by one recent publication (Zeng *et al.*, 2012b). Instead, *huMETCAM* increased *in vivo* tumorigenesis of the two luminal-like human breast cancer cell lines in immunodeficient mouse models. The reason for the observed results of Shih *et al.* may be due to the artifact of including fetal bovine serum in their injection mixtures, as extensively discussed in our published paper (Zeng *et al.*, 2011). The studies of the effect of *huMETCAM* on *in vivo* tumorigenesis of the two basal-like human breast cancer cell lines and are currently in progress. The study of the effect of *huMETCAM* on *in vivo* tumorigenesis of the human breast cancer cell line,

MCF-7, in the presence of estrogen supplement has been recently performed and published, in which *huMETCAM* also increased *in vivo* tumorigenesis of the human breast cancer cell line, MCF-7, in immunodeficient SCID mice (Zeng *et al.*, 2012b), consistent with our conclusion as described above.

3   METCAM and Breast Cancer Metastasis

We also used the overly expressed clones of *MCF-7* and *SK-BR-3* cells, which were transfected with the *huMETCAM* gene, for *in vitro* motility and invasiveness studies. We found the over-expression of *huMETCAM* significantly increased *in vitro* motility and invasiveness of these cells and this augmentation effect was significantly reduced in the presence of the anti-*huMETCAM* antibodies, suggesting that *huMETCAM* directly increases these *in vitro* processes in the two breast cancer cell lines and also is consistent with the two recently published papers, in which they showed that over-expression of *huMETCAM* promotes the epithelial-mesenchymal transition (EMT) of *MCF-7* cells (Zeng *et al*, 2012b; Imbert *et al.*, 2012). Since the two basal-like cell lines, *MDA-MB-231* and *MDA-MB-468*, already express *huMETCAM,* we also directly used them for the similar studies. We found the motility and invasiveness of the two basal-like cell lines were also significantly reduced by the anti-*huMETCAM* antibodies (Zeng *et al.*, 2011; Zeng *et al.*, 2012a). From these results, we suggest that the expression of *METCAM* promotes the motility and invasiveness of the four breast cancer cell lines. However this result contradicts the findings of Ouhtit *et al.* (Ouhtit *et al.*, 2009), who found that over-expression of *huMETCAM* inhibited the *in vitro* invasiveness of *MDA-MB-231* cells, supporting the notion of Shih *et al*. Nevertheless, our results are consistent with the recently published results from three groups (Zabouo *et al.*, 2009; Zeng *et al.*, 2012b; Imbert *et al.*, 2012). Thus majority of the observations strongly support our conclusion. To be consistent with *in vitro* studies, one group used the human breast cancer cell line *MCF-7* for the metastasis studies in a mouse model in the presence of estrogen supplement and found that over-expression of *huMETCAM* could induce the metastasis of *MCF-7* cells in *SCID/Beige* mice (Zeng *et al.*, 2012b).

In conclusion, more evidence appears to support that *huMETCAM* plays a positive role in the progression of human breast cancer cells, similar to melanoma, prostate cancer, and osteosarcomas (Wu, 2005; Wu, 2012).

4   Mechanisms of METCAM-Mediated Tumorigenesis and Metastasis

How does *METCAM* mediate or regulate tumorigenesis and metastasis of cancer cells? By deducing knowledge learned from the tumorigenesis of other tumors (Chambers *et al.*, 2002; Vogelstein & Kinzler, 2004; Christofori, 2006; Gupta & Massague, 2006; Hanahan & Weinberg, 2011) and the *huMETCAM*-mediated progression of melanoma (Li *et al.*, 2003; Melnikova *et al.*, 2009; Melnikova *et al.*, 2010) and angiogenesis (Anfosso *et al.*, 2001; Bardin *et al.*, 2001; Kang *et al.*, 2006; Yan *et al.*, 2003), we may be able to find some common clues to begin understanding its mechanisms.

First, the transcriptional expression of *huMETCAM* gene may be regulated by *PKA/CREB* (cAMP-responsive element binding protein), *AP-2α* (Melnikova *et al.*, 2009; Melnikova *et al.*, 2010) and other transcription factors, such as *SP-1, c-Myb, N-Oct2, ETs, CArG, Egr-1,* and transcription factors binding to insulin response elements in a minimal promoter region of *huMETCAM* gene, as shown in Fig. 6 (Wu, 2005).

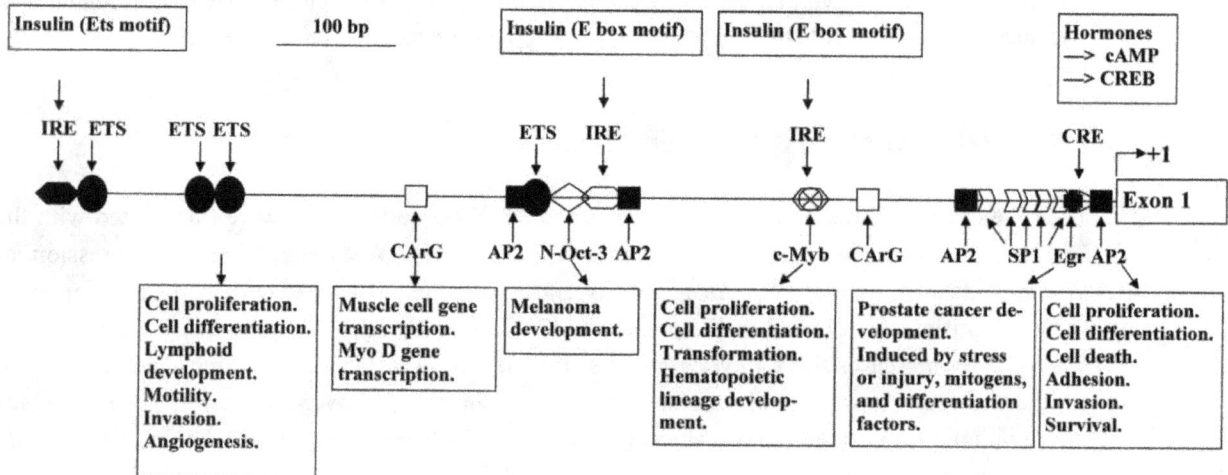

Figure 6: The minimal promoter of the *huMETCAM* gene. The locations of various transcriptionally regulatory elements are shown in the 900 bp promoter region of the *huMETCAM* gene. The possible function of each element is also indicated. The promoter contains four AP-2 (activator protein-2, GCCNNNGGC), one CRE (cAMP response element, TGACGTCA), one Egr (early growth response element, CCCTG), five SP-1 (CCGCCC), two CArG (CC(A/t)6GG), three IRE (two insulin responsive elements with E-box motif, CANNTG, and one with Ets motif, ACGGAT), one c-Myb (coincided with one IRE with E-box motif, CACCTG), one N-Oct-3 (or brn-2, GCCTGAAT), and four Ets elements (GGAA).

Among these potential regulators, it is well documented that the *AP-2α* transcription factor plays a crucial tumor suppressor role in the progression of melanoma, prostate and breast cancer (Melnikova *et al.*, 2010). It has been shown that *PKA/CREB* plays a positive role in the progression of melanoma, and perhaps also applicable to breast cancer, as well as other cancers, by inhibiting the expression of AP-2α and increasing the expression of *huMETCAM* (Melnikova *et al.*, 2010). However, the expression level of *AP-2α* in other cancers has not been explored. The roles of other transcription regulators, tissue specific enhancers and repressors, epigenetic control, and control at the level of chromatin remodeling of the gene have still yet to be investigated by using a longer DNA fragment that contains tissue specific regulators for the gene (Wu, 2005).

Second, since the cytoplasmic tail of *huMETCAM* contains consensus sequences potentially to be phosphorylated by *PKA*, *PKC*, and *CK2*, it may manifest its functions by cross-talk with various signaling pathways mediated by these protein kinases (Wu, 2005). For example, *huMETCAM* expression in melanoma cells is reciprocally regulated by *AKT*, in which *AKT* up-regulates the level *huMETCAM* and over-expression of *huMETCAM* activates endogenous *AKT*, which in turn inhibits apoptosis and increases survival ability (Li *et al.*, 2003). However it is not clear if a similar mechanism is also used in breast cancers. Also the detailed mechanism of how *AKT* up-regulates the expression of *METCAM* has not been worked out. *PKA*, *PKC*, and *CK2* may phosphorylate the cytoplasmic tail of *METCAM*, which then facilitates its interaction with *FAK,* thus promoting cytoskeleton remodeling. Alternatively, after phosphorylation of its cytoplasmic tail by these protein kinases, *huMETCAM* may interact with the downstream effectors of *Ras*, activating *ERK* and *JNK,* which in turn may transcriptionally activate the expression of *AKT* or other genes that promote the proliferation and angiogenesis of tumor cells. Though *huMETCAM* has not been shown to be a substrate of *CK2,* which has been shown to phosphorylate other *CAMs*, such as *CD44*, *E-cadherin*, and *L1-CAM*, and one of integrin-receptors in the extracellular matrix protein, *vitronectin*, it is also likely that *CK2* may be able to phosphorylate *huMETCAM* (Maggio &Pinna, 2003) and link it to *AKT* to affect the proliferation, survival and other tumorigenesis-related functions of tumor cells (Datta *et al.*, 1999).

Third, after the engagement of *huMETCAM* with the ligand(s) or extracellular matrix, it may transmit the outside-in signals into tumor cells by activating *FAK* and the downstream signaling components, promoting cytoskeleton remodeling and increasing tumor cell motility and invasiveness (Anfosso *et al.*, 2001; Wu, 2005). This is consistent with the recent findings that METCAM may promote EMT of breast cancer cells via activation of RhoA and up-regulation of slug (Zeng *et al.*, 2012b).

Fourth, from what we know about the roles of other *CAM*s in the progression of other tumors (Vogelstein & Kinzler, 2004; Christofori, 2006; Gupta & Massague, 2006; Wong *et al.*, 2012), it is logical to postulate that *METCAM* may affect cancer cell progression by cross-talk with signaling pathways that affect apoptosis, survival and proliferation, angiogenesis, and energy metabolism of tumor cells (Wu, 2005; Cavallaro & Christofori, 2005; Kang *et al.*, 2006; Fritz & Fajas, 2010; Hanahan & Weinberg, 2011). Thus *huMETCAM* may affect tumorigenesis and metastasis by altering the expression of various indexes in apoptosis, survival signaling, proliferation signaling, angiogenesis, and aerobic glycolysis. Consistent with this notion, we have found that *huMETCAM* may promote the progression of breast cancer cells by rendering the cells with increased anti-apoptotic and survival ability by elevating levels of *Bcl2*, with increased angiogenic ability by elevating levels of *VEGF* and *VEGFR2,* and increased proliferation via aerobic glycolysis by elevating levels of LDH-A; but it has no effect on the process of apoptosis (Zeng *et al.*, 2012a). Further systematic studies by using specific RNAi's to knockdown the downstream effectors one-by-one in the *METCAM*-expressing clones may be necessary to further understand this aspect of mechanism.

Fifth, *huMETCAM* may mediate hematogenous spreading of melanoma cells, which had been implicated by its expression in endothelial cells, as well as in malignant melanoma cells (Sers *et al.*, 1994) and further shown to be present in the junctions of endothelial cells (Bardin *et al.*, 2001; Kang *et al.*, 2006) and essential for tumor angiogenesis in at least three tumor cell lines (Yan *et al.*, 2003) and human prostate cancer *LNCaP* cells (Wu & Son, 2006). It is highly likely that *huMETCAM* expression may promote hematogenous spreading of breast cancer cells, similar to melanoma and prostate cancer cells (Wu, 2011; Wu *et al.*, 2004). However, it is not known if *huMETCAM* also plays a role in the lymphatic spread of cancer cells. Recent results from one group showed that *huMETCAM* is one of the lymphatic metastasis-associated genes, which is up-regulated in malignant mouse hepatocarcinoma (Song *et al.*, 2005), suggesting that *huMETCAM* may also play a role in promoting lymphatic metastasis of cancer cells. However, the details of how *huMETCAM* mediates hematogenous or lymphatic spreading of cancer cells have still yet to be investigated. Labeling the cells with viable dyes and following the process in real time by using a newly developed non-intruding, but highly photo-penetrating imaging method of photoacoustic tomography (PAT) (Zhang *et al.*, 2008; Wang, 2008) may be useful for monitoring each step in the *huMETCAM*-mediated progression of breast cancer cells in hair-less nude mice.

Sixth, *huMETCAM* has been shown to express in normal mesenchymal cells (smooth muscle, endothelium, and Schwann cells) in the tissue stroma and be a marker for the mesenchymal stem cells (Sorrentino *et al.*, 2008), *huMETCAM* may play an important role in regulating tumor dormancy or awakening, driving or preventing cancer cells to pre-metastatic niche, and formatting a microenvironment for favorable or unfavorable tumor growth in secondary sites (Wu, 2005; Hanahan & Weinberg, 2011; Wong *et al.*, 2012; Wu, 2012).

Seventh, *huMETCAM* may affect the progression of cancer cells by interactions with the host immune system, which however has been shown to have a paradoxical role in tumor progression (deVisser *et al.*, 2006; Hanahan & Weinberg, 2011). Recently one group has shown that a subset of host B lymphocytes may control melanoma metastasis through *huMETCAM*-dependent interaction (Staqyuicini *et al.*, 2008). Since human breast cancer cells can only grow as xenografts in immunodeficient mouse models, the role of B and T cells in the progression of human breast cancer cells may not be explored in these mouse models. But the investigation of the effect of *huMETCAM* expression on the mediation of NK cells in this process may be possible in athymic nude mouse models. The surface *huMETCAM* expressed in breast cancer cells may have a homophilic interaction with the *NK* cells, which also express *huMETCAM*, and enhance cytotoxic functions of *NK* cells (Despoix *et al.*, 2008). This hypothesis should be testable by studying the *huMETCAM*-mediated metastasis of *huMETCAM*-expressing breast cancer cells by injecting cells into nude mice pre-treated with anti-NK surface markers antibodies to deplete NK cells.

Eighth, malignant progression of cancer cells has been shown to associate with an abnormal glycosylation, resulting in expression of altered carbohydrate determinants (Kannagi *et al.*, 2004). Thus, the glycosylated status of *huMETCAM* in breast cancer types may be different from normal cells, thus manifesting positive or negative effect on the progression of different cancer types. This aspect of the *huMETCAM*-mediated cancer progression has not been well-studied, but is especially intriguing since *huMETCAM* possesses six conserved N-glycosylation sites in the extracellular domain (Wu, 2005; Wu *et al.*, 2001a).

We should always keep in mind that mechanisms of *huMETCAM*-mediated cancer progression may be slightly different in different breast cancer cell lines due to their different intrinsic properties, which provides different co-factors and/or different ligand(s) that may modulate the *huMETCAM*-mediated tumorigenesis and metastasis. To further understand the role of *huMETCAM* in these processes, it is essential to diligently identify the co-factors and the *huMETCAM*-cognate heterophilic ligand(s), which modulate the biological functions of *huMETCAM*. The endeavor in this direction appears to be promising from our preliminary attempts that we may have successfully found a possible candidate of *huMETCAM*'s heterophilic ligand in *huMETCAM*-expressing human prostate cancer cells (Wu, 2005).

5   Conclusions and Clinical Applications

Taken together, over-expression of *huMETCAM* is very likely to promote tumor progression of both luminal-like and basal-like human breast cancer cells. The results of Shih *et al.* (Shih *et al.*, 1997), which suggested a tumor-suppressive effect of *huMETCAM* on human breast cancer cells, can not be reproduced by using standard injection methods in animal studies. The positive role of *huMETCAM* in the progression of breast cancer is very likely to be similar to that in melanoma and prostate cancer (Wu, 2005; Wu, 2011; Wu, 2012). Since the role of *huMETCAM* in the progression of breast cancer has been resolved, *huMETCAM* may be a potential therapeutic target for an alternative treatment of breast cancer. These established mouse model systems can also serve as model systems for studies on the effect of over-expression of an immunoglobulin-like CAM on the progression of breast cancer cells and for further mechanical studies on the progression of breast cancer. In addition, these mouse systems should serve as an excellent preclinical model for designing immunotherapeutic means to arrest this dreadful cancer. For example, a fully humanized anti-*METCAM* antibody against melanoma growth and metastasis may also be used against breast cancer (Leslie *et al.*, 2007). Alternatively, small soluble peptides derived from *huMETCAM* may also be useful for blocking the tumor formation and tumor angiogenesis (Satyamoothy *et al.*, 2001; Hafner *et al.*, 2002; Wu & Son, 2006). The attachment of these reagents to nanoparticles may be another alternative for therapeutic use (Nie, 2006).

Acknowledgement

This work has been supported by the seed money of Department of Bioscience Technology, CYCU, Taiwan and a grant from National Science Council in Taiwan.

References

Aldovini, D., Demichelis, F., Doglioni, C., Di Vizio, D., Galligioni, E., Brugnara, S., Zeni, B., Griso, C., Pegoraro, C., Zannoni, M., Garibold, M., Balladore, E., Mezzanzanica, D., Canevari, S., & Barbareschi, M. (2006). M-CAM expression as marker of poor prognosis in epithelial ovarian cancer. *International Journal of Cancer, 119(8),* 1920-1926.

Anfosso. F., Bardin, N., Vivier, E., Sabatier, F., Sampol, J., & Dignat-George, F. (2001). Outside-in signaling pathway linked to CD146 engagement in human endothelial cells. *Journal of Biological Chemistry, 276,* 1564-1569.

Bardin, N., George, F., Mutin, M., Brisson, C., Horschowski, N., Frances, V., Lesaule, G., & Sampol, J. (1996). S-endo1, a pan-endothelial monoclonal antibody recognizing a novel human endothelial antigen. *Tissue Antigens, 48,* 531-539.

Bardin, N., Anfosso, F., Masse, J., Cramer, E., Sabatier, F., LeBivic, A., Sampol, J., Dignat-George, F. (2001). Identification of CD146 as a component of the endothelial junction involved in the control of cell-cell adhesion. *Blood, 98,* 3677-3684.

Cavallaro, U. & Christofori, G. (2005). Cell adhesion and signaling by cadherins and Ig-CAMs in cancer. *Nature Reviews/Cancer, 4,* 118-132.

Chambers, A., Groom, A. C., & MacDonald, I. C. (2002). Dissemination and growth of cancer cells in metastatic sites. *Nature Reviews/Cancer, 2,* 563-572.

Charafe-Jauffret, E., Geinestier, C., Monville, F., Finetti, P., Adelaide, J., Cervera, N., Fekairi, S., Xerri, L., Jacquemier, J., Birnbaum, D., & Bertucci, F. (2006). Gene expression profiling of breast cell lines identifies potential new basal markers. *Oncogene, 25,* 2273-2284.

Christofori, G. (2006). New signals from the invasive front. *Nature, 44,* 444-450.

Datta, S. R., Brunet, A., & Greenberg, M. E. (1999). Cellular survival: a play in three AKTs. *Genes and Development, 13,* 2905-2927.

Despoix, N., Walzer, T., Jouve, N., Blot-Chabaud, M., Bardin, N., Paul, P., Lyonnet, L., Vivier, E., Dignat-George, F., & Vely, F. (2008). Mouse CD146/MCAM is a marker of natural killer cell maturation. *European Journal of Immunology, 38,* 2855-2864.

deVisser, K. E., Eichten, A., Coussens, L. M. (2006). Paradoxical roles of the immune system during cancer development. *Nature Review/Cancer, 6:*24-37.

Fritz, V. & Fajas, L. (2010). Metabolism and proliferation share common regulatory pathways in cancer cells. *Oncogene, 29,* 4369-4377.

Garcia, S., Dales, J. P., Charafe-Jauffret, E., Carpentier-Meunier, S., Andrac-Meyer, L., Jacquemier, J., Andonian, C., Lavaut, M. N., Allasia, C., Bonnier, P., & Charpin, C. (2007). Poor prognosis in breast carcinomas correlates with increased expression of targetable CD146 and c-Met and with proteomic basal-like phenotype. Human Pathology, 38, 830-841.

Gupta, G. P. & Massague, J. (2006). Cancer metastasis: building a frame work. Cell, 127, 679-695.

Hafner, C., Samwald, U., Wagner, S., Felici, F., Heere-Ress, E., Jensen-Jarolim, E., Wolff, K., Scheiner, O., Pehamberger, H., & Breiteneder, H. (2002). Selection of mimotopes of the cell surface adhesion molecule of Mel-CAM from a random pVIII-28aa phage peptide library. Journal of Investigative Dermatology, 119, 865-869.

Hanahan, D. and Weinberg, R. A. (2011). The hallmarks of cancer: the next generation. Cell, 144, 646-674.

Imbert, A. –M., Garulli, C., Choquet, E., Koubi, M., Aurrand-Lions, M., & Chabaccon, C. (2012) CD146 expression in human breast cancer cell lines induces phenotypic and functional changes observed in epithelial to mesenchymal transition. PLOS One, 7(8), e43752, 8 pages.

Kang, Y., Wang, F., Feng, J., Yang, D., Yang, X., & Yan, X. (2006). Knockdown of CD146 reduces the migration and proliferation of human endothelial cells. Cell Research, 16, 313-318.

Kannagi, R., Izawa, M., Koike, T., Miyazaki, K., Kimura, N. (2004). Carbohydrate-mediated cell adhesion in cancer metastasis and angiogenesis. Cancer Science, 95(5), 377-384.

Lehmann, J. M., Reithmuller, G., & Johnson J. P. (1989). MUC18, a marker of tumor progression in human melanoma. Proceedings of National Academy of Science USA, 86, 9891-9895.

Leslie, M. C., Zhao, Y. J., Lachman, L. B., Hwu, P., Wu, G. –J., & Bar-Eli, M. (2007). Immunization against MUC18/MCAM, a novel antigen that drives melanoma invasion and metastasis. Gene therapy, 14, 316-323.

Li, G., Kalabis, J., Xu, X., Meier, F., Oka, M., Bogenrieder, T., & Herlyn, M. (2003). Reciprocal regulation of MelCAM and AKT in human melanoma. Oncogene, 22, 6891-6899.

Lin, J. C., Chiang, C. - F., Wang, S. - W., Wang, W. Y., Kwan, P. C., & Wu, G. –J. (2014). Significance and expression of human METCAM/MUC18 in nasopharyngeal carcinoma (NPC) and metastatic lesions. Asian Pacific J of Cancer Prevention, 15 (1), 245-252.

Maggio, F. & Pinna, L. A. (2003). One-thousand-and-one substrates of protein kinase CK2? FASEB Journal, 17, 349-368.

Melnikova, V. O., Balasubramanian, K., Villares, G. J., Debroff, A. S., Zigler, M., Wang, H., Petersson, F., Price, J. E., Schroit, A., Prieto, V. G., Hung, M. C., & Bar-Eli, M. (2009). Crosstalk between protease-activated receptor1 and platelet-activating factor receptor regulates melanoma cell adhesion molecule (MCAM/MUC18) expression and melanoma metastasis. Journal Biological Chememistry, 284(42), 28845-28855.

Melnikova, V. O., Debroff, A. S., Zigler, M., Villares, G. J., Braeuer, R., Wang, H., Huang, L., & Bar-Eli, M. (2010). CREB inhibits AP-2a expression to regulate the malignant phenotype of melanoma. PLoS One, 5, e12452.

Neve, R. M., Chin, K., Fridlyand, J., Yeh, J., Baehner, F. L., Fevr, T., Clark, L., Bayani, N., Coppe, J. P., Tong, F., Speed, T., Spellman, P. T., DeVries, S., Lapuk, A., Wang, N. J., Kuo, W. L., Stilwell, J. L., Pinkel, D., Albertson, D. G., Waldman, F. M., McCormick, F., Dickson, R. B., Johnson, M. D., Lippman, M., Ethier, S., Gazdar, A., Gray, J. W. (2006). A collection of breast cancer cell lines for the study of functionally distinct cancer subtypes. Cancer Cell, 10, 515-527.

Nie, S. (2006). Nanotechnology for personalized and predictive medicine. Nanomedicine, 2(4), 305.

Ouhtit, A., Gaur, R. L., Abd Elmageed, Z. Y., Fernando, A., Thouta, R., Trappey, A. K., Abdraboh, M. E., El-Sayyad, H. I., Rao, P., & Raj, M. G. H. (2009). Towards understanding the mode of action of the multifaceted cell adhesion receptor CD146. Biochimica et Biophysica Acta, 1795, 130-136.

Perou, C. M., Sorlie, T., Eisen, M. B., van de Rijn, M., Jeffrey, S. S., Rees, C. A., Pollack, J. R., Ross, D. T., Johnson, H., Aksien, L. A., Fluge, O., Pergamenschikov, A., Williams, C., Zhu, S. X., Lenning, P. E., Borrensen-Dale, A., Brown, P. O., & Botstein, D. (2000). Molecular portraits of human breast tumours. Nature, 406, 747-52.

Satyamoothy, K., Muyrers, J., Meier, F., Patel, D., & Herlyn, M. (2001). Mel-CAM-specific genetic suppressor elements inhibit melanoma growth and invasion through loss of gap junction communication. Oncogene, 20, 4676-4684.

Schlagbauer-Wadl, H., Jansen, B., Muller, M., Polteraeur, P., Wolff, K., Eichler, H. G., Pehamberger, H., Konak, E., & Johnson, J. P. (1999). Influence of MUC18/MCAM/CD146 expression on human melanoma growth and metastasis in SCID mice. International Journal of Cancer, 81, 951-955.

Sers, C., Riethmuller, G., Johnson, J. P. (1994). MUC18, a melanoma-progression associated molecule, and its potential role in tumor vascularization and hematogenous spread. Cancer Research, 54, 5689-5694.

Shih, I. –M., Elder, D. –E., Hsu, M. Y., & Herlyn, M. (1994). Regulation of Mel-CAM/MUC18 expression on melanocytes of different stages of tumor progression by normal keratinocytes. American Journal of Pathology, 145, 837-845.

Shih, I. –M., Elder, D. E., Speicher, D., Johnson, J. P, & Herlyn, M. (1994). Isolation and functional characterization of the A32 melanoma-associated antigen. Cancer Research, 54, 2514-2520.

Shih, I. –M., Hs, M. Y., Palazzo, J. P., & Herlyn, M. (1997). The cell-cell adhesion receptor MEL-CAM acts as a tumor suppressor in breast carcinoma. American Journal of Pathology, 151, 745-751.

Shih, I. - M. (1999). The role of CD146 (MelCAM), in biology and pathology. Journal of Pathology, 189, 4 -11.

Song, B., Tang, J. W., Wang, B., Cui, X. N., Zhou, C. H., & Hou, L. (2005). Screening for lymphatic metastasis-associated genes in mouse hepatocarcinoma cell lines Hca-F and Hca-P using gene chip. Chinese Journal of Cancer, 24(7):774-780.

Sorrentino, A., Ferracin, M., Castelli, G., Biffoni, M., Tomaselli, G., Baiocchi, M., Fatica, A., Negrini, M., Peschle, C., & Valtieri, M. (2008). Isolation and characterization of CD146+ multipotent mesenchymal stromal cells. Experimental Hematology, 36, 1035-1046.

Sorlie, T., Perou, C. M., Tibshirani, R., Aas, T., Geisler, S., Johnsen, H., Hastie, T., Eisen, M. B., van de Rijn, M., Jeffrey, S. S., & Botstein, D. (2001). Gene expression patterns of breast carcinomas distinguish tumor subclasses with clinical implications. Proceedings of National Academy of Science USA, 98, 10869-74.

Staquicini, F., Tandle, A., Libutti, S. K., Sun, J., Zigler, M., Bar-Eli, M., Aliperti, F., Perez, E. C., Gershenwald, J. E., Mariano, M., Pasqualini, R., Arap, W., & Lopes, J. D. (2008). A subset of host B lymphocytes controls melanoma metastasis through a melanoma cell adhesion molecule/MUC18-dependent interaction: evidence from mice and humans. Cancer Research, 68(20), 8419-8428.

Vogelstein, B. & Kinzler, K. W. (2004). Cancer genes and the pathways they control. Nature Medicine, 10, 789-799.

Wang, L. V. (2008). Prospects of photoacoustic tomography. Medical Physics, 35(12), 5758-5767.

Wong, C. W., Dye, D. E., & Coombe, D. R. (2012). The role of immunoglobulin superfamily cell adhesion molecules in cancer metastasis. International Journal of Cell Biology, 2012, Article ID 340296, 9 pages.

Wu, G. –J., Wu, M. –W. H, Wang, S. –W., Liu, Z., Peng, Q., Qu, P., Yang, H., Varma, V. A., Sun, Q., Petros, J. A., Lim, S., & Amin, M. B. (2001a). Isolation and characterization of the major form of human MUC18 cDNA gene and correlation of MUC18 over-expression in prostate cancer cells and tissues with malignant progression. Gene, 279, 17-31.

Wu, G. –J., Varma, V. A., Wu, M. –W. H., Wang, S. –W., Qu, P., Liu, Z., Petros, J. A., Lim, S., & Amin, M. B. (2001b), Expression of a human cell adhesion molecule, MUC18, in prostate cancer cells and tissues. Prostate, 48, 305-315.

Wu, G. –J. (2004). Chapter 7: The role of MUC18 in prostate carcinoma in Immunohistochemistry and in situ hybridization of human carcinoma. In Vol 1. Molecular pathology, lung carcinoma, breast carcinoma, and prostate carcinoma. Hayat, M.A. (Ed.), Elsevier Science/Academic Press, pp. 347-358.

Wu, G. –J., Peng, Q., Fu, P., Chiang, C. -F., Wang, S. –W., Dillehay, D. L., Wu, M. - W. H. (2004). Ectopical expression of human MUC18 increases metastasis of human prostate cancer LNCaP cells. Gene, 327, 201-213.

Wu, G. –J. (2005). METCAM/MUC18 expression and cancer metastasis. Current Genomics, 6, 333-349.

Wu, G. –J. & Son, E. L. (2006). *Soluble METCAM/MUC18 blocks angiogenesis during tumor formation of human prostate cancer cells. In The proceedings of the 97th Annual Meeting of American Association for the Cancer Research, 47, #252.*

Wu, G. –J., Fu, P., Wang, S. –W., & Wu, MWH: (2008). *Enforced expression of MCAM/MUC18 increases in vitro motility and invasiveness and in vivo metastasis of two mouse melanoma K1735 sublines in a syngeneic mouse model. Molecular Cancer Research, 2008, 6(11), 1666-1677.*

Wu, G. –J. (2011). *Chapter 11: Dual roles of the melanoma CAM (MelCAM/METCAM) in malignant progression of melanoma. In "Research on Melanoma: a glimpse into current directions and future trends" INTECH Open Access Publisher, pp. 229-242.*

Wu, G. - J. (2012). *Dual roles of METCAM in the progression of different cancers. Journal of Oncology, 2012, ID 853797, 13 pages.*

Wu, G. -J. & Dickerson, E. B. (2014). *Frequent and increased expression of human METCAM/MUC18 in cancer tissues and metastatic lesions associates with the clinical progression of human ovarian carcinoma. Taiwanese J Obstetrics & Gynecology, (in press).*

Wu, G. –J. & Wu, M. –W. H. (2014). *Ectopic expression of MCAM/MUC18 increases in vitro motility and invasiveness, but decreases tumorigenesis and metastasis of a mouse melanoma K1735-9 subline in a syngeneic mouse model. (submitted).*

Xie, S., Luca, M., Huang, S., Gutman, M., Reich, R., Johnson, J. P., Bar-Eli, M. (1997). *Expression of MCAM/MUC18 by human melanoma cells leads to increased tumor growth and metastasis. Cancer Research, 57, 2295-2303.*

Yan, X., Lin, Y., Tang, D., Shen, Y., Yuan, M., Zhang, Z., Li, P., Xia, H., Li, L., Luo, D., Liu, Q., Mann, K., & Bader, B. L. (2003). *A novel anti-CD146 monoclonal antibody, AA98, inhibits angiogenesis and tumor growth. Blood, 102, 184-191.*

Yang, H., Wu, M. –W. H., Wang, S. W., Liu, Z., & Wu, G. –J. (2001). *Isolation and characterization of murine MUC18 cDNA, and correlation of its expression in murine melanoma cell lines with their metastatic ability. Gene, 265, 133-145.*

Zabouo, G., Imbert, A. M., Jacquemier, J., Finetti, P., Moreau, T., Esterni, B., Birnbaum, D., Bertucci, F., & Chabannon, C. (2009). *CD146 expression is associated with a poor prognosis in human breast tumors and with enhanced motility in breast cancer cell lines. Breast Cancer Research, 11, R1 (doi:10.1186/bcr2215).*

Zeng, G., Cai, S., & Wu, G. –J. (2011). *Up-regulation of METCAM/MUC18 promotes motility, invasiveness and tumorigenesis of human breast cancer cells. BMC Cancer, 11, 113.*

Zeng, G., Cai, S., Liu, Y., & Wu, G. –J. (2012a). *METCAM/MUC18 augments promotes migration, invasion and tumorigenicity of human breast cancer SK-BR-3 Cells. Gene, 492, 229-238.*

Zeng, Q., Li, W., Lu, D., Wu, Z., Duan, H., Luo, Y., Feng, J., Yang, D., Fu, L., & Yan, X. (2012b) *CD146, an epithelial-mesenchymal transition inducer, is associated with triple-negative breast cancer. Proceedings of National Academic of Science USA, 109 (4), 1127-1132.*

Zhang, Q., Liu, Z., Carney, P. R., Yuan, Z., Chen, H., Roper, S. N., & Jiang, H. (2008). *Non-invasive imaging of epileptic seizures in vivo using photoacoustic tomography (PAT). Physical Medical Biology 53, 1921-1931.*

Neu Implications in Breast Cancer

Gerald M. Higa
Schools of Pharmacy and Medicine
West Virginia University, Morgantown, USA

1   *Neu* Introduction

The *HER2* proto-oncogene is also designated as *neu*, the origin of which has been linked to a neuroblastoma cell line established in rats (Coussens *et al.*, 1985). Moreover, *neu* appeared to be related to a gene found in the avian erythroblastosis virus (v-*ErbB)* that encoded epidermal growth factor receptor (EGFR) (Vennstrom & Bishop, 1982), a conclusion supported by the substantial homology that exists between the two onco-proteins. Hence, this was how HER (Human EGFR-Related) 2 derived its name; and the rather mundane way the other three members of the ErbB family, HER1 (EGFR), HER3, and HER4 are identified (Figure 1).

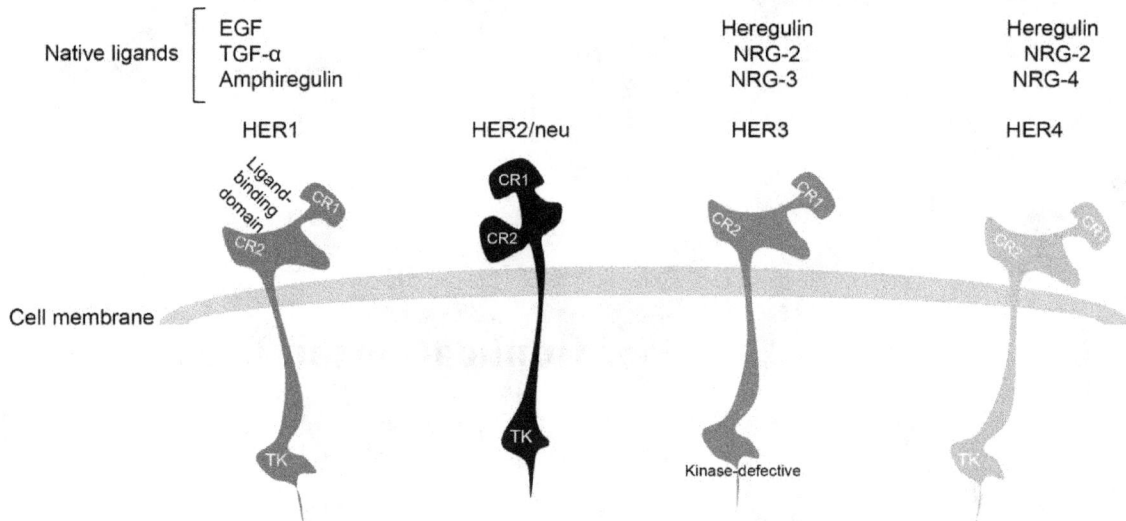

Figure 1: Structural configuration of monomeric ErbB family members. Each member has a ligand-binding extracellular, a trans-membrane, and an intracellular kinase domain. Ligand-binding has been localized to a site between CR1 and CR2. In contrast to the "closed" position of HER2, the "open" or extended conformer exhibited by HER1, HER3, and HER4 appears to allow ligand access. Two items of note – no endogenous ligand for HER2 has been identified and the defective or deficient kinase activity of HER3.

The HER family of receptor tyrosine kinases (RTKs) is physiologically and functionally important as signals emanating from each receptor appear to have profound implications in human development as evidenced by the wide distribution of the receptors (Miettinen *et al.*, 1995; Lee *et al.*, 1995). In breast tissue, studies suggest each receptor has a different function in normal mammary gland development. For example, whereas HER1 contributes to ductal growth, HER2 promotes lobuloalveolar differentiation and lactation (Jones & Stern, 1999). That much less is known about HER3 in the normal development of breast tissue may be partly related to an inherent defect in the kinase domain of the receptor (Guy *et al.*, 1994). Even though HER3 cannot be activated on its own, the receptor can be trans-phosphorylated by other members of the HER family. The significance of this finding in breast cancer will be discussed later. Finally, HER4 provides striking evidence of the signaling diversity among the ErbB family members. Coupled to the activated intracellular domain is an array of cellular responses including differentiation of epithelial cells, reduction in proliferation, and activation of apoptotic pathways, all of which suggest the presence of HER4 may *antagonize* the activity of over-expressed HER2 (Sartor *et al.*, 2001; Barnes *et al.*, 2005).

The primary focus of this chapter is the biology of *neu* in breast cancer. However, where appropriate, additional information has been included in order to elucidate and further clarify the impact other components may have on the HER2-signaling pathway. And because of the relatively poor prognosis, a comprehensive discussion of novel therapeutic agents that are currently approved (or in clinical trials) for the treatment of HER2-positive breast cancer is also provided. The final sections relate to two important issues that highlight our increased, though by no means complete, understanding of *neu* – first, potential mechanisms that may contribute to tumor resistance; and second, numerous uncertainties that persist despite the bona-fide progress made in treating this particular subtype of breast cancer.

2   *Neu* Biology

Localized to the long arm of chromosome 17(q21), the *HER2* gene encodes a 185 kDa protein (p185^{HER2}) RTK (Barnes *et al.*, 1986). All HER receptors have a structural configuration that includes a short membrane-spanning region that connects the extracellular receptor-binding portion to the intracellular catalytic kinase domain (Figure 1) (van der Geer *et al.*, 1994). Ligand binding, which promotes receptor dimerization, is considered the initial event in activating the internal signal transduction pathway. However, newer information suggests that receptor conformation, rather than phosphorylation, is the major determinant of kinase activation (Zhang *et al.*, 2006). Nonetheless, the ultimate cellular response depends on a complex process involving recruitment and activation of additional protein kinases located downstream of the receptor, more of which will be discussed in detail later.

3   *Neu* Expression

While receptors, in general, are essential for regulating normal tissue development, they could also be a liability to the cell. This paradox, especially with regards to HER2, is strongly supported by evidence which links neu to a specific breast cancer subtype. It should be emphasized that HER2 expression alone neither identifies nor correlates with this unique tumor phenotype. Instead, gene amplification and/or receptor over-expression confers the only accepted designation of HER2-positivity, a diagnostic subtype of approximately 20% of all breast cancers (Hynes & Stern, 1994; McCann *et al.*, 1991; Menard *et al.*, 2001). An extension of the importance of this genetic and molecular abnormality has been validated in three ways. First, the clear association between receptor over-expression, adverse tumor features, and poor clinical prognosis; second, confirmation that amplified *neu* has both predictive and prognostic significance; and third, development of a sophisticated technique that could reliably assess *HER2* oncogene amplification (Wolff *et al.*, 2007). And now, more than two decades later, accumulated knowledge resulted in two additional noteworthy observations. One, and arguably the most important, identification of the receptor provided an enterprising stimulus towards developing inhibitors that specifically target the receptor (Slamon *et al.*, 2001); and two, incorporation of *HER2* and other associated genes into a genomic complex used to identify patients most likely to benefit from administration of adjuvant chemotherapy (Paik *et al.*, 2004).

4   *Neu* Generation of Therapies

In September 1998, trastuzumab became the first targeted agent approved for use in patients with HER2-positive breast cancer. Nearly a decade later, lapatinib (in combination with capecitabine) received FDA approval for treatment of HER2-positive disease progressing on trastuzumab. The recent approval of pertuzumab represents the third target-specific agent for *neu*-amplified breast cancer. And based on results of the EMILIA study presented at the 2012 Annual Meeting of the American Society of Clinical Oncology, it is now anticipated that trastuzumab emtansine, a novel antibody-drug conjugate (ADC), will be the fourth approved therapeutic compound. Expanded discussion of these agents, as well as neratinib, is provided below using unofficial-labeled generations. Although arbitrary, separation in this manner helps delineate not only the developmental time course but also the purported mechanisms and differences of the HER2-targeted agents.

4.1   First Generation

4.1.1   Trastuzumab

Marketed as Herceptin™ (Genentech), trastuzumab is a recombinant humanized monoclonal antibody that recognizes and binds with high affinity to an epitope located on the extracellular portion of HER2 (Figure 2). One interesting anomaly relates to the observation that while at least seven endogenous ligands differentially bind HER1, HER3 and HER4, none of these molecules has affinity for HER2. However, the latter finding does not necessarily preclude the presence of naturally occurring HER2-specific ligands. The reason why identification remains elusive could be partly related to the receptor itself. Analysis of the crystal structure of HER2 exposed a pair of clarifying facets about the receptor: 1) the "closed" conformation of monomeric HER2 may hinder binding of any HER-like peptide (Figure 1) (Burgess *et al.*, 2003); and 2) structural defects at the ligand-binding site appear to be the result of un-conserved or altered amino acid residues (Di Fiore *et al.*, 1987). Hence, binding of trastuzumab likely occurs at a location distinct from the receptor's native ligand-binding site.

4.1.2   Clinical Impact

While overall response rates (ORR) of 12% - 26% achieved in early phase 2 studies do not appear to be overwhelmingly positive, it is of note that these disease outcomes were achieved with monotherapy trastuzumab in a cohort of subjects, many of who had received extensive prior treatment (Baselga *et al.*, 1996; Cobleigh *et al.*, 1999; Vogel *et al.*, 2002). Moreover, these percentages were restricted to traditional objective responses and not clinical benefit rate (CBR), an endpoint of most, in not all, studies involving molecular targeted agents. Hence, if patients who achieved stable disease were added to those with complete and partial responses, the CBR would be approximately 50%. It is also conceivable that the use of immunohistochemistry (IHC) to assess HER2 status could have misclassified true receptor positivity. Evidence to support the latter concern is the difference in response rates of 35% *vs.* 0% in patients with 3+ *vs.* 2+ over-expression, respectively (Vogel *et al.*, 2002).

Response rates (RR) were also higher when trastuzumab, either alone (Burstein *et al.*, 2003) or with chemotherapy, is used as first-line therapy. Results of two phase 2 clinical trials compared trastuzumab with or without chemotherapy. One study compared trastuzumab plus docetaxel versus docetaxel alone in 186 patients with HER2-positive (primarily determined by IHC) metastatic breast can-

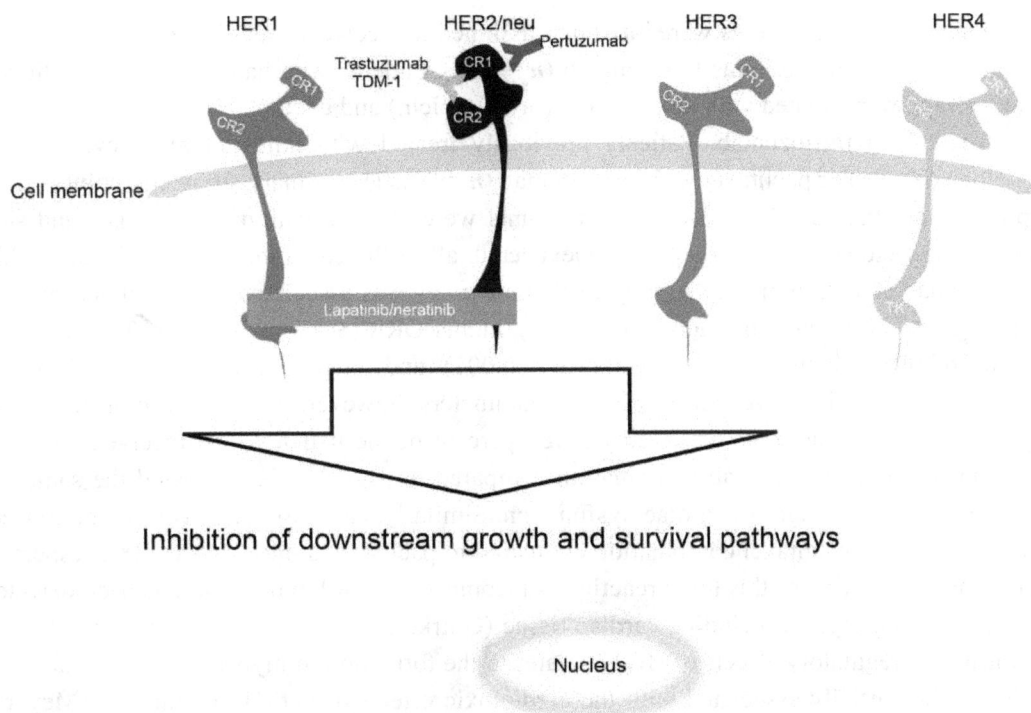

Figure 2: HER2-targeted agents. The monoclonal antibodies bind to a site on the extracelluar domain of the receptor. However, pertuzumab appears to bind to a site distinct from trastuzumab and TDM-1. As such, pertuzumab is able to "sterically" hinder HER2 from dimerizing with other HER family members. This property may result in an additive or synergistic effect when pertuzumab is combined with any other HER2-targeted agent. One feature that distinguishes neratinib from lapatinib is its ability to also inhibit VEGFR-2 and Src.

cer (Marty *et al.*, 2005). Significantly superior outcomes favoring the combination arm were observed in all efficacy parameters including RR (61% *vs.* 34%; $p = 0.0002$), median duration of survival (31.2 *vs.* 22.7 months; $p = 0.0325$), median time to progression (TTP, 11.7 *vs.* 6.1 months; $p = 0.0001$), median time to treatment failure (9.8 *vs.* 5.3 months; $p = 0.0001$), and median duration of response (11.7 *vs.* 5.7 months; $p = 0.009$). With stable disease (SD) observed in 27% of the patients, the CBR for the combination was 88%. Toxicity, primarily related to myelosuppression, was slightly higher among subjects receiving docetaxel plus the antibody. Another study involving 118 assessable patients with advanced, HER2-positive (2+ and 3+ IHC scores) breast cancer evaluated the activity of weekly paclitaxel with or without trastuzumab (Gasparini *et al.*, 2007). Overall response rate, the primary study objective was significantly improved with the addition of trastuzumab (75% *vs.* 56.9%; $p = 0.037$). Moreover, the ORR was even higher with the combination (84.5% *vs.* 47.5%; $p = 0.0005$) in the subset of IHC 3+ patients. This same group of patients also had a significantly longer median TTP (369 *vs.* 272 days; $p = 0.03$). Importantly, multivariable analysis indicated that only IHC score retained statistically significant predictive value for response ($P = 0.0035$). No patients developed grade 4 hematologic toxicity; cardiac toxicity was not observed.

Arguably the most important clinical trial was conducted in women with previously untreated metastatic breast cancer that over-expressed (central laboratory-confirmed 2+ and 3+ by IHC) HER2 (Table

1). Four hundred sixty-nine patients were randomly assigned to receive standard chemotherapy alone (n = 234) or standard chemotherapy plus trastuzumab (n = 235). Patients who had not received adjuvant an-thracycline therapy were treated with doxorubicin (or epirubicin) and cyclophosphamide with (n n = 143) or without (n = 138) trastuzumab. Patients previously treated with adjuvant anthracycline received paclitaxel alone (n = 96) or paclitaxel with trastuzumab (n = 92). The primary study end point was time to disease progression. Pre-specified secondary endpoints were ORR, duration of response, and survival. Data were locked October 1999. Perhaps not unexpected, all of the endpoints favored the arm which in-cluded trastuzumab. Addition of the antibody to chemotherapy was associated with a longer median time to disease progression (7.4 *vs.* 4.6 months; $p < 0.001$), higher ORR (50% *vs.* 32%, $p < 0.001$), longer me-dian duration of response (9.1 *vs.* 6.1 months; $p < 0.001$), and longer median survival (25.1 *vs.* 20.3 months; $p = 0.046$). The improvement in efficacy parameters, however, was achieved at the expense of relatively significant cardiac toxicity. Twenty-seven percent of the patients who received the anthracy-cline/cyclophosphamide/trastuzumab combination compared to 8% of patients treated the same chemo-therapy regimen alone had signs of cardiac dysfunction. Similarly, cardiotoxicity occurred more frequent-ly with the trastuzumab/paclitaxel combination compared to paclitaxel alone, 13% *vs.* 1%, respectively.[16] Although our understanding of this toxic reaction is incomplete, HER2 expression has been detected in a number of developing organs, including cardiac tissue (Quirke *et al.*, 1989). In the myocardium, one of the more intriguing regulatory effects of HER2 relates to the formation of myocardial ventricular trabecu-lae, which may be partially associated with the cardiotoxic effects of anti-HER2 therapy (Meyer *et al.*, 1995).

The beneficial effects of trastuzumab in the advanced disease setting led to the design and conduct of five clinical trials in patients with HER2-positive early breast cancer. Results of the three largest stud-ies with a median follow up of at least 2 years indicated addition of trastuzumab, either to or following adjuvant chemotherapy, was associated with a significant improvement in disease-free survival (DFS), the primary study endpoint (Romond *et al.*, 2005; Piccart-Gebhart *et al.*, 2005; Slamon *et al.*, 2011). In-vestigators of two of the studies also reported findings related to the drug's effect on overall survival (OS). At a median follow up of 65 months In the Breast Cancer International Research Group (BCIRG) 006 study, the overall survival rate for the patients receiving anthracycline- and taxane- based chemother-apy plus trastuzumab compared to the same chemotherapy regimens alone was 92% *vs.* 87%, respectively (hazard ratio [HR], 0.63; $p < 0.001$) (Slamon *et al.*, 2011). Similarly, analysis of OS performed on an in-tent-to-treat basis in the Herceptin Adjuvant (HERA) study indicated a 34% lower risk of death with trastuzumab compared with observation alone (unadjusted HR, 0.66; 95% CI, 0.47 to 0.91; $p = 0.0115$) after a median follow-up of 2 years (Table 1). Of equal importance was the lower incidence of cardiac toxicity observed in all three studies, a finding most likely attributable to the avoidance of concomitant administration of trastuzumab and an anthracycline (Smith *et al.*, 2007).

A number of phase 2 clinical trials have also been conducted to evaluate the impact of adding trastuzumab to chemotherapy when used in the pre-operative (i.e. neo-adjuvant) setting (Bines *et al.*, 2003; Tripathy *et al.*, 2007; Coudert *et al.*, 2007; Burstein *et al.*, 2003). The primary endpoint in most, if not all, of the studies was pathological complete response (pCR), which appears to be a reliable predictor of survival. And in spite of the small numbers of subjects enrolled, the reported pCR ranged between 14% and 52%, higher than previous reports in HER2-unselected patients. Two randomized phase 3 clini-cal studies also demonstrated significantly higher pCR among patients who had trastuzumab added to their chemotherapy regimen. In one of the studies, the difference in pCR so substantially favored the trastuzumab arm (65% *vs.* 26%, $p = 0.016$) that the study was stopped with only 25% of the pre-

Design	Treatment schema	Primary outcomes
Phase 3, randomized study involving 469 patients with previously untreated metastatic HER2- positive (2+ or 3+ by IHC) breast cancer[16]	"AC" = doxorubicin, 60 mg/m^2 + cyclophosphamide, 600 mg/m^2) + trastuzumab ($n = 107$) "EC" = epirubicin, 75 mg/m^2 + cyclophosphamide, 600 mg/m^2) + trastuzumab ($n = 36$) AC/EC alone ($n = 138$) or Paclitaxel, 175 mg/m^2 + trastuzumab ($n = 92$) or Paclitaxel alone ($n = 96$)	1^0 end points a. time to disease progression significantly favored addition of trastuzumab ($p < 0.001$) b. adverse events: cardiac dysfunction occurred more frequently in the trastuzumab-added groups 2^0 end points (significantly favored addition of trastuzumab) a. objective response rate ($p < 0.001$) b. duration of response ($p < 0.001$) c. death rate at 1 year ($p = 0.008$) d. overall survival ($p = 0.046$)
Phase 3, open-label, randomized study involving 5,081 women with early-stage HER2-positive (IHC 3+ and FISH-positive) breast cancer[28] Note: randomization to trastuzumab performed after loco-regional therapy and a minimum of four courses of adjuvant, neo-adjuvant, or both adjuvant and neo-adjuvant therapy.	Stratification based on world region, age, nodal status, hormone-recetor status, and type of chemotherapy, then randomized to one of 3 groups a. trastuzumab for 1 year, b. trastuzumab for 2 years c. observation only	1^0 end point (results relate to one year treatment with trastuzumab or observation) a. disease-free survival favored trastuzumab ($p<0.0001$) 2^0 end points a. overall survival (p=NS). b. cardiac safety (severe cardiotoxicity occurred in <1% of patients receiving trastuzumab)
Open-label randomized study with planned enrollment of 528 subject with HER2-positive metastatic breast cancer progressing on trastuzumab-based therapy[42]	Assignment performed in a 1:1 ratio to: a. lapatinib, 1250 mg daily on a continuous basis + capecitabine, 2000 mg/m^2 in two divided doses, days 1-14 of a 21-day cycle or b. capecitabine, 2500 mg/m^2 in two divided doses, days 1-14 of a 21-day cycle	1^0 end point (specified criteria for early reporting of the data was based on superiority in the combination arm) a. time to progression favored lapatinib containing regimen ($p<0.001$)
Phase 3, randomized double-blind study involving 808 treatment-naïve subjects with advanced HER2-positive breast cancer[70]	Randomization to one of 2 groups a. trastuzumab + docetaxel + pertuzumab or b. trastuzumab + docetaxel	1^0 end point a. progression-free survival favored the pertuzumab-containing regimen ($p < 0.001$) 2^0 end points (interim analysis) a. overall survival indicated a trend in favor of the pertuzumab-containing regimen. b. safety profile (grade $\geq$3 febrile neutropenia and diarrhea higher in the pertuzumab-containing regimen)

| Phase 3, randomized study of second-line therapy involving 978 treated patients with disease progressing on trastuzumab-based therapy[78] | Randomization to one of 2 groups
a. TDM-1, or
b. lapatinib + capecitabine | 1^0 endpoints(analysis performed at median duration of follow up ~12.5 months)
a. PFS favored T-DM1 ($p<0.0001$)
b. median overall survival not reached in TDM-1 group ($p=0.0005$);
c. safety (no unexpected issues; thrombocytopenia, increased AST and ALT in TDM-1 group) |

Table 1: Selected clinical trials of HER2-targeted agents

established population enrolled (Buzdar *et al.*, 2007). Interim analysis of the other study showed a near doubling of the pCR in patients who received trastuzumab (43% *vs.* 23%, p = 0.002) (Gianni *et al.*, 2007).

The antibody's substantial impact notwithstanding, it is sobering to note that trastuzumab resistance develops in all patients treated in the metastatic setting; disease relapse also occurs with adjuvant trastuzumab; and the antibody is inactive in some tumors despite HER2-positivity. All of these findings emphasize the need for alternative treatment options for patients with disease progressing on, or refractory to, trastuzumab. This concern is extremely important because of the inference that HER2 remains a viable target despite the apparent loss of antibody activity. The latter belief is supported by evidence showing that continuation of trastuzumab with different chemotherapy in patients whose breast cancers progressed during treatment resulted in longer median TTP compared to chemotherapy alone, 8,2 *vs.* 5.6 months, respectively (HR, 0.69; 95% CI, 0.48 to 0.97; p = 0.0338) (von Minckwitz *et al.*, 2009). Overall response rates in the same two groups were 48.1% and 27.0% (odds ratio, 2.50; p = 0.0115), respectively. These data suggest that tumor resistance to prior trastuzumab-chemotherapy regimens is not necessarily due to HER2-mediated mechanisms alone. Although these outcomes were statistically and clinically significant, trastuzumab failure was the major stimulus for developing other agents that could target the receptor.

4.2   Second Generation

4.2.1   Lapatinib

Tykerb[TM], GLAXOSMITHKLINE is a potent, reversible, small molecule inhibitor of HER1 and HER2 (Figure 2). Structured crystal analysis of the lapatinib/HER1 complex revealed that lapatinib dissociates much slower from the receptor compared to erlotinib, which correlates with the prolonged time tyrosine phosphorylation in down-regulated in tumor cells (Wood *et al.*, 2004). Similar crystallographic and stoichimetric studies of lapatinib's interaction with HER2 have not been published, though substantial evidence indicate that receptor phosphorylation is similarly depressed (Xia *et al.*, 2004).

Limited data from a phase I study are available which show a relationship between serum concentration and anti-tumor activity (Burris *et al.*, 2005). Four of the 67 heavily pretreated subjects achieved a partial response (PRs). All of the responding patients had breast cancers that over-expressed HER2. Tumor responses appeared to correlate with median daily lapatinib dosages of 1200 mg and C_{min} serum concentration between 0.3 ug/mL - 0.6 ug/mL. These values also correspond to the inhibitory effect on HER1 and HER2 kinase activity *in-vitro* (Burris, 2004). Interestingly, the incidence and severity of diarrhea and rash, the most frequently reported side effects, did not correlate with trough drug concentrations.

4.2.2   Clinical Impact

Lapatinib was the first new drug to demonstrate significant clinical benefits in patients with HER2-positive, advanced breast cancer progressing on trastuzumab. The results of a pivotal phase III clinical trial involving women with advanced, HER2-positive, trastuzumab- and chemotherapy-refractory breast cancer, have been published (Table 1) (Geyer *et al.*, 2006). It is important to note that the study was terminated early when a pre-planned interim analysis performed by an independent data monitoring committee showed a significant benefit for subjects randomized to the lapatinib arm. At that time, 324 patients had been randomized (1:1) to capecitabine plus lapatinib (163) or capecitabine alone (161). On the basis of 121 events, 49 in the combination and 72 in the monotherapy groups, median TTP was nearly twice as long among patients receiving the lapatinib-containing regimen compared to capecitabine alone, 8.4 months and 4.4 months, respectively, $p < 0.001$. Progression-free survival was also improved in the group treated with the two agents (HR, 0.47; 95% CI, 0.33 to 0.67; $p < 0.001$). Equally noteworthy was the observation that the development of brain metastasis was lower with the lapatinib-containing regimen compared to capecitabine alone, 2 versus 11 cases, respectively, $p = 0.0445$. An update of the data continued to show that the addition of lapatinib to capecitabine results in superior efficacy compared to capecitabine alone (Cameron *et al.*, 2008). Time to tumor progression was increased by 43% (HR, 0.57; 95% CI, 0.43 to 0.77; $p < 0.001$) and the incidence of central nervous system (CNS) involvement was decreased (4 *vs.* 13 cases, $p = 0.045$).

Two salient issues add credence to the results of this clinical trial. First, despite an earlier study (Burris, 2005) of lapatinib which suggested that clinical responses may be higher in breast tumors that co-expressed HER1, the absence of HER1 expression was not an exclusion criterion. Second, the fact that nearly two-thirds of the patients received trastuzumab within the previous eight weeks led to the speculation that a portion of the positive outcomes were related to a synergistic effect between residual amounts of trastuzumab and recently administered lapatinib (Sonpavde, 2007). However, analysis of data in women who received lapatinib and prior trastuzumab (≤ 8 wk versus > 8 wk) indicated that the contribution of residual trastuzumab appeared to be minimal (Geyer *et al.*, 2007).

The issue regarding CNS metastasis deserves further comment. A small, but significant, number of patients (approximately 15%) with advanced breast cancer develop symptomatic brain metastasis (DiStefano *et al.*, 1979). The observation that CNS disease as the site of first relapse occurs more frequently in a subset of patients treated with trastuzumab compared to patients who receive standard chemotherapy alone appears to be a troubling anomaly (Clayton *et al.*, 2004; Bendell *et al.*, 2003). Attempts to reconcile this finding include two plausible reasons. One relates to the demonstrated effectiveness of trastuzumab in that prolongation of survival may also translate to an increased risk of eventually developing cerebral metastasis. Another consideration is the blood-brain barrier may create a sanctuary for tumor cells by restricting or limiting penetration of the large molecular-sized antibody. Hence, it is conceivable that one of the advantages of small molecule inhibitors such as lapatinib may relate to its ability to cross into the CNS and lower the frequency of, or even treat, brain metastasis. Although modest, clinical evidence of the latter effect has been published (Lin *et al.*, 2009).

Few reports of lapatinib as first-line therapy of HER-2 positive breast cancer have been published. One, a randomized, open-label study compared the efficacy and safety of two different lapatinib dosages and administration schedules, 1,500 mg once daily and 500 mg twice daily (Gomez *et al.*, 2008). The ORR was 24% in the intent-to-treat population consisting of 138 subjects; an additional 7% of the patients had stable disease. The median time to response was approximately 8 weeks. The most common lapatinib-related adverse events (AEs), primarily grade 1 or 2) were diarrhea, rash, pruritus, and nausea. There were no apparent differences in either clinical activity or the AE profile between the two arms.

At least three phase III studies of lapatinib in combination with a taxane are ongoing. However, one of the most intriguing clinical trials in progress compares an aromatase inhibitor with or without lapatinib in women with estrogen receptor (ER)-positive tumors regardless of HER2 status (Johnston *et al.*, 2009). The rationale for this clinical trial was based on laboratory findings that bi-directional crosstalk between ER and HER2 could enhance tumor cell proliferation and cell survival (Shou *et al.*, 2004). In this study, 1171 postmenopausal women with ER-positive metastatic breast cancer were randomly assigned to receive daily doses of letrozole (2.5 mg orally) plus lapatinib (1,500 mg orally) or letrozole (same dose) and placebo. Only 19% (n = 219) of the enrolled subjects were also HER2-positive. The primary end point was progression-free survival (PFS). Among the cohort of women who had hormone and HER2 receptor-positive tumors, the combination of agents was associated with a 29% reduction in risk of disease progression compared to those receiving the placebo, (HR, 0.71; 95% CI, 0.53 to 0.96; p = 0.019); median PFS was 8.2 *vs.* 3 months, respectively. Clinical benefit rate (complete response [CR} + partial response [PR] + SD $\geq$ 6 months) was also significantly greater for lapatinib-letrozole versus letrozole-placebo (48% *vs.* 29%, respectively; p = 0.003). Arguably, the relative importance of the two receptors relates not only to the superior disease-related outcomes achieved with combination therapy (which could have been anticipated) but also their presence provided biological targeted-proof of principle.

Perhaps, and not without regard for HER1, targeting the intracellular HER2 kinase domain has been an effective therapeutic option for patient with disease progressing on trastuzumab (Geyer *et al.*, 2006; Stein *et al.*, 2005). More intriguing, however, is whether trastuzumab and lapatinib, each poised at two different HER2 domains, are better than either agent given alone. This is an important question as mechanistic differences between the two classes of drugs could have significant clinical implications. Therefore, an opportunity exists to assess whether targeting HER2 from the "outside" and "inside" concurrently has additive or perhaps even synergistic activity in patients with HER2-overexpressing breast cancers. One small study was designed to test this hypothesis (Blackwell *et al.*, 2010). Two hundred ninety-six subjects with HER2-positive metastatic breast cancer with disease progression on prior trastuzumab therapy were randomly assigned to receive either lapatinib alone or in combination with trastuzumab. The primary end point was PFS; secondary end points included CBR and OS. Results in the intention-to-treat population indicated a superior PFS with the combination of lapatinib and trastuzumab compared to lapatinib alone, (HR, 0.73; 95% CI, 0.57 to 0.93; p = 0.008); CBR 24.7% and 12.4% in the same two arms, respectively; p = 0.01; and a trend towards improved OS with combination therapy. The incidence of diarrhea, one of the most frequent AEs, was higher in the combination arm (p = 0.03). Symptomatic and asymptomatic cardiac events with the combination were 2% and 3.4%, respectively; the incidence of similar cardiac events with lapatinib alone was 0.7% and 1.4%.

A common practice in oncology is to conduct clinical trials of an agent with demonstrated activity in the advanced-disease setting in patients with early-stage disease. Because the primary endpoint or goal of therapy in the latter is cure, an important consideration is the potential impact of a drug's adverse effect profile. In contrast to most adjuvant therapy which is usually of short duration (i.e., $\leq$ 6 months), adjuvant anti-HER2 therapy has been investigated as long as 24 months. Thus, the development of toxicities such as congestive cardiomyopathy becomes an important consideration. There is some evidence that lapatinib alone does not confer a high risk of developing heart failure. Analysis of cardiac function in a large cohort of patients (n = 3,558) treated with lapatinib either as monotherapy or in combination with cytotoxic agents indicated an incidence of 1.6% with confirmed decreases in left ventricular ejection fraction (LVEF) (Perez *et al.*, 2006). However, only seven of the 58 patients (0.2%) were symptomatic. However, the answer related to this issue is not absolute as the possibility of selection bias and the relatively short observation period could impact future outcomes. While cardiac monitoring is mandatory in patients receiving lapatinib, it is also important to note that asymptomatic decreases in LVEF have been reported to be two to four fold higher than in the general population (Kannel, 2000).

A phase III clinical trial called Adjuvant Lapatinib and/or Trastuzumab Treatment Optimization (ALTTO) was conducted to evaluate the comparative effectiveness of lapatinib against trastuzumab in patients with HER2-overexpressing early breast cancer. In order to meet the primary endpoints of OS and TTP, investigators planned to enroll approximately 8,400 women who would be followed for 10 years after randomization. Essentially non-inferiority in design, the trial investigated four treatment arms following surgery: 1) trastuzumab for one year, 2) lapatinib for one year, 3) both agents for one year, or 4) trastuzumab for 12 weeks, followed sequentially by a six week therapy-free period, then lapatinib for 34 weeks. Begun in June of 2007, the accrual goal was met in July 2011. Because early analysis of data indicated that lapatinib was not expected to meet the criterion of non-inferiority, the lapatinib monotherapy arm was closed. As such, trastuzumab remains the only HER2-targeted agent approved for use in the adjuvant setting.

A companion study known as NeoALTTO was conducted between January 2008 and May 2010 to test the hypothesis that same two anti-HER2 agents given concurrently would be better than single-agent therapy (ClinicalTrials.gov, NCT00553358.) This randomized, open-label, phase 3 study involved approximately 450 women with HER2-positive primary breast cancer with tumours exceeding 2 cm. Subjects were randomly assigned to monotherapy lapatinib or trastuzumab, or the combination. Neoadjuvant anti-HER2 therapy was given for the first 6 weeks; weekly paclitaxel was then added to the regimen for an additional 12 weeks followed by definitive surgery. After surgery, patients received adjuvant chemotherapy followed by the same targeted therapy as in the neo-adjuvant phase to complete one year of treatment. The primary endpoint was the rate of pCR. The results indicated that the pCR rate was significantly higher in the group treated with both agents (51.3%; 95% CI, 43.1 to 59.5]) than the groups given trastuzumab alone (29.5%; 95% CI, 22.4 to 37.5) or lapatinib alone (24.7%; 95% CI, 18.1 to 32.3); $p =$ 0.0001. No major cardiac events were observed. Again, the frequency of grade 3 diarrhea was higher with lapatinib, either alone (23·4%) or in combination with trastuzumab (21.1%) compared to trastuzumab alone (2.0%).

The approval of lapatinib for the treatment of trastuzumab-resistant advanced breast cancer can be viewed as a substantial therapeutic advance. In some respects, results of the randomized phase III study strengthen this perception as lapatinib in combination with capecitabine significantly reduced the risk of disease progression and improved the overall response rates. Furthermore, the addition of lapatinib to chemotherapy was not related to increases in rates of adverse events or withdrawal due to serious toxicity. Another perspective is that the dual kinase inhibitor may not be superior to the humanized antibody as results of the ALTTO trial indicate. However, these observations should not be inferred that there is little or nothing to be gained by inhibiting HER1 in breast cancer. Although the somewhat disappointing outcomes may be related to antagonistic pharmacologic and/or molecular mechanisms, the findings indirectly raise the question of how much of lapatinib's effect can be attributed to inhibition of HER1.

4.2.3 Neratinib

While some may argue that neratinib should not be considered a second generation HER2 antagonist, it is discussed here because of some features it shares with lapatinib. Not yet approved by the FDA, this tyrosine kinase inhibitor has a broader spectrum of inhibitory activity than lapatinib. When tested, neratinib inhibited HER1 and HER2, and to a lesser extent, vascular endothelial growth factor receptor (VEGFR)-2 and Src (Figure 2) (Rabindran, 2004). What likely contributes to the greater potency of this small molecule compared to lapatinib is a chemical modification known as the Michael addition, which results in irreversible binding and thus, inhibition of the receptors (Mather *et al.*, 2006; Yun *et al.*, 2008). Preclinical data also suggest that neratinib can overcome resistance that HER1 acquires after initially responding to either gefitinib or erlotinib treatment.[59] Results of a phase I trial involving patients with metastatic HER1- or HER2-positive cancers that had failed standard therapy were recently published (Wong *et al.*, 2009). Dose-limiting diarrhea occurred at 400 mg given once daily; constitutional symptoms such as fatigue and asthenia were also observed frequently. Notably, PRs were achieved in 8 (32%) of 25 evaluable patients with breast cancer.

4.2.4 Clinical Impact

Preliminary results of efficacy and safety have also been reported from three clinical trials. The first, a two part phase 1/2 open-label study was conducted to evaluate the combination of neratinib and paclitaxel (Chow *et al.*, 2009). Part 1 was designed to assess the safety of neratinib at 160 mg or 240 mg daily when given with weekly paclitaxel in patients with advanced solid tumors. The second part of the study evaluated the ORR of the combination at their maximum tolerated doses in patients with HER2-positive metastatic breast cancer. Of the 99 evaluable patients enrolled in part 2 (and based on investigator assessment), 68 (69%) patients achieved an objective response (5 CRs; 63 PRs). Interestingly, the percent of patients achieving either a CR or PR was nearly identical regardless if it was given as first-line or second-line therapy. Thirteen additional patients had SD ≥ 24 weeks as their best outcome. Only six patients developed progressive disease (PD). Of the 28 patients who received prior trastuzumab and the 14 patients previously treated with lapatinib, 18 (64%) and 10 (71%), respectively, achieved an objective response. Median PFS for all patients with HER2-positive breast cancer was approximately 52 weeks (95% CI, 47.7 to NE). The confidence interval can be interpreted to mean that while the lower boundary represents a median PFS of 47.7 weeks, the upper boundary is non-estimable (i.e., NE). The probable explanation for the NE status is likely because many of the patients have not yet "progressed".

The results of a second phase 1/2 trial have recently been reported (Awada *et al.*, 2009). Similar in design to the previous study, neratinib was given concomitantly with vinorelbine to 34 patients with advanced HER2-positive breast cancer, all of who received prior trastuzumab and taxane therapy. Twenty-two patients were also treated previously with an anthracycline. At the time of their report, 18 patients were evaluable, 4 of who received prior trastuzumab and lapatinib. Although there were no CRs, seven (68%) patients achieved at least a PR; SD ≥ 24 weeks was observed in three additional patients. The third study included 136 women with locally advanced (stage IIIB and IIIC) and metastatic HER2-positive breast cancer (Burstein *et al.* 2010). This phase 2 study was designed to evaluate neratinib as a single agent. The study's primary end point was 16-week PFS rate; secondary end points included safety, ORR, and CBR. Based on prior trastuzumab therapy, two study arms were created; arm A included patients who received at least 6 weeks of prior trastuzumab therapy while arm B consisted of patients who never received treatment with any HER2-targeted agent. Of the 136 patients, 127 were included in the efficacy analysis; 63 in arm A and 64 in arm B. The median 16-week PFS rates in arm A and arm B were 59% and 78%, respectively; the median PFS times were 22.3 weeks and 39.6 weeks, respectively. Stable disease ≥ 24 weeks was observed 6 and 8 patients in Arms A and B, respectively. The ORR and CBR were 24% (all PRs) and 33% compared to 56% (one of which was a CR) and 69% in the two respective arms.

Accumulated clinical data indicate that diarrhea is the most frequently occurring toxicity associated with neratinib therapy. Although nearly all patients develop this adverse effect, up to 25% of the patients may have grade ≥ 3 diarrhea. Interestingly, while this toxic reaction usually occurs early (median onset of 3 days) in patients treated with single agent neratinib, the frequency and severity of this toxicity appears to decrease with increasing duration of therapy (Burstein *et al.*, 2010). Neratinib-induced diarrhea can be managed with standard supportive therapy; in some instances dose interruptions and/or reductions may have to be implemented. The low incidence of cardiac toxicity suggests that small molecule inhibitors of the HER2 tyrosine kinase may be relatively safer than antibodies. Nevertheless, the cardiac safety profile for neratinib must be regarded as preliminary.

4.3   Third Generation

4.3.1   Pertuzumab

Pharmacologically, pertuzumab (Perjeta^{TM}, Genentech, a member of the Roche Group) is a humanized monoclonal antibody that also recognizes and binds HER2, but at a site distinct from trastuzumab (Figure 2). This notion is supported by structural evidence showing that contact between extracellular domains I and III (i.e., the principal HER ligand-binding site) produces an "extended conformation" of the receptor, which limits ligand access (Figure 1) (Burgess *et al.*, 2003). This peculiar conformational status may also explain why HER2 is the preferential dimeric partner for all other family members (Graus-Porta *et al.*, 1997). Although both pertuzumab and trastuzumab are monoclonal antibodies that inhibit HER2-mediated signaling, a number of notable differences do exist. First, each agent recognizes discrete extracellular epitopes (Cho *et al.*, 2003), a finding that could have important therapeutic ramifications. Second, the unique binding site of pertuzumab induces structural aberrations that sterically prevent the process of homo- and hetero-dimerization. In effect, pertuzumab could inhibit HER2 signaling initiated by ligand-actived HER1 or HER3 and thus provide even greater inhibition of HER2 than trastuzumab (Agus *et al.*, 2002). Notable also is the finding that the Fab fragment of pertuzumab is just as effective as the intact antibody in blocking HER2 signaling. This finding has two possible implications: 1) inhibitory effect not mediated solely by an antibody-dependent cell-mediated cytotoxicity mechanism and 2) potential activity in breast tumors that do not over-express HER2 or signaling driven by the HER2 dimeric partner.

4.3.2   Clinical Impact

Based on their unique binding sites, as well as preclinical data showing enhanced activity with combined antibody therapy (Scheuer *et al.*, 2009), a phase II clinical trial was performed to assess the effectiveness of the pertuzumab/trastuzumab doublet in patients with advanced HER2-positive breast cancer progressing on prior trastuzumab therapy (Baselga *et al.*, 2010). In this single arm study, women with HER2 over-expressing metastatic breast cancer were treated with standard weekly or three-weekly doses of trastuzumab plus pertuzumab, 420 mg every three weeks following an 840 mg loading dose. The primary endpoints were RR and CBR. The first eight cycles constituted the main treatment period with tumor assessment occurring prior to cycles 3, 5, 7, and 9. For those who continued therapy, response status was evaluated every three months thereafter. Treatment was continued until disease progression or unacceptable toxicity. The most important secondary endpoint was safety, especially cardiac events. Despite the relatively long median duration of prior trastuzumab therapy (i.e., 16.2 months) among the 66 patients enrolled in the study, the ORR was 24.2% (5 CRs and 11 PRs); the CBR was 50%. Of note, some patients exhibited delayed tumor responses as several patients with SD eventually achieved an objective response. Furthermore, clinical benefit appeared to be quite durable with median PFS of approximately 5½ months.

Because of the purported regulatory role of HER2 in the development of cardiac myocytes, myocardial function was evaluated after cycles 1, 2, 4, 6, and 8. Based on predetermined criteria, three patients had evidence of cardiac dysfunction although none were symptomatic. Left ventricular ejection function returned to normal in two patients, even though cancer therapy was not interrupted. The third patient withdrew from the study because of disease progression. Overall, the mean LVEF remained stable during the first eight cycles. The most frequently reported adverse effect was diarrhea which occurred in 64% of the patients; however, this toxic reaction was classified as grade 3 and 4 in only two patients.

Results of another phase II clinical trial of pertuzumab were recently reported (Gianni *et al.*, 2010). The study was restricted to patients with metastatic, HER2-negative breast cancer, who received no more than two prior anthracycline-containing chemotherapy regimens. Maximum cumulative doses of doxorubicin and epirubicin could not exceed 360 mg/m^2 and 720 mg/m^2, respectively; prior therapy with any agent targeting HER2 was also an exclusion criterion. Patients were randomly assigned to receive either 420 mg (following an 840 mg loading dose, Arm A) or 1,050 mg (Arm B) every three weeks. The primary objective was response rate as determined by RECIST (Response Evaluation Criteria in Solid Tumors) and safety. The study also investigated the role of predictive tumor biomarkers and the pharmacokinetics of the antibody. Of the 78 evaluable patients only two achieved a PR, while four others had SD $\geq$ 24 weeks as their best outcomes. Although previously treated and HER2-negative by FISH (fluorescent in situ hybridization), 74 (95%) of the patients had low level expression (i.e., 1+ or 2+) of HER2 by IHC. Hence, these data do not support the notion that pertuzumab would be active in breast tumors that do not over-express HER2. Diarrhea, rash, and fatigue were the most common drug-related adverse events observed. Cardio-toxic events occurred in eight patients, all of who experienced $\geq$ 10% decreases in LVEF. Although most of the cardiac events were asymptomatic, one patient developed congestive heart failure and was removed from the study. Another patient developed syncope, shortness of breath and loss of consciousness, all of which were transient. Upon resolution, treatment was continued.

The results of a double-blind, randomized, placebo-controlled phase III clinical trial (CLEOPATRA) was recently published (Table 1) (Baselga *et al.*, 2012). The acronym, CLEOPATRA, is derived from CLinical Evaluation Of Pertuzumab And TRAstuzumab. This study involved 808 patients with HER2-positive metastatic breast cancer who were randomized to receive the combination of trastuzumab plus docetaxel without (control arm) or with pertuzumab (experimental arm) until disease progression or the development of toxicity that could not be effectively managed. The primary end point was an independent assessment of PFS. Secondary end points included OS, investigator-assessed PFS, RR, and safety. The median PFS in the control and experimental arms were 12.4 months and 18.5 months, respectively (HR, 0.62%; 95% CI, 0.51 to 0.75; $p < 0.001$); interim analysis of OS indicated a trend in favor of the pertuzumab-containing regimen. The safety profile was generally similar in the two groups, with no increase in left ventricular systolic dysfunction. However, the rates of grade $\geq$ 3 febrile neutropenia and diarrhea were higher in the pertuzumab group compared to the control group.

Based on these findings, the Food and Drug Administration (FDA) approved pertuzumab in June of 2012 for clinical use in combination with trastuzumab and docetaxel for treatment-naïve patients with HER2-positive metastatic breast cancer.

4.4   Fourth Generation

4.4.1   Trastuzumab-DM1

One of the most significant limitations of cytotoxic chemotherapy is the lack of tumor selectivity. As such, chemotherapy doses have traditionally been determined by what is deemed to be "tolerable" toxicity to normal cells. Coupling target specificity with the observation that trastuzumab's modest anti-tumor effect was substantially improved by the addition of chemotherapy led to the idea that antibodies could be used to deliver chemotherapy rather selectively to tumor cells. However, the efficacy of antibody-chemotherapy (drug) conjugates (ADCs) has historically been limited by variable expression of the target antigen, defective tumor cell uptake mechanisms, and unwieldy linkers used in the conjugation process.

A novel therapeutic entity known as trastuzumab-DM1 (T-DM1, ImmunoGen, Genentech, and Roche) has been developed that appears to have resolved all of the above issues (Figure 2). For example, maytansine (Remillard *et al.*, 1975), a natural product derived from the Ethiopian shrub *Maytenus serrata,* is a potent anti-microtubule agent (Bhattacharyya & Wolff, 1977). However, significant neurological and gastrointestinal toxicities observed in clinical trials of the agent precluded further testing in humans (Eagan *et al.*, 1978); In order to improve the therapeutic index, it was hypothesized that targeted delivery of maytansine could reduce, or even prevent, some drug-associated toxicities. Because HER2 is over-expressed in approximately 20% of breast cancers, trastuzumab was identified as a reasonable vehicle for drug delivery. To achieve this, a maytansine derivative (i.e., emtansine, DM1) was synthesized. The resulting maytansinoid was configured to have an easily cleavable methyl disulfide "handle" linked to trastuzumab (Chari *et al.*, 1992). Notable also, DM1 was shown to be up to 10-fold more potent than the parent compound. Hence, T-DM1 has the potential not only of retaining the anti-tumor properties of the individual agents but also maintaining a tolerable side effect profile.

Investigators of a dose-finding phase I study reported dose-limiting thrombocytopenia occurred at 4.8 mg/kg (given every three weeks) (Krop *et al.*, 2010). Platelet nadirs were observed approximately a week after drug administration with recovery occurring seven days later. None of the patients had clinically significant bleeding. No other grade 4 adverse event and no cardiac-specific toxicity have been observed. Other frequently occurring side effects included liver function test abnormalities, fatigue, nausea and anemia. However, none of these adverse events were greater than grade 2. Although not an efficacy study, the clinical benefit rate, which included five objective responses, was 73% among 15 patients treated at 3.6 mg/kg, the maximum tolerated dose.

4.4.2   Clinical Impact

Two phase 2 studies have been conducted in women with HER2-positive metastatic breast cancer progressing on previous HER2-therapy and chemotherapy. All patients were treated with T-DM1 at a dose of 3.6 mg/kg once every three weeks. Even though the median follow-up period of the first study only slightly exceeded four months, image-confirmed objective responses (CRs and PRs) were achieved in 29 of 108 evaluable patients; the median PFS was 4.6 months. Notably, 24% of 66 subjects who received prior therapy with both trastuzumab and lapatinib achieved an objective response (Vogel *et al.*, 2009). Preliminary results of another phase 2 study were presented at the 2009 San Antonio Breast Cancer Symposium (Krop *et al.*, 2009). The study included 110 patients, 109 of who had received prior anthracycline, taxane, capecitabine, trastuzumab and lapatinib, with disease progressing on the last treatment regimen. The median duration of prior trastuzumab therapy for metastatic disease was 19.4 months; and 6.9 months for lapatinib. The primary endpoint was ORR assessed by independent review. Median follow-up was 8.3 months (range 0.7–13.1). Thirty-six (32.7%) of the enrolled patients achieved a PR as their best tumor outcome; disease stabilization occurred in 51 additional patients; the CBR was 44.5%. The major reason for discontinuation of therapy was disease progression.

The most encouraging results emanated from a phase 3 clinical trial known as EMILIA which compared T-DM1 against the combination of lapatinib plus capecitabine as second-line therapy for patients with HER2-positive breast cancer progressing on trastuzumab and a taxane (Table 1) (Blackwell *et al.*, 2012). T-DM1 was given at 3.6 mg/kg once every three weeks or capecitabine, 1000 mg/m^2 twice daily for 14 days every three weeks plus lapatinib, 1,250 mg daily until disease progression or unmanageable toxicity. Primary end points were PFS (by independent review), OS and tolerability. A total of 991 patients were enrolled, 978 of who received assigned treatment. Median duration of follow-up was approximately one year. Compared to the capecitabine/lapatinib, TDM-1 reduced the risk of disease progression or death by 35% (6.4 mo *vs.* 9.6 mo; HR, 0.650 [95% CI, 0.549 to 0.771]; $p < 0.0001$). Median OS for patients in the TDM-1 arm was not reached at the time the date were analyzed compared to 23.3 months for the combination arm (HR, 0.621; 95% CI, 0.475 to 0.813; $p = 0.0005$). The most common grade $\geq$ 3 AEs which were higher in the TDM-1 arm included thrombocytopenia (12.9% *vs.* 0.2%), increased AST (4.3% *vs.* 0.8%), and increased ALT (2.9% *vs.* 1.4%) while diarrhea (20.7% *vs.* 1.6%), hand-foot syndrome (16.4% *vs.* 0) and vomiting (4.5% *vs.* 0.8%) occurred more frequently in those receiving capecitabine/lapatinib.

Two other studies are worthy of mention. Having met their accrual goal, results of a phase 2 trial involving patients who have not received any treatment of advanced HER2-positive disease were reported in 2011 (Hurvitz *et al.*, 2011). Designed to evaluate the efficacy and safety of T-DM1 versus a standard combination of trastuzumab and docetaxel, median PFS was significantly longer with TDM-1 compared to standard therapy, 14.2 months and 9.2 months, respectively; $p = 0.0353$. Equally important was the finding that grade $\geq$ 3 AEs occurred in 89% and 32% of the patients in the standard treatment and TDM-1 arms, respectively. A third clinical trial of note is an ongoing multi-national, three-arm, phase 3 study designed to evaluate the combination of TDM-1 with or without pertuzumab and trastuzumab/taxane combination as first-line therapy for metastatic breast cancer. The primary endpoint is PFS; secondary endpoints include safety, ORR, OS, duration of response, and quality of life. Enrollment began in July 2010; the accrual goal is 1092 patients. An independent Data Monitoring Committee which assessed safety data recently recommended continuation of the study without modification. The results are highly anticipated.

5   *Neu* Resistance

Despite accumulating published data, it is humbling to note that only a small portion of the receptor's complete biology is apparently known. What appears certain is the eventual development of tumor resistance. This conclusion is supported by the observation that nearly all patients with HER2-positive metastatic breast cancer become refractory, usually within 12 months after initially responding to trastuzumab (Montemurro *et al.*, 2006). The finding that most of the patients (with tumors resistant to trastuzumab) exhibit disease progression after six months of treatment with lapatinib indicates that resistance also develops against small molecule inhibitors; and possibly by a mechanism distinct from trastuzumab. Even when used in the adjuvant setting, disease relapse has occurred following antibody therapy (Romond *et al.*, 2005; Piccart-Gebhart *et al.*, 2005). This lack of understanding undermines our ability to explain why anti-HER2 therapy is not effective in all tumors that over-express the receptor or to apply strategies that overcome, prevent, or delay the development of resistance.

Elucidating the mechanistic basis of HER2-resistance is speculative at best and made even more difficult because the receptor is, arguably, the most enigmatic member of the ErbB family. Although over-expression of HER2 results in formation of constitutively active homodimers (Di Fiore *et al.*, 1987), it is conceivable that the pathologic significance and the development of resistance are due, in part, to HER2's dimeric partner (Figure 3) (Graus-Porta *et al.*, 1997). For example, it has been shown that the dimerization partner and its activating ligand play essential roles in determining not only which receptor sites are phosphorylated, but also which downstream proteins are recruited (Olayioye *et al.*, 1998). These data provide a possible explanation why neither monomeric HER2 (ligand-less) nor HER3 (kinase-impaired) can support linear signaling alone, yet the combination appears to possess the most potent mitogenic properties (Alimandi *et al.*, 1995). Similarly, tumorigenic signals emanating from the HER1/HER2 heterodimer are stronger compared to either homodimer alone (Kokai *et al.*, 1989). Based on these findings, it is rational to develop and test agents which block signaling through HER1, HER2, and HER3; the contribution of HER4 to the tumorigenic process is less well appreciated.

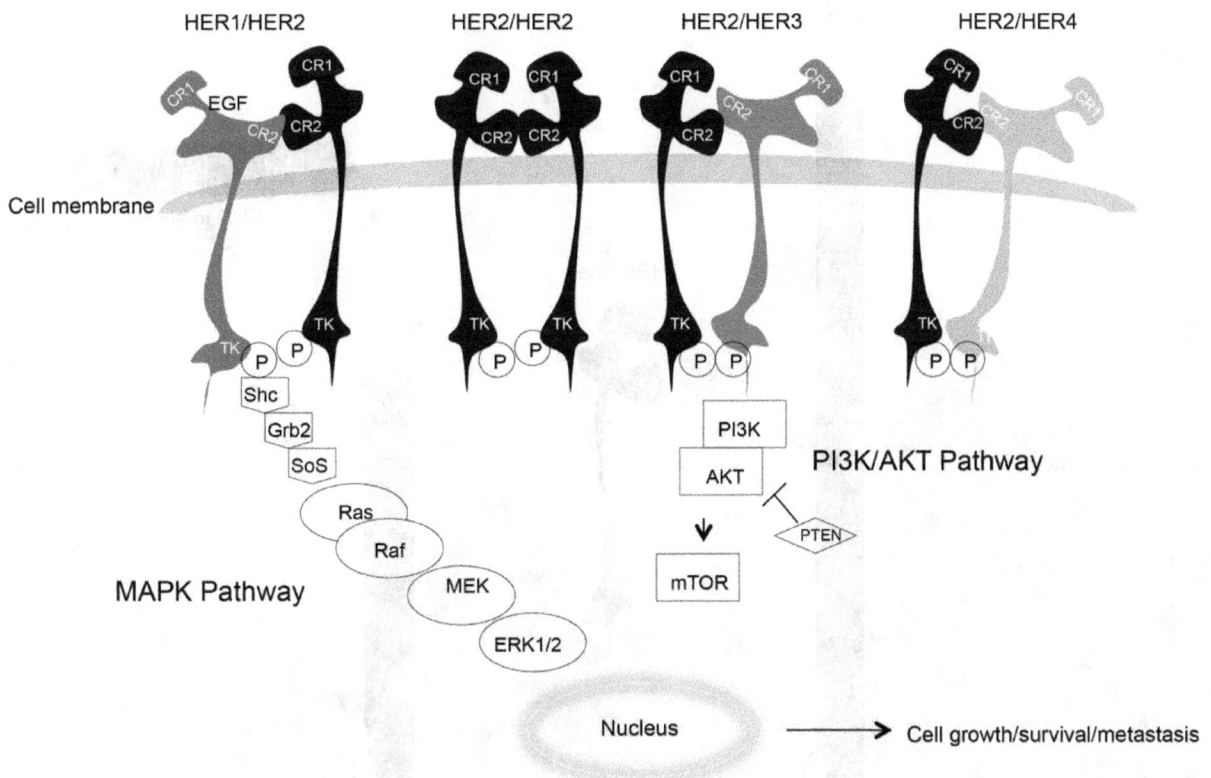

Figure 3: HER2 signaling pathways. HER2 is the preferential partner in four possible dimers. EGF (epidermal growth factor)-bound HER1 can form a heterodimer with HER2. As a result, the MAPK (mitogen-activated protein kinase) pathway can be activated. Ras is engaged following recruitment of Shc and Grb2 (growth-factor receptor bound protein 2. Grb2 forms a complex with son of sevenless (SoS). Downstream of Ras include soluble Raf, MEK (mitogen activated protein kinase kinase), and ERK (extracellular signal-regulated kinase). The HER2 homodimer is constitutively activated. HER3 preferentially signals through the PI3K (phosphatidylinositol 3 kinase) survival pathway. Akt blocks cell death by inhibiting pro-apoptotic proteins or up-regulating anti-apoptotic proteins. Akt can also promote angiogenesis via mTOR (mammalian target of rapamycin). PTEN (phosphatase and tensin homolog) is a negative regulator of Akt.

HER2 resistance may also be biochemically mediated. Molecularly, full-length HER2 (p185^{ErbB2}) undergoes proteolytic cleavage resulting in a deceptively shortened receptor (p95^{ErbB2}) with increased autokinase activity (Figure 4) (Segatto *et al.*, 1988). The truncated receptor is notable for two other reasons. First, it preferentially dimerizes with HER3; and second, trastuzumab does not inhibit receptor phosphorylation (due to loss of the drug-binding epitope) (Xia *et al.*, 2004). Even though elevated serum levels of the dissociated extracellular domain (ECD) have been correlated with poorer responses to therapy as well as lymph node metastasis (Molina *et al.*, 2002), this finding may also be of value as a biologic marker of increased sensitivity to small molecule kinase inhibitors. The latter notion also provides a partial explanation for the effectiveness of lapatinib (in patients who fail trastuzumab) in tumors that overexpress EGFR with high circulating levels of the ECD.

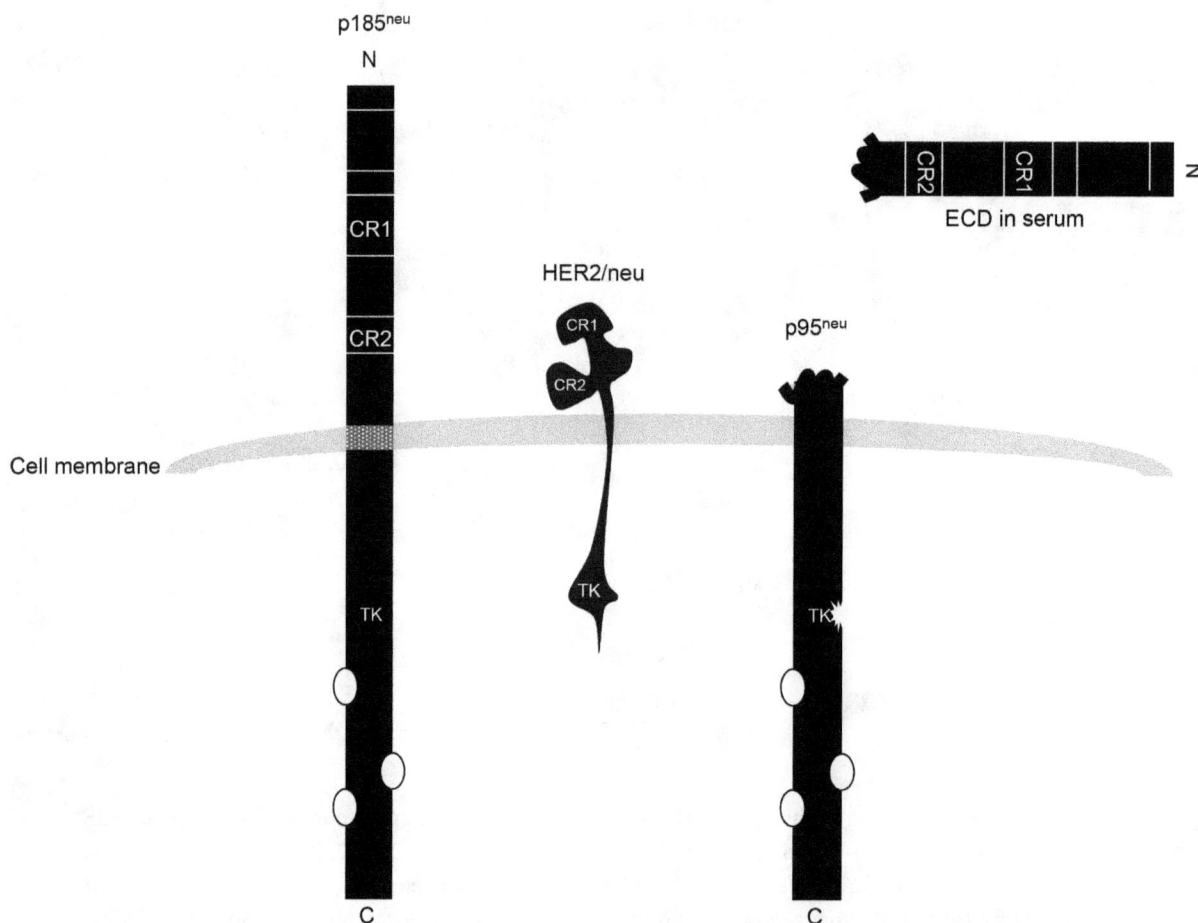

Figure 4: Possible mechanisms of HER2 resistance. In addition to the belief that resistance may be due to HER2 heterodimers (see Figure 3), another plausible reason may relate to the formation of the truncated receptor, which has three notable properties: 1) devoid of the antibody binding site, 2) constitutively active, and 3) HER3-preferred partner. Gene/protein defects in the ATP binding site of the internal tyrosine kinase domain may also confer resistance to some of the small molecule inhibitors. As seen in Figure 3, mutation of members of the MAPK and PI3K pathways may result in constitutively activated downstream molecules that can also account for HER2 resistance.

Preclinical and clinical evidence also suggest that insulin-like growth factor-1 receptor (IGF-1R) may be another mechanism of HER2 resistance. Using human breast cancer cell lines that over-express HER2 and IGF-1R, investigators observed only modest inhibition of tumor cell proliferation with trastuzumab. However, a three-fold greater decrease in tumor growth occurred when the same cells were treated with trastuzumab plus an IGF-1R antagonist (Lu *et al.*, 2001). In addition, expression of (IGF-1R) in HER2-positive breast tumors was independently associated with significantly lower responses to neo-adjuvant trastuzumab-containing chemotherapy (Harris *et al.*, 2007). Thus, rather than the co-receptor concept characterized by formation of HER2 heterodimers, IGF-1R appears to be an important membrane protein with the promiscuous ability to induce HER2 phosphorylation (Nahta *et al.*, 2005). It is also possible that signaling through the IGF-1R pathway may confer resistance to trastuzumab separately by modulating the same downstream complex (i.e., cyclin E/Cdk2) in opposite ways (Lai *et al.*, 2001). These findings suggest that concomitant inhibition of tumors that express both HER2 and IGF-1R would improve tumor outcomes. However rational this approach appears to be may not necessarily translate into any therapeutic benefit. The primary reason is based on the sound knowledge that while HER2 gene amplification is used to guide the application of anti-HER2 therapy, genetic aberrations have yet to be reported for IGF-1R.

HER2 may be at the focus of yet another malevolent relationship, one that involves the estrogen receptor (ER). Although the connection could be a manifestation of genetic evolution, it is more likely to be one that has been genetically conserved since growth factor pathways have been demonstrated to influence, and be influenced by, E α signaling (Nicholson *et al.*, 2004). Compelling evidence suggest that estrogen deprivation strategies are associated with over-expression of heregulin (Tang *et al.*, 1996), as well as HER1 and HER2, which may contribute to the development of resistance to endocrine therapies in breast cancer (Nicholson *et al.*, 2004). Furthermore, relative endocrine resistance has been observed in hormone receptor-positive tumor cells that co-express HER2 (Massarweh *et al.*, 2006). Results from two phase III clinical studies suggest that this is indeed true. Progression-free survival in postmenopausal women with ER- and HER2-positive breast cancer was significantly improved among patients treated with either anastrozole or letrozole plus anti-HER2 therapy compared to an aromatase inhibitor alone (Johnston *et al.*, 2009; Mackey *et al.*, 2009).

In-vitro data showing that HER2 up-regulates the expression of a number of pro-angiogenic growth factors including vascular endothelial growth factor (VEGF), and that tumor expression of both proteins likely contribute to the poorer prognosis associated with HER2-overexpression provides a biological rationale for conducting clinical trials involving combined anti-HER2 and anti-angiogenic therapy (Konecny *et al.*, 2004; Yen *et al.*, 2000). Final results of one study indicate that dual therapy with bevacizumab and trastuzumab as first-line chemotherapy-naïve treatment for advanced HER2-positive breast cancer resulted in an ORR of 48% (Hurvitz *et al.*, 2009). Objective responses, including 2 CRs, were documented in 24 of the 50 enrolled patients; 15 other patients had SD, 6 of which lasted ≥ 6 months for a CBR of 60%. The median time to progression was 9.2 mos (95% C, 5.4 to 20.5); median OS was 43.8 months. The most frequently reported drug-associated related AEs (grade ≥ 3) included hypertension, infusion reactions, headache, epistaxis, fatigue, and proteinuria. One patient dies of a perforated bowel. One grade 4 cardiac event was reported in a patient previously treated with doxorubicin. The investigators concluded that the combination could be feasibly given and active even in the absence of chemotherapy in this patient population.

What have also been elucidated are the many pathways downstream of the receptor that may be linked to the aberrant behavior of HER2-positive tumor cells. Mutations involving PI3K (phospatidylinositol 3-kinase), Akt, and mTOR (mammalian target of rapamycin) may result in constitutive activation of these effectors as well as tumor resistance. Even more intriguing is the possibility that targeted inhibition of essential regulatory components of the cell such as histone deacetylases can, by altering gene expression, induce cell differentiation, cell cycle arrest, and cell death (Marks *et al.*, 2000). Heat shock proteins (HSPs) are another intracellular component with key regulatory functions. Present under normal conditions and up-regulated during stress, some of these proteins (i.e., HSP 90) appear to confer HER2-resistance possibly by blocking receptor degradation (Chandarlapaty *et al.*, 2010). In essence, these somewhat unexpected targets, like the 26S proteasome in myeloma, appear to contradict the dogma that aberrant proteins drive all phases of the neoplastic process. In hindsight, perhaps targeting the obvious, the aberrant molecules, has been a masterful diversion of tumor cells.

As many of the targeted agents have very acceptable toxicity profiles, we should expect economic toxicities to dramatically influence their clinical application. Therefore, it will be essential that new therapeutic goals include: 1) elucidation of relevant molecular targets tumors are partially or completely dependent on; 2) determination of the optimal biologic dose which results in complete and selective target inhibition; 3) identification of appropriate surrogate markers that correlate target inhibition with anti-tumor activity; 4) recognition of appropriate clinical trial endpoints that reflect drug efficacy; and 5) incorporation of genomics and proteomics which hold additional promise in diagnosing, profiling, and possibly individualizing treatment of cancers.

6   *Neu* Uncertainties

Despite all of the accumulated information, the clarity of a number of important aspects linking the therapeutic agents with the receptor still remains ill-defined. For example, an area of intense inquiry involves the precise mechanism of trastuzumab's anti-tumor effect. Although uncertain, a number of hypotheses have been proposed. One involves perturbation of critical signal transduction pathways following receptor internalization and subsequent proteolysis (Figure 3). As such, signaling through key molecules located "downstream" of the receptor, including phosphatidylinositol 3 kinase (PI3K) and mitogen-activated protein kinase (MAPK), is disrupted (Wang *et al.*, 2005; Yakes *et al.*, 2002). In addition to the purported effects on tumor proliferation, the antibody may also impact tumor survival pathways such as angiogenesis by modulating the release of pro-angiogenic and anti-angiogenic factors (Izumi *et al.*, 2002; Petit *et al.*, 1997).

Tumor cells treated with trastuzumab also exhibit growth arrest in G_1 phase which appears to be due to reduced concentrations of proteins involved in the separation of p27[kip1] and the cyclin E/cdk2 complex (Lane *et al.*, 2000). Two other anti-tumor mechanisms include inhibition of DNA repair, an effect partially mediated by modulating p21[WAF1] and decreased formation of the constitutively active truncated form of HER2 by blocking proteolytic cleavage of the extracellular domain (ECD) (Pietras *et al.*, 1998). Furthermore, because HER2 can be recycled to the cell membrane in its functional state, part of trastuzumab's anti-tumor mechanism may involve recruitment of a protein known as c-Cbl which enhances lysosomal-enhanced degradation of the receptor (Yeon & Pegram, 2005).

Nonetheless, controversy exists regarding these proposed mechanisms. Some investigators contend that cell surface receptor down-regulation is not an important anti-tumor mechanism of trastuzumab

(Austin *et al.*, 2004; Yeon & Pegram, 2005) as they demonstrate that the antibody does not alter any of the previous findings, even the ability to cause apoptosis as the terminal event (Gennari *et al.*, 2004). An alternative, though not necessarily mutually exclusive, explanation of the function of trastuzumab involves the recruitment of an immune component. Suggestive, though not absolute, evidence indicate that the antibody binds and activates Fc receptors expressed on immunocompetent lymphocytes and NK cells resulting in antibody dependent cellular cytotoxicity (ADCC) (Clynes *et al.*, 2000). However, even the phenomenon of ADCC may not be important as inhibition of tumor growth has been observed with antibodies that lack the Fc fragment (Fan *et al.*, 1993). What is absolutely certain is that mere binding of trastuzumab to the receptor alone provides only a superficial explanation of how the antibody elicits its effect.

Another nuance relates to the relative importance of HER1 and HER3 in the disease. Although high level HER1 expression has been found in breast cancer, specific anti-HER1 blockade has not translated into anti-tumor efficacy (Baselga *et al.*, 2005). On the other hand, an even more intriguing phenomenon relates to HER3. Despite the absence of, or at least weakened, intrinsic kinase activity, the presence of HER3 in breast cancer appears to have prognostic relevance (Bieche *et al.*, 2003; Witton *et al.*, 2003) Hence, what appears to be a plausible conclusion is that the lack of homodimer HER1 and HER3 dependence can be overcome by heterodimer formation with HER2. Finally, it remains uncertain whether the pathologic alterations of the receptor occur very early (i.e., atypical hyperplasia) or later (i.e., neoplasia) in the tumorigenic process. The determination of when this functional abnormality occurs may be crucial as earlier detection may improve the prognosis of a significant number of patients.

It is somewhat perplexing when the considerable knowledge gained is coupled with the substantial progress made, especially with regards to targeting HER2, that there are still perceptibly large gaps in our understanding of the receptor. More than likely, some of the current voids will be filled in the not too distant future. As such, HER2 will continue to be the subject of periodic reviews.

References

Agus DB, Akita RW, Fox WD, et al. *Targeting ligand-activated ErbB2 signaling inhibits breast and prostate tumor growth. Cancer Cell 2002; 2:127-137.*

Akiyama T, Sudo C, Ogawara H, Toyoshima K, Yamamoto T. *The product of the human c-erbB-2 gene: a 185 kilodalton glycoprotein with tyrosine kinase activity. Science 1986; 232:1644-1646.*

Alimandi M, Romano A, Curia MC, et al. *Cooperative signaling of erbB3 and erbB2 in neoplastic transformation and human mammary carcinomas. Oncogene 1995; 10:1813-1821.*

Austin CD, De Maziere AM, Pisacane PI, et al. *Endocytosis and sorting of ErbB2 and the site of action of cancer therapeutics trastuzumab and geldanamycin. Mol Biol Cell 2004;15:5268-5282.*

Awada A Dirix L, Beck J, et al. *Safety and efficacy of neratinib (HKI-272) in combination with vinorelbine in ErbB2+ metastatic breast cancer. Cancer Res 2009; 69 (Suppl.). Abstract 5095.*

Barnes NL, Khavari S, Boland GP, Cramer A, Knox WF, Bundred NJ. *Absence of HER-4 expression predicts recurrence of ductal carcinoma in situ of the breast. Clin Cancer Res 2005; 11:2163-2168.*

Baselga J, Albanell J, Ruiz A, et al. *Phase II and tumor pharmacodynamic study of gefitinib in patients with advanced breast cancer. J Clin Oncol 2005; 23:5323-5333.*

Baselga J, Cortés J, Kim S-B, et al. *Pertuzumab plus trastuzumab plus docetaxel for metastatic breast cancer. N Engl J Med 2012; 366:109-119.*

Baselga J, Gelmon KA, Verma S, et al. Phase II trial of pertuzumab and trastuzumab in patients with human epidermal growth factor receptor 2-positive metastatic breast cancer that progressed during prior trastuzumab therapy. J Clin Oncol 2010; 28:1138-1144.

Baselga J, Tripathy D, Mendelsohn J, et al. Phase II study of weekly intravenous recombinant humanized anti-p185HER2 monoclonal antibody in patients with HER2/neu-overexpressing metastatic breast cancer. J Clin Oncol 1996; 14:737-744.

Bendell JC, Domchek SM, Burstein HJ, et al. Central nervous system metastasis in women who receive trastuzumab-based therapy for metastatic breast carcinoma. Cancer 2003; 97:2972–2977.

Bhattacharyya B, Wolff J. Maytansine binding to the vinblastine sites of tubulin. FEBS Lett 1977; 75:159-162.

Bieche I, Onody P, Tozlu S, Driouch K, Vidaud M, Lidereau R. Prognostic value of ERBB family mRNA expression in breast carcinoma. Int J Cancer 2003; 106:758-765.

Bines J, Murad A, Lago S, et al. Primary treatment with weekly docetaxel (Taxotere) and trastuzumab (Herceptin) for HER-2 overexpressing locally advanced breast cancer. Eur J Cancer 2003; 1(5 Suppl.):S114. Abstract 370.

Blackwell KL, Burstein HJ, Storniolo A-M, et al. Randomized study of lapatinib alone or in combination with trastuzumab in women with erbB2-positive, trastuzumab-refractory metastatic breast cancer. J Clin Oncol 2010; 28:1124-1130.

Blackwell KL, Miles D, Gianni L, et al. Primary results from EMILIA, a phase III study of trastuzumab emtansine (T-DM1) versus capecitabine (X) and lapatinib (L) in HER2-positive locally advanced or metastatic breast cancer (MBC) previously treated with trastuzumab (T) and a taxane. J Clin Oncol 2012; 30 (suppl). Abstract LBA1.

Burgess AW, Cho HS, Eigenbrot C, et al. An open-and- shut case? Recent insights into the activation of EGF/ErbB receptors. Mol Cell 2003; 12:541-552.

Burris HA III, Hurwitz HI, Dees EC, et al. Phase I study, pharmacokinetics, and clinical activity study of lapatinib (GW572016), a reversible dual inhibitor of epidermal growth factor receptor tyrosine kinases, in heavily pretreated patients with metastatic carcinomas. J Clin Oncol 2005; 23:5305-5313.

Burris HA III. Dual kinase inhibition in the treatment of breast cancer: initial experience with the EGFR/ErbB-2 inhibitor lapatinib. Oncologist 2004; 9(suppl 3):10-15.

Burstein HJ, Harris LN, Gelman R, et al. Preoperative therapy with trastuzumab and paclitaxel followed by sequential adjuvant doxorubicin/cyclophosphamide for HER2 overexpressing stage II and III breast cancer: a pilot study. J Clin Oncol 2003; 21:46-53.

Burstein HJ, Sun Y, Dirix LY, et al. Neratinib, an irreversible erbB receptor tyrosine kinase inhibitor, in patients with advanced erbB2-positive breast cancer. J Clin Oncol 2010; 28:1301-1307.

Buzdar AU, Valero V, Ibrahim NK, et al. Neoadjuvant therapy with, paclitaxel followed by 5-fluorouracil, epirubicin, and cyclophosphamide chemotherapy and concurrent trastuzumab in human epidermal growth factor receptor 2-positive operable breast cancer: an update of the initial randomized study population and data of additional patients treated with the same regimen. Clin Cancer Res 2007; 13:228–233.

Cameron D, Casey M, Press M, et al. A phase III randomized comparison of lapatinib plus capecitabine versus capecitabine alone in women with advanced breast cancer that has progressed on trastuzumab: updated efficacy and biomarker analyses. Breast Cancer Res Treat 2008; 112:533-543.

Chandarlapaty S, Scaltriti M, Angelini P, et al. Inhibitors of HSP90 block p95-HER2 signaling in trastuzumab-resistant tumors and suppress their growth. Oncogene 2010; 29:325-334.

Chari RV, Martell BA, Gross JL, et al. Immunoconjugates containing novel maytansinoids: promising anticancer drugs. Cancer Res 1992; 52:127-131.

Cho HS, Mason K, Ramyar KX, et al. Structure of the extracellular region of HER2 alone and in complex with the Herceptin Fab. Nature 2003; 421:756-760.

Chow L, Gupta S, Hershman DL, et al. Safety and efficacy of neratinib (HKI-272) in combination with paclitaxel in ErbB2+ metastatic breast cancer. Cancer Res 2009; 69 (Suppl.). Abstract 5081.

Clayton AJ, Danson S, Jolly S, et al. Incidence of cerebral metastasis in patients treated with trastuzumab for metastatic breast cancer. Br J Cancer 2004; 91:639–643.

Clynes RA, Towers TL, Presta LG, Ravetch JV. Inhibitory Fc receptors modulate in vivo cytoxicity against tumor targets. Nat Med 2000; 6::443-446.

Cobleigh MA, Vogel CL, Tripathy D, et al. Multinational study of the efficacy and safety of humanized anti-HER2 monoclonal antibody in women who have HER2-overexpressing metastatic breast cancer that has progressed after chemotherapy for metastatic disease. J Clin Oncol 1999; 17:2639-2648.

Coudert B, Largillier R, Arnould L, et al. Multicenter phase II trial of neoadjuvant therapy with trastuzumab, docetaxel, and carboplatin for human epidermal growth factor receptor-2-overexpressing stage II or III breast cancer: results of the GETN (A)-1 trial. J Clin Oncol 2007; 25:2678–2684.

Coussens L, Yang-Fen TL, Liao Y-C, et al. Tyrosine kinase receptor with extensive homology to EGF receptor shares chromosomal location with neu oncogene. Science 1985; 230:1132-1139.

Di Fiore PP, Pierce JH, Kraus MH, Segatto O, King CR, Aaronson SA. erbB-2 is a potent oncogene when overexpressed in NIH/3T3 cells. Science 1987; 237:178-182.

DiStefano A, Yap HY, Hortobagyi GN, Blumenschein GR. The natural history of breast cancer patients with brain metastasis. Cancer 1979; 44:1913-1918.

Eagan RT, Ingle JN, Rubin J, Frytak S, Moertel CG. Early clinical study of an intermittent schedule for maytansine (NSC-153858): brief communication. J Natl Cancer Inst 1978; 60:93-96.

Fan Z, Masui H, Altas I, Mendelsohn J. Blockade of epidermal growth factor receptor function by bivalent and monovalent fragments of C225 anti-epidermal growth factor receptor monoclonal antibodies. Cancer Res 1993; 53:4322-4328.

Gasparini G, Gion M, Mariani L, et al. Randomized phase II trial of weekly paclitaxel alone versus trastuzumab plus weekly paclitaxel as first-line therapy of patients with Her-2 positive advanced breast cancer. Breast Cancer Res Treat 2007; 101:355-365.

Gennari R, Menard S, Fagnoni F, et al. Pilot study of the mechanism of action of preoperative trastuzumab in patients with primary operable breast tumors overexpressing HER2. Clin Cancer Res 2004;10:5650-5655.

Geyer CE, Forster J, Cameron MD. Lapatinib plus capecitabine in breast cancer. N Engl J Med 2007; 356:1471-1472.

Geyer CE, Forster J, Lindquist D, et al. Lapatinib plus capecitabine for HER2-positive advanced breast cancer. N Engl J Med 2006; 355:2733-2743.

Gianni L, Llado A, Bianchi G, et al. Open-label, phase II, multicenter, randomized study of the efficacy and safety of two dose levels of pertuzumab, a human epidermal growth factor receptor 2 dimerization inhibitor, in patients with human epidermal growth factor receptor 2-negative metastatic breast cancer. J Clin Oncol 2010; 28:1131-1137.

Gianni L, Semiglazov V, Manikhas GM, et al. Neoadjuvant trastuzumab (Herceptin) in locally advanced breast cancer (NOAH): antitumor and safety analysis. J Clin Oncol 2007; 25(18S). Abstract 532.

Gomez HL, Doval DC, Chavez MA, et al. Efficacy and safety of lapatinib as first-line therapy for ErbB2-amplified locally advanced or metastatic breast cancer. J Clin Oncol 2008; 26:2999-3005.

Graus-Porta D, Beerli RR, Daly JM, Hynes NE. ErbB-2, the preferred heterodimerization partner of all ErbB receptors, is a mediator of lateral signaling. EMBO J 1997; 16:1647-1655.

Guy PM, Platko JV, Cantley LC, Cerione RA, Carraway KL. Insect cell-expressed p180erbB3 possesses an impaired tyrosine kinase activity. PNAS 1994; 91:8132-8136.

Harris LN, You F, Schnitt SJ, et al. Predictors of resistance to preoperative trastuzumab and vinorelbine for HER2-positive early breast cancer. Clin Cancer Res 2007; 13:1198-1207.

Hurvitz S, Dirix L, Kocsis J, et al. Trastuzumab emtansine (T-DM1) vs. trastuzumab plus docetaxel (H+T) in previously-untreated HER2-positive metastatic breast cancer (MBC): primary results of a randomized, multicenter, open-label phase II study (TDM4450g/B021976). Eur J Cancer 2011; 47S. Abstract 5001.

Hurvitz S, Pegram M, Lin L, et al. Final results of a phase II trial evaluating trastuzumab and bevacizumab as first line treatment of HER2-amplified advanced breast cancer. Cancer Res 2009; 69(24 Suppl). Abstract 6094.

Hynes NE, Stern DF. The biology of erbB-2/neu/HER-2 and its role in cancer. Biochim Biophys Acta Rev Cancer 1994; 1198:165-184.

Izumi Y, Xu L, di Tomaso E, Fukumura D, Jain RK. Tumour biology: herceptin acts as an anti-angiogenic cocktail. Nature 2002;416(6878):279-280.

Johnston S, Pippen J Jr, Pivot X, et al. Lapatinib combined with letrozole versus letrozole and placebo as first-line therapy for postmenopausal hormone receptor-positive metastatic breast cancer. J Clin Oncol 2009; 27:5538-5546.

Jones FE, Stern DF. Expression of dominant-negative ErbB2 in the mammary gland of transgenic mice reveals a role in lobuloaveolar development and lactation. Oncogene 1999; 18:3481-3490.

Kannel WB. Incidence and epidemiology of heart failure. Heart Fail Rev 2000; 5:167-173.

Kokai Y, Myers JN, Wada T, et al. Synergistic interaction of p185c-neu and the EGF receptor leads to transformation of rodent fibroblasts. Cell 1989; 58:287-292.

Konecny GE, Meng YG, Michael Untch, et al. Association between HER-2/neu and vascular endothelial growth factor expression predicts clinical outcome in primary breast cancer patients. Clin Cancer Res 2004; 10:1706–1716.

Krop I, LoRusso P, Miller KD, et al. A phase II study of trastuzumab-DM1 (T-DM1), a novel HER2 antibody–drug conjugate, in HER2+ metastatic breast cancer patients previously treated with conventional chemotherapy, lapatinib, and trastuzumab. Cancer Res 2009; 69 (Suppl 3). Abstract 710.

Krop IE, Beeram M, Modi S, et al. Phase I study of trastuzumab-DM1, an HER2 antibody-drug conjugate, given every 3 weeks to patients with HER2-positive metastatic breast cancer. J Clin Oncol 2010; 28:2698-2704.

Lai A, Sarcevic B, Prall OWJ, Sutherland RL. Insulin/insulin-like growth factor-I and estrogen cooperate to stimulate cyclin E-Cdk2 activation and cell cycle progression in MCF-7 breast cancer cells through differential regulation of cyclin E and p21WAF1/Cip. J Biol Chem 2001; 276:25823-25833.

Lane HA, Beuvink I, Motoyama AB, Daly JM, Neve RM, Hynes NE. ErbB2 potentiates breast tumor proliferation through modulation of p27(Kip1)-Cdk2 complex formation: receptor overexpression does not determine growth dependency. Mol Cell Biol 2000;20(9):3210-3223.

Lee KF, Simon H, Chen H, Bates B, Hung MC, Hauser C. Requirement for neuregulin receptor erbB2 in neural and cardiac development. Nature 1995; 378:394-398.

Lin NU, Diéras V, Paul D, et al. Multicenter phase II study of lapatinib in patients with brain metastases from HER2-positive breast cancer. Clin Cancer Res 2009; 15:1452-1459.

Lu Y, Zi X, Zhao Y, Mascarenhas D, Pollak M. Insulin-like growth factor-1 receptor signaling and resistance to trastuzumab. J Natl Cancer Inst 2001; 93:1852-1857.

Mackey JR, Kaufman B, Clemens M, et al. Trastuzumab plus anastrozole versus anastrozole alone for the treatment of postmenopausal women with human epidermal growth factor receptor 2-positive, hormone receptor-positive metastatic breast cancer: results from the randomized phase III TAnDEM study. J Clin Oncol 2009; 27:5529-5537.

Marks PA, Richon VM, Rifkind RA. Histone deacetylase inhibitors: inducers of differentiation or apoptosis of transformed cells. J Natl Cancer Inst 2000; 92:1210-1216.

Marty M, Cognetti F, Maraninchi D, et al. Randomized phase II trial of the efficacy and safety of trastuzumab combined with docetaxel in patients with human epidermal growth factor receptor 2–positive metastatic breast cancer administered as first-line treatment: The M77001 Study Group. J Clin Oncol 2005; 23:4265-4274.

Massarweh S, Osborne CK, Jiang S, et al. Mechanisms of tumor regression and resistance to estrogen deprivation and fulvestrant in a model of estrogen receptor-positive, HER-2/neu-positive breast cancer. Cancer Res 2006; 66:8266-8273.

Mather B, Viswanathan K, Miller K, Long T. Michael addition reactions in macromolecular design for emerging technologies. Progress Polymer Science 2006; 31:487-531.

McCann AH, Dervan PA, O'Regan M, et al. Prognostic significance of c-erbB-2 and estrogen receptor status in human breast cancer. Cancer Res 1991;51:3296–3303.

Menard S, Fortis S. Castiglioni F, Agresti R, Balsari A. HER2 as a prognostic factor in breast cancer. Oncology 2001; 61 (Suppl 2): 67-72.

Meyer C, Birchmeier C. Multiple essential functions of neuregulin in development. Nature 1995; 378:386-390.

Miettinen PJ, Berger JE, Meneses J, et al. Epithelial immaturity and multiorgan failure in mice lacking epidermal growth factor receptor. Nature 1995; 376:337-341.

Molina MA, Saez R, Ramsey, et al. NH(2)-terminal truncated HER-2 protein but not full-length receptor is associated with nodal metastasis in human breast cancer. Clin Cancer Res 2002; 8:347-353.

Montemurro F, Donadio M, Clavarezza M, et al. Outcome of patients with HER2-positive advanced breast cancer progressing during trastuzumab-based therapy. Oncologist 2006; 11:318-324.

Nahta R, Yuan LXH, Bing Zhang, Kobayashi R, Esteva FJ. Insulin-like growth factor-1 receptor/human epidermal growth factor receptor 2 heterodimerization contributes to trastuzumab resistance of breast cancer cells. Cancer Res 2005; 65:11118-11128.

Nicholson RI, Hutcheson IR, Knowlden JM, et al. Nonendocrine pathways and endocrine resistance; observations with antiestrogens and signal transduction inhibitors in combination. Clin Cancer Res 2004; 10:346-354s.

Nicholson RI, Staka C, Boyns F, Hutcheson IR, Gee JM. Growth factor-driven mechanisms associated with resistance to estrogen deprivation in breast cancer: new opportunities for therapy. Endocr Relat Cancer 2004; 11:623-641.

Olayioye MA, Graus-Porta D, Beerli RR, Rohrer J, Gay B, Hynes NE. ErbB-1 and erbB-2 acquire distinct signaling properties dependent upon their dimerization partner. Mol Cell Biol 1998; 18:5042-5051.

Paik S, Shak S, Tang G, et al. A multigene assay to predict recurrence of tamoxifen-treated, node-negative breast cancer. N Engl J Med 2004; 351:2817-2826.

Perez EA, Byrne JA, Hammond IW, et al. Cardiac safety experience in 3127 patients treated with lapatinib. Ann Oncol 2006; 17(suppl 9):1420.

Petit AM, Rak J, Hung MC, et al. Neutralizing antibodies against epidermal growth factor and ErbB-2/neu receptor tyrosine kinases down-regulate vascular endothelial growth factor production by tumor cells in vitro and in vivo: angiogenic implications for signal transduction therapy of solid tumors. Am J Pathol 1997;151(6):1523-1530.

Piccart-Gebhart MJ, Procter M, Leyland-Jones B, et al. Trastuzumab after adjuvant chemotherapy in HER2-positive breast cancer. N Engl J Med. 2005; 353(16):1659–1672.

Pietras RJ, Pegram MD, Finn RS, Maneval DA, Slamon DJ. Remission of human breast cancer xenografts on therapy with humanized monoclonal antibody to HER-2 receptor and DNA-reactive drugs. Oncogene. 1998; 17:2235-2249.

Quirke P, Pickles A, Tuzi NL, Mohamdee O, Gullick WJ. Pattern of expression of c-erbB2 oncoprotein in human fetuses. Br J Cancer 1989; 60:64-69.

Rabindran SK, Discafani CM, Rosfjord EC, et al. Antitumor activity of HKI-272, an orally active, irreversible inhibitor of the HER-2 tyrosine kinase. Cancer Res 2004; 64:3958-3965.

Remillard S, Rebhun LI, Howie GA, Kupchan SM. Antimitotic activity of the potent tumor inhibitor maytansine. Science 1975; 189:1002-1005.

Romond EH, Perez EA, Bryant J, et al. Trastuzumab plus adjuvant chemotherapy for operable HER2-positive breast cancer. N Engl J Med.2005; 353:1673–1684.

Sartor CI, Zhou H,Kozlowska E, et al. Her4 mediates ligand-dependent antiproliferative and differentiation responses in human breast cancer cells. Mol Cell Biol 2001;21:4265–75.

Scheuer W, Friess T, Burtscher H, Bossenmaier B, Endl J, Hasmann M. *Strongly enhanced antitumor activity of trastuzumab and pertuzumab combination treatment on HER2-positive human xenograft tumor models. Cancer Res 2009; 69:9330-9336.*

Segatto O, King CR, Pierce JH, DiFiore PP, Aaronson SA. *Different structural alterations upregulate in vitro tyrosine kinase activity and transforming potency of the erbB-2 gene. Mol Cell Biol 1988; 8:5570-5574.*

Shou J, Massarweh S, Osborne CK, et al. *Mechanisms of tamoxifen resistance: increased estrogen receptor-HER2/neu crosstalk in ER/HER0-posivitive breast cancer. J Natl Cancer Inst 2004; 96:926-935.*

Slamon D, Eiermann W, Robert N, et al. *Adjuvant trastuzumab in HER2-positive breast cancer. N Engl J Med 2011; 365:1273-1283.*

Slamon DJ, Leyland-Jones B, Shak S, et al. *Use of chemotherapy plus a monoclonal antibody against HER2 for metastatic breast cancer that overexpresses HER2. N Engl J Med 2001; 344:783-792.*

Smith I, Procter M, Gelber RD, et al. *2-year follow-up of trastuzumab after adjuvant chemotherapy in HER2-positive breast cancer: a randomized controlled trial. Lancet 2007; 369:29-36.*

Sonpavde G. *Lapatinib plus capecitabine in breast cancer. N Engl J Med 2007; 356:1471-1472.*

Stein SH, Gomez HL, Chavez MA, et al. *Interim results of a phase II randomized study of lapatinib (GW572016) as first-line treatment for patients with FISH-amplified advanced or metastatic breast cancer. Eur J Cancer 2005; 3(suppl):78.*

Tang CK, Perez C, Grunt T, Waibel C, Cho C, Lupu R. *Involvement of heregulin-beta2 in the acquisition of the hormone-independent phenotype of breast cancer cells. Cancer Res 1996; 56:3350-3358.*

Tripathy D, Moisa C, Gluck S, et al. *Neoadjuvant capecitabine plus docetaxel ± trastuzumab therapy for recently diagnosed breast cancer: phase II results. Breast Cancer Res 2007; 106(Suppl. 1). Abstract 5059.*

van der Geer P, Hunter T, Lindberg RA. *Receptor protein-tyrosine kinases and their signal transduction pathways. Annu Rev Cell Biol 1994; 10:251-337.*

Vennstrom B, Bishop JM. *Isolation and characterization of chicken DNA homologous to the two putative oncogenes of avian erythroblastosis virus. Cell 1982; 28:135-143.*

Vogel CL, Burris HA, Limentani S, et al. *A phase II study of trastuzumab-DM1 (T-DM1), a HER2 antibody-drug conjugate (ADC), in patients with HER2+ metastatic breast cancer (MBC): Final results. J Clin Oncol 2009; 27 (15S). Abstract 1017.*

Vogel CL, Cobleigh MA, Tripathy D, et al. *Efficacy and safety of trastuzumab as a single agent in first-line treatment of HER2-overexpressing metastatic breast cancer. J Clin Oncol 2002; 20:719-726.*

von Minckwitz G, du Bois A, Schmidt M, et al. *Trastuzumab beyond progression in human epidermal growth factor receptor 2–positive advanced breast cancer: A German Breast Group 26/Breast International Group 03-05 Study. J Clin Oncol 2009; 27:1999-2006.*

Wang CX, Koay DC, Edwards A, et al. *In vitro and in vivo effects of combination of trastuzumab (Herceptin) and tamoxifen in breast cancer. Breast Cancer Res Treat 2005; 92:251-263.*

Witton CJ, Reeves JR, Going JJ, Cooke TG, Bartlett JM. *Expression of the HER1-4 family of receptor tyrosine kinases in breast cancer. J Pathol 2003; 200:290-297.*

Wolff AC, Hammond EH, Schwartz JN, et al. *American Society of Clinical Oncology/College of American Pathologists guideline recommendations for human epidermal growth factor receptor 2 testing in breast cancer. J Clin Oncol 2007; 25:118-145.*

Wong KK, Fracasso PM, Bukowski RM, et al. *A phase I study with neratinib (HKI-272), an irreversible pan ErbB receptor tyrosine kinase inhibitor, in patients with solid tumors. Clin Cancer Res 2009; 15:2552-2558.*

Wood ER, Truesdale AT, McDonald OB, et al. A unique structure for epidermal growth factor receptor bound to GW572016 (Lapatinib): relationships among protein conformation, inhibitor off-rate, and receptor activity in tumor cells. Cancer Res 2004; 64:6652-6659.

Xia W, Liu L-H, Ho P, Spector NL. Truncated ErbB2 receptor (p95ErbB2) is regulated by heregulin through heterodimer formation with ErbB3 yet remains sensitive to the dual EGFR/ErbB2 kinase inhibitor GW72016. Oncogene 2004; 23:646-653.

Yakes FM, Chinratanalab W, Ritter CA, King W, Seelig S, Arteaga CL. Herceptin-induced inhibition of phosphatidylinositol-3 kinase and Akt Is required for antibody-mediated effects on p27, cyclin D1, and antitumor action. Cancer Res 2002; 62:4132-4141.

Yen L., You XL, Al Moustafa AE, et al. Heregulin selectively upregulates vascular endothelial growth factor secretion in cancer cells and stimulates angiogenesis. Oncogene 2000; 19:3460-3469.

Yeon CH, Pegram MD. Anti-erbB-2 antibody trastuzumab in the treatment of HER2-amplified breast cancer. Invest New Drugs 2005;23(5):391-409.

Yun C-H, Mengwasser KE, Toms AV, et al. The T790M mutation in EGFR kinase causes drug resistance by increasing the affinity for ATP. Proc Acad Sci USA 2008; 105:2070-2075.

Zhang X, Gureasko J, Shen K, Cole PA, Kuriyan J. An allosteric mechanism for activation of the kinase domain of epidermal growth factor receptor. Cell 2006; 125:1137-1149.

Estrogen Receptor Coregulators and Breast Cancer

Laura Buffa

Sylvester Comprehensive Cancer Center
University of Miami, USA

Zafar Nawaz

Sylvester Comprehensive Cancer Center and Dept. of Biochemistry and Molecular Biology
University of Miami, USA

1   Estrogen Signaling and Breast Cancer

Breast cancer is the second most common type of cancer diagnosed in women and is the leading cause of death among U.S. women aged 40 to 79. According to the National Cancer Institute, it is estimated that, for 2012, there will be 229,000 new cases of breast cancer and 39,900 deaths.

Sex steroid hormones, testosterone in males and estrogen and progesterone in women, play an important role in development, sexual behavior and reproductive functions, including the normal development of the breast in women. Their effect is achieved, in responsive cells, through specific hormone receptors that initiate signal cascades ultimately leading to regulation of cell proliferation and differentiation (Edwards, 2005).

The same hormones however, play also a role in the development and progression of different kind of cancers (Deroo & Korach, 2006; Yager, 2000). Estrogen, in particular, is strongly implicated in breast cancer development and progression. In fact, inhibition of estrogen production and/or action is a major strategy for the prevention and treatment of breast cancer. This approach, however, can be used only if the tumors maintain their estrogen responsiveness: these are cancers that are estrogen receptor positive (about 50-70% of the total number of breast cancers) and are also associated with a better prognosis compared to cancers which are estrogen receptor negative (Bai & Gust, 2009; Sommer & Fuqua, 2001).

In this chapter we will describe the mechanisms by which estrogen can exert its role in estrogen-responsive cells, focusing on specific aspects of estrogen receptor signaling, which have been investigated in our lab. Furthermore we will show how some of the proteins involved in estrogen receptor signaling can be used as predictive markers in breast cancer and we will describe a proposed clinical study related to the combined use of two drugs (bortezomib and tamoxifen) as therapeutic agents for estrogen receptor negative breast cancers.

2   Estrogen Receptor

The effect of estrogens is mediated, in responsive tissues, byspecific receptors called estrogen receptors (ER). Two different ERs have been identified, ERα and ERß, codified by two different genes (Greene *et al.*, 1984; Mosselman *et al.*, 1996). They both belong to the steroid hormone receptor family (SHR) superfamily, whose members are ligand (hormone)-dependent transcription factors: the receptor can bind to its ligand and consequently regulate transcription (Carson-Jurica *et al.*, 1990; Mangelsdorf*et al.*, 1995; Novac & Heinzel, 2004). In this chapter, we will focus on ERα signaling, as this isoform is the one that is more relevant to breast cancer (Sommer & Fuqua, 2001).

SHR are modular in structure and accommodate6 domains (Figure 1): A/B contains the hormone independent activation function 1, that synergizes with the activation function 2 to regulate gene expression; C is the DNA binding domain; D is the hinge region, a flexible linker important for dimerization and interaction with heat shock proteins; E contains the ligand binding domain (LBD) which containsthehormone dependent activation function 2, for regulation of gene expression; F is important for dimerization. Upon hormone binding the LBD undergoes conformational changes contributing to the dimerization of the receptor and creating a cleft for the interaction of the receptor with regulatory proteins (Nilsson *et al.*, 2001).

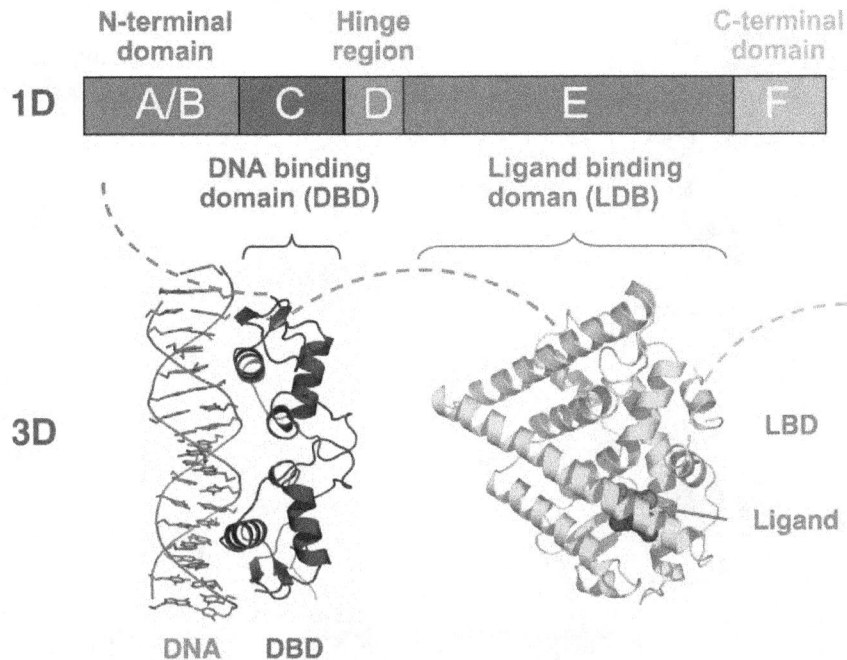

Figure 1: Top, schematic (1D) structure of ERα. Bottom, 3D structure of ERα DNA binding domain (DBD) when bound to the DNA and of ERα ligand binding domain (LBD) when bound to the ligand. All nuclear receptors share similar structure.

2.1   Genomic Function of ERα

ERα has been shown to exert both genomic and non-genomic functions.Genomic functions of ERα indicate the processes by which, upon hormone interaction, ERα translocates to the nucleus and regulates gene transcription. More specifically, upon estrogen binding, ERαundergoes conformational changes: it dissociates from heat shock proteins (Hsp) that maintain ERα in the cytoplasm, it dimerizes and translocates to the nucleus. At that location,the dimer binds, through its DNA-binding domain, to specific DNA sequences called estrogen response elements (ERE), mainly on the promoters (and sometimes at enhancers) of genes, which are for these reason defined estrogen responsive genes. Finally, through its transactivation domains, ERα aids the basal transcriptional machinery (RNA polymerase II and general transcription factors) in gene transcription.Follow degradation of ERα and of some of the components of the basal transcription machinery through a multiprotein complex called the proteasome, to clear the promoter, and initiate, eventually, another round of transcription (Carson-Jurica *et al.*, 1990; Dahlman-Wright *et al.*, 2006). This mechanism is common to all SHRs (Figure 2).

2.2   Non-genomic Function of ERα

Despite the most studied effects of estrogen happen through the mechanism described above, some estrogen effects occur through a so-called non-genomic mechanism, which does not involve the binding of ERα to the DNA.A small fraction of ERα is localized indeed to the plasmamembrane; upon estrogen binding, membrane-associated ERa, through protein-protein interactions, can rapidly and transitorily activate the Src/Erk/Ras signaling pathways (Levin, 2001). Genomic and non-genomic actions of ERα can

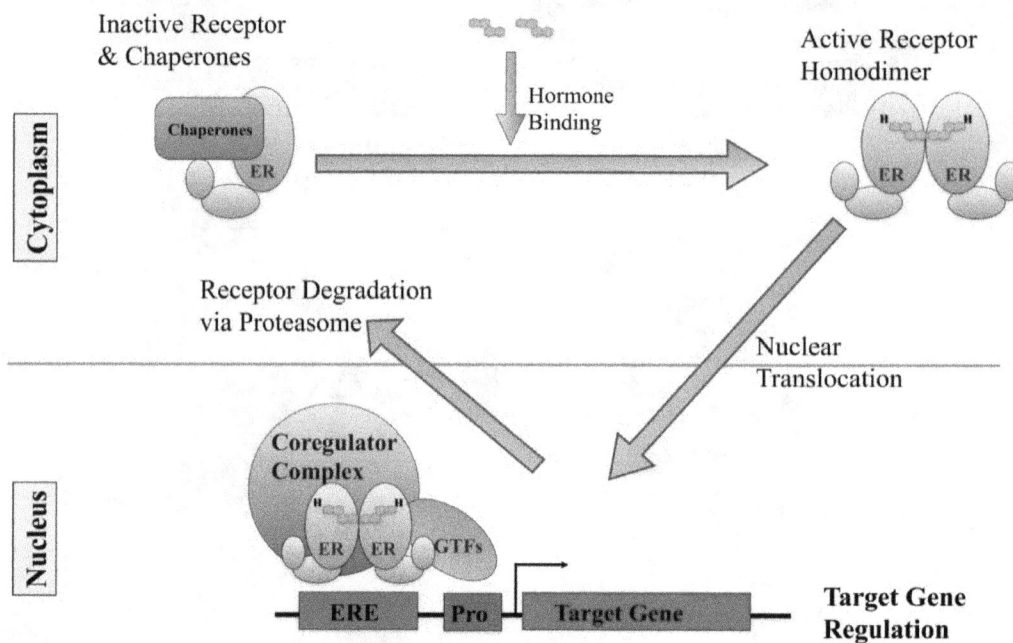

Figure 2: Scheme about the genomic function of estrogen receptor. See text for details. ER: estrogen receptor; H: hormone; GTFs: general transcription factors; ERE: estrogen responsive element; Pro: promoter.

overlap in what has been defined as "transcriptional cross-talk", a mechanism by which, signal transduction initiated by membrane-bound- ERα ultimately influences gene expression (Bjornstrom & Sjoberg, 2005; Pedram *et al.*, 2002). Non-genomic functions of ERα have been recently associated to cancer (Cabodi *et al.*, 2004). However, these pathways are not investigated in our lab, and will no be further described in this chapter.

3   ERα Coregulators

As mentioned above, genomic effects of ERα indicate its capability to bind DNA and regulate gene transcription, whose ultimate effect is the synthesis messenger RNA (mRNA) by RNA polymerase II (Pol-II). Modulation of transcription is one of the ways each cell of an organism can control its gene expression. This is an extremely dynamic process, in order to continuously adapt gene expression to the actual needs of the cell/organism.Transcription is tightly regulated in all its phases: initiation, elongation and/or termination. A continuously growing number of proteins (transcription factors and coregulators) and RNAs (non-coding RNAs) are involved in the in the modulation of mRNA transcription (Fuda *et al.*, 2009; Guenther *et al.*, 2007; Pan *et al.*, 2009, 2010). One important aspect of this control is the regulation of DNA accessibility by the transcriptional machinery. Decades of seminal work have thought us that in eukaryotic cells DNA is indeed packaged into chromatin, through its interaction with histones and other proteins. Highly packaged DNA is not easily accessible for transcription, while loosely packaged DNA is transcriptionally active. In this contest, any factor, which contributes in loosening the chromatin structure, contributes also in activating gene transcription. On the contrary, if a factor causes a more extensive or tighter packaging of chromatin, it represses transcription (Jenuwein & Allis, 2001; Leader *et al.*, 2006; Berger, 2007; Kouzarides, 2007; Cohen*et al.*, 2011). A more complex and, as of today, not fully understood aspect of this topic is how, in the first place, factors which modulate transcription can interact with their binding sites on the DNA, if they are packaged in the chromatin. It has been postulated the existence of "pioneer transcription factors" which can interact with their target sequences even in the contest of highly packaged chromatin, and initiate the process of loosening its structure (Bell*et al.*, 2011; Zaret & Carroll, 2011).

Coregulators play a key role in the regulation of steroid receptortransactivation functions. Coregulators can be classified into two classes, coactivators, which activate gene transcription and corepressors, which repress gene transcription. As of today, more than 350 different coregulators of hormone receptors have been identified; they are essential for the proper function of the latter, allowing fine-tuning of gene expression (Lonard & O'Malley B, 2007; McKenna & O'Malley, 2002; York & O'Malley, 2010).

Transcriptional coactivators regulate the expression of target genes by indirect binding to their target gene promoters and other *cis*-regulatory elements (such as enhancers and locus control regions) (Forsberg *et al.*, 1999; Li *et al.*,2002; McKenna *et al.*, 1999). Coactivators can bind transcription factors or RNA polymerase II influencing their activities, or help the recruitment of chromatin modifying enzymes, or act as chromatin modifiers themselves. In such ways, coactivators act as regulators in multiple processes, and are able to generate tissue-, cell- and promoter-specific effects (Gao *et al.*, 2002; Lonard & O'Malley B, 2007; Naar *et al.*, 2001; Perissi *et al.*, 2004). Despite the largenumber of estrogen receptor coactivators, in this chapter, we will focus only on two of them, WBP-2 (WW domain binding protein-2) and E6-AP (E6-associated protein) whose function in relation to ERα has been investigated in our laboratory.

It is of fundamental importance to fully understand the mechanism of action of ERα coregulators: the sequential and combinatorial assembly of transcription factors and coregulators at promoters allows indeed for fine-tuning of gene expression of the genes that are regulated by ERα. This step-wise knowledge of gene expression in cancer cells, not only contributes to our understanding of the basic mechanisms involved in ERα signaling, but could also provide new future points of intervention for therapeutic purposes. Our ultimate goal is indeed to employ the knowledge we acquire in the laboratory to ultimately prevent and/or treat breast cancer. It is the direct medical relevance of these fundamental questions that is our motivation to work in this area.

4   WBP-2[1]

One of the coactivators currently investigated in our laboratory is the protein WBP-2 (WW-domain binging protein 2). WBP-2has been identified as a binding partner of Yes kinase associated protein (YAP) (Chen & Sudol, 1995). YAP is a transcriptional regulator and a component of the so-called "Hippo pathway", important for regulation of cell growth, proliferation and tumorigenesis (Komuro *et al.*, 2003; Overholtzer *et al.*, 2006). The binding between WBP-2 and YAP occurs through interaction between WW-domains (two in YAP) and PPXY-motifs (three in WBP-2) (McDonald *et al.,* 2011). The WW-

---

[1] Details in the experimental procedures to obtain the data here reported are fully described in the cited primary publication.

domain is a small module that forms a binding pocket for the PPXY-motif; the name refers to two signature tryptophan (W) residues 20-22 amino acids apart in most of the WW-domains. The PPXY-motif (P, proline, X, any amino acid, Y, tyrosine) is a short motif located within a proline rich domain, and is the cognate ligand of WW-domains (Sudol, 1996; Sudol *et al.*, 1995; Sudol & Hunter, 2000) (Figure 3).

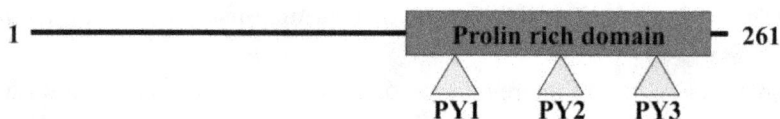

Figure 3: Schematic representation of WW-domain binding protein 2 (WBP-2). PY: PPXY motif.

Through a similar interaction, WBP-2 interacts with the following proteins: TAZ (transcriptional co-activator with PDZ-binding motif), similar to YAP and also a component of the Hippo pathway (Harvey & Tapon, 2007; Wang *et al.*, 2009); the tumor suppressor WW-domain containing oxidoreductase 1 (WWOX1) (Bednarek, *et al.*, 2000; Del Mare *et al.*, 2011); the ubiquitin-protein ligase Nedd4 (Jolliffe *et al.*, 2000). WBP-2 can also interact with proteins that do not contain WW-domains, as in the case of Pax8 (Paired box gene 8), a thyroid-specific transcription factor (Nitsch *et al.*, 2004), or E6-AP, an E3 ubiquitin ligase and a coactivator of ERα (Dhananjayan *et al.*, 2006). In this case the interaction does not require the PPXY motifs of WBP-2.

4.1   Molecular Mechanism of WBP-2 Action

Our laboratory has conducted important studies to understand the *in vivo* functions of WBP-2, with focus on ERα signaling. The first hint that WBP-2 could be involved in ERα action came from the finding that it interacts with E6-AP, which, as will be discussed later in detail, is by itself a coactivator for ERα (Dhananjayan *et al.*, 2006). To investigate the possibility that WBP-2 potentiatesERα transactivation function, we conducted luciferase reporter gene assays. In this *in vitro* assay cells are transfected with a plasmid in which the luciferase gene is under the control of an artificial promoter containing the binding sites for the general transcription machinery and multiple copies of the estrogen response element. Cells are also transfected with a plasmid encoding for the protein whose transcriptional effects are being studied. The analyzed protein acts as an ERα coactivator if, in presence of estrogen, it causes an increase in luciferase activity (measured through a luminometer) compared to the samples where the same protein is absent. Figure 4A shows that WBP-2 significantly enhances the hormone-dependent transcriptional activity of ERα.

We also explored the role of WBP-2 in regulating endogenous ERα target genes (Buffa *et al.*, 2012). For this purpose, we examined the effects of WBP-2 down regulation on ERα-mediated gene transcription using a breast cancer cells as a model. To determine if WBP-2 aidsERαfunction, we knocked down WBP-2expression in cells by RNA interference. This technique allows the downregulation of the product of specific genes within the cells, by transfecting small interfering RNA (siRNA), which are approximately 20 nucleotides long and are complimentary to a short stretch of the mRNA of the target gene. By exploiting a mechanism naturally existing in the cells, this leads to degradation of the target mRNA and consequent down regulation of the protein it codifies for.

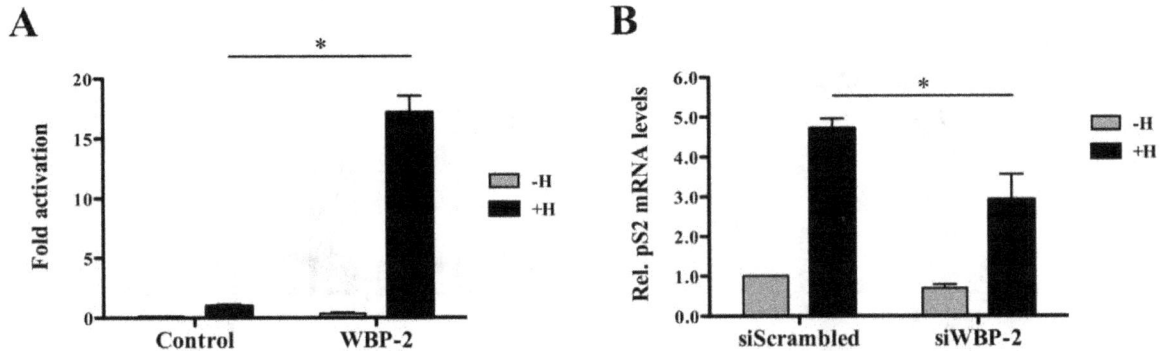

Figure 4: WBP-2 is a novel ERα coactivator. A: Luciferase reporter gene assay: HeLa cells were transfected with a plasmid expressing WBP-2 or a control plasmid, together with a luciferase reporter plasmid (see text for details). Later, cells were treated with either vehicle (-H) or estrogen (+H), harvested and assayed for luciferase activity. Data is plotted as fold induction. The activity in the presence of hormone and absence of WBP-2 serve as reference and is set as 1. Error bars are the standard deviation (STD) from 3 independent experiments. Student's t-test was used to calculate significant differences (*P<0.05) between the indicated datasets. B: MCF-7 cells were transfected with control (siScrambled) or siWBP-2 siRNAs. After 72 hours, cells were treated either with vehicle (-H) or estrogen (+H) for 12 hours and mRNA was isolated. pS2 mRNA levels was analyzed by qPCR. Results are normalized against 36B4 transcripts. Data is plotted as relative mRNA level, where vehicle-treated control siRNA transfected cells serve as the reference sample and are set as 1. Error bars are the STD from 3 independent experiments. Student's t-test was used to calculate significant differences (*P<0.05) between the indicated datasets.

We transfected cells either with WBP-2 specific siRNA (siWBP-2) or with control siRNA (called siScrambled) and, after estrogen starvation, we treated cells either with vehicle (-H) or with hormone (+H). Total mRNA was isolated and subjected to quantitative PCR (qPCR) focusing on the estrogen-regulated gene pS2, a widely used as a model gene to investigate ERα genomic functions (Barkhem et al., 2002) (Figure 4B). Notably, WBP-2 knockdown resulted in reduced mRNA levels of the ERα-target gene pS2, in the presence of hormone suggesting that WBP-2 is essential for ERα functions. This phenomenon appears to be gene specific, as similar results were obtained for the mRNA levels of GREB1 (growth regulation by estrogen in breast cancer 1) but not of PR (progesterone receptor), that are also well-studied ERα target genes.

To better understand WBP-2 function, we performed chromatin immunoprecipitation (ChIP) assays. This technique allows determiningif proteins or protein complexes are bound to specific DNA sequences. Proteins and associated DNA in the chromatin are first linked together; chromatin is then sheared in small fragments. Specific protein/DNA complexes are immunoprecipitated by incubating the sheared chromatin with an antibody (specific for the protein investigated). Finally theprecipitated DNA is purified and subjected to amplification (qPCR) with specific primers, in our case primer sets specific for the pS2 promoter, the gene we decided to focus on (Figure 5).

We found that WBP-2 binds to pS2 promoter upon estrogen treatment (Figure 5A), which agrees with the idea that WBP-2 is an ERα coactivator. Along with this, knockdown of WBP-2 resulted in reduced occupancy of the phosphorylated form of RNA polymerase II (pPol-II) at the same promoter. This modified form of RNA polymerase II is associated with a state of productive elongation of mRNA (Ahn

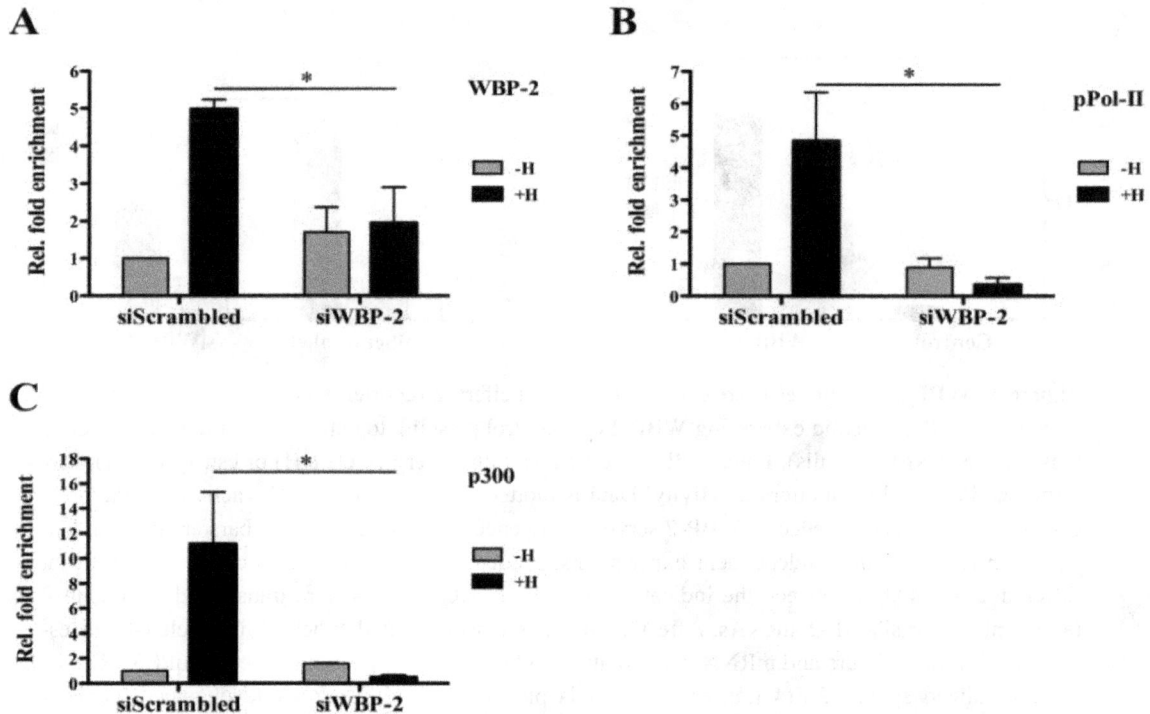

Figure 5: WBP-2 knockdown affects pPol-II and p300 recruitment at the pS2 promoter. MCF-7 cells were transfected with control (siScrambled) or siWBP-2 siRNAs. After 72 hours of estrogen starvation, cells were treated either with vehicle (-H) or estrogen (+H). Then, chromatin was prepared and subjected to chromatin. Antibodies used for IPs were specific for WBP-2 (A), pPol-II (B) or p300 (C); immunoprecipitated DNA was analyzed by qPCR. Data reported are a representative of three independent experiments. Data is plotted as relative fold enrichment, where (for a specified protein whose binding is being investigated) vehicle-treated control siRNA transfected cells serve as the reference sample and are set as 1. Data show mean and standard deviation of triplicates measurements within one experiment. Student's t-test was used to calculate significant differences (*P<0.05) between the indicated datasets.

et al., 2004; Kim*et al.*, 2004). Therefore WBP-2 is associated with active transcription of our model gene. Finally, in the search for a possible cause for decreased transcription at the pS2 promoter in the context of WBP-2 knockdown, we found that WBP-2 is required for the recruitment of the p300 (an enzyme that acetylate histones and protein complexes) to the pS2 promoter (Figure 5C): knockdown of WBP-2 is indeed associated with decreased recruitment of p300 to the pS2 promoter. This finding is critical, as p300 is a histone modifier enzyme that, upon histone acetylation, favors a relaxed chromatin structure, permissive of transcription (Chen & Li, 2011). We believe that WBP-2 helps transcription at some ERα target genes, by promoting the recruitment/stabilization of p300 at these promoters. Our findings have therefore shed important mechanistic insight into WBP-2 coactivation function in estrogen receptor signaling. They might also lay the basis for therapeutic intervention, in the event we develop a strategy for selectively blocking WBP-2 action and therefore potentiation of ERα signaling. This could be achieved by identifying small molecules-drugs capable of blocking/interfering with WBP-2 action. A particularly attractive possibility could also be the development of an RNA interference based intervention to knockdown

WBP-2 in living organisms. In this case, siRNAs specific for WBP-2 would be delivered, in specific cell-types (breast cells) through viral vectors. We hope that the understanding of the basic biology of WBP-2 function can contribute, in the not-so far future, to this kind of applications.

5   E6-AP[2]

Protein degradation allows for removal of unwanted or damaged proteins from the cell and is one of the means cellular processes are regulated. One of the ways proteins are degraded is through a complex multiprotein structure called proteasome. Proteins are tagged for proteasome degradation upon the addiction of a series of the small molecule ubiquitin. The tagging reaction is catalyzed by the successive action of three enzymes (E1 andE2-ubiquitin conjugating enzymes and E3 ubiquitin ligases) (Pickart, 2001).

Our laboratory and others have demonstrated that ERα degradation is an important aspect of its transcriptional action (Nawaz & O'Malley, 2004). More specifically, after ERα binds to its target gene promoters and regulates transcription, it is ubiquitinilated and targeted to degradation through the proteasome pathway (Dennis *et al.*, 2005; Rochette-Egly, 2005). ERα undergoes ubiquitination and degradation during each round of transcription. Clearance of ERα from target promoters is essential for sustained transcription: failure in its removal and degradation leads to inhibition of ERα transactivation functions (Nawaz & O'Malley, 2004). This phenomenon allows for the possibility of quick regulation in ERα transactivation function in response to variation in estrogen abundance.

Over the past 15 years our laboratory has extensively studied a critical player in ERα turnover: E6-associated protein (E6-AP). This protein was originally identified as an E3 ubiquitin protein ligase that interacts with the E6 protein of the human papilloma virus. The complex E6/E6-AP targets p53 for degradation through the proteasome (Hatakeyama *et al.*, 1997; Huibregtse*et al.*, 1993). Loss of a functional E6-AP is also associated the Angelman syndrome (Kishino *et al.*, 1997), a neuro-genetic disorder characterized by intellectual and developmental impairment, seizures, and frequent (inappropriate) laughter/smiling. The role of E6-AP in Angelman syndrome is beyond the scopeof this book chapter, and will therefore not be discussed here.

We have demonstrated that E6-AP is one of the E3 ubiquitin ligases important for ERα ubiquitinilation and degradation. The catalytic function of E6-AP resides in the carboxyl-terminal of the protein, within the so-calledhect domain (domain homologous to E6-AP carboxyl terminus). Its action is not limited to ERα; E6-AP is also involved in the degradation of other SHR as well, such as androgen receptor (AR) and progesterone receptor (PR) (Gao *et al.*, 2005).

5.1   Coactivation Function of E6-AP

Importantly, we have discovered that E6-AP also functions as a coactivator for several SHR, including ERα, PR and androgen receptor (Nawaz *et al.*, 1999). In luciferase reporter gene assays, we found that E6-AP enhances the transcriptional activity of multiple steroid hormone receptors. For example, in the presence of estrogen, E6-AP increases ERα-dependent transcription of approximately 3 fold (Figure 6). For this reason E6-AP has been defined as a dual function coactivators of steroid hormone receptors. We have also determined that the coactivator function of E6-AP is independent of its ligase function. Indeed,

---

[2] Details in the experimental procedures to obtain the data here reported are fully described in the cited primary publication.

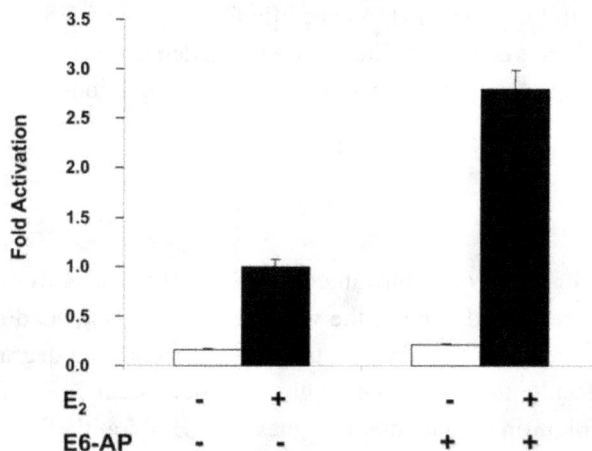

Figure 6: E6-AP is an ERα coactivator. Luciferase reporter gene assay: HeLa cells were transfected with a plasmid expressing E6-AP or a control plasmid, together with a luciferase reporter plasmid. Later, cells were treated with either vehicle (-H) or estrogen (+H), harvested and assayed for luciferase activity. Data is plotted as fold induction. The activity in the presence of hormone and absence of E6-AP serve as reference and is set as 1. Error bars are the standard deviation (STD) from 3 independent experiments. Student's t-test was used to calculate significant differences (*$P < 0.05$) between the indicated datasets.

in luciferase reporter gene assays with deletion mutants of E6-AP instead of the full-length protein, we found that loss of the E3 ligase activity (because of a mutation of the catalytic domain) is not accompanied by loss of its coactivation function (Nawaz *et al.*, 1999).

In studies similar to those described above for WBP-2, we have analyzed the molecular mechanism governing E6-AP transactivating function. Like WBP-2, E6-AP recruits p300 to some ERα target genes, favoring an open chromatin structure, permissive of transcription (Catoe & Nawaz, 2011). WBP-2 and E6-AP, which interact with each other, recruit the same histone modifying enzyme to the chromatin: this points to a macromolecular complex with at least four components: ERα, E6-AP, WBP-2 and p300. In this regard, E6-AP and WBP-2 function partially overlaps. Because knockdown of either of the two proteins is associated with a similar phenotype in cells, we believe that they can act independently in helping the recruitment/stabilization of p300 to gene promoters. We are currently investigating whether they act synergistically (potentiating each other), or interchangeably. A possibility is that in some physiological conditions only one of the two coactivators is required, while in other conditions both act to help ERα and maybe recruit some other protein(s) to promoters.

6   E6-AP and Breast Cancer

Because of E6-AP activity on ERα and PR, and considering the role of the latters in breast development, we decided to further dissect the role of E6-AP in mammary gland development (Ramamoorthy *et al.*, 2010). To this purpose, we generated transgenic mouse lines that either overexpressed wild type E6-AP (E6-AP^{WT}) or an ubiquitin ligase defective E6-AP (E6-AP^{C833S}) that cannot target ERα for degradation, and compared the development of the mammary glands in these mice with that of E6-AP knock-out mice (E6-AP^{KO}) (Figure 7).

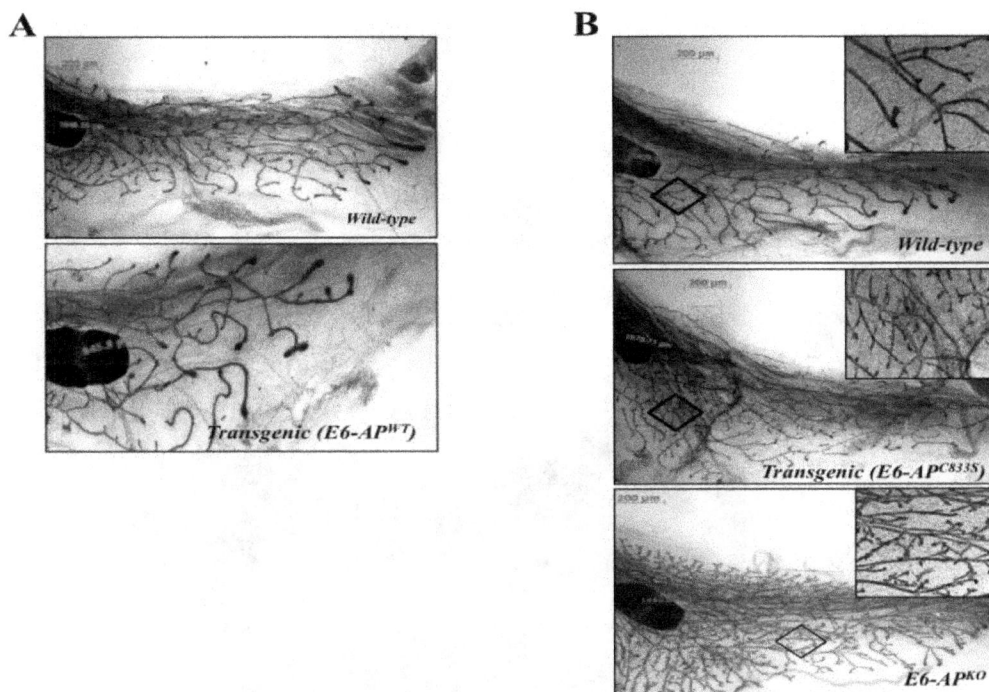

Figure 7: E6-AP is involved in mammary gland development. A: overexpression of E6-APWT results in impaired elongation and branching of mammary ducts. B: overexpression of E6-APC833S or lack of E6-AP result in increased elongation and branching of mammary ducts.

We assessed the branching of mammary glands by carmine alum staining of whole mammary glands, which were embedded in paraffin for sectioning. We found that overexpression of E6-AP^{WT} results in impaired mammary gland development (Figure 7A). On the contrary, overexpression of E6-AP^{C833S} results in increased branching and buds formation in the breast. The same phenotype was observed in E6-AP^{KO} mice (Figure 7B). Therefore, E6-AP, important for the degradation of ERα and PR, seems to counteract mammary gland development. In the same study, we actually demonstrated that the main role of E6-AP in mammary gland development is exerted through the degradation of PR, specifically of the isoform PR-B, which is a target of ERα.

To understand the significance of E6-AP in breast cancer, we also analyzed the expression profile of E6-AP in human breast cancers in two different studies (Gao *et al.*, 2005; Ramamoorthy *et al.*, 2012). We compared the expression of E6-AP in normal breast tissue, ductal carcinoma in situ (not invasive and that can be considered as an intermediate state in carcinoma development) and invasive ductal carcinoma. We found that the protein levels of E6-AP are decreased in invasive carcinoma, compared to normal tissue (Figure 8A). Our expression studies also reveal that the protein levels of ERα are inversely correlated with that ofE6-AP (Figure 8B). This result supports the idea that, by promoting ERα degradation, E6-AP has a negative role on breast cancer development and/or progression.

Furthermore, we examined the association between loss of E6-AP and survival in patients with breast cancer (Figure 8C): E6-AP negative patients had worse survival rate, if compared to E6-AP positive patients R. Therefore E6-AP can also be used as a predictive marker in breast cancer.

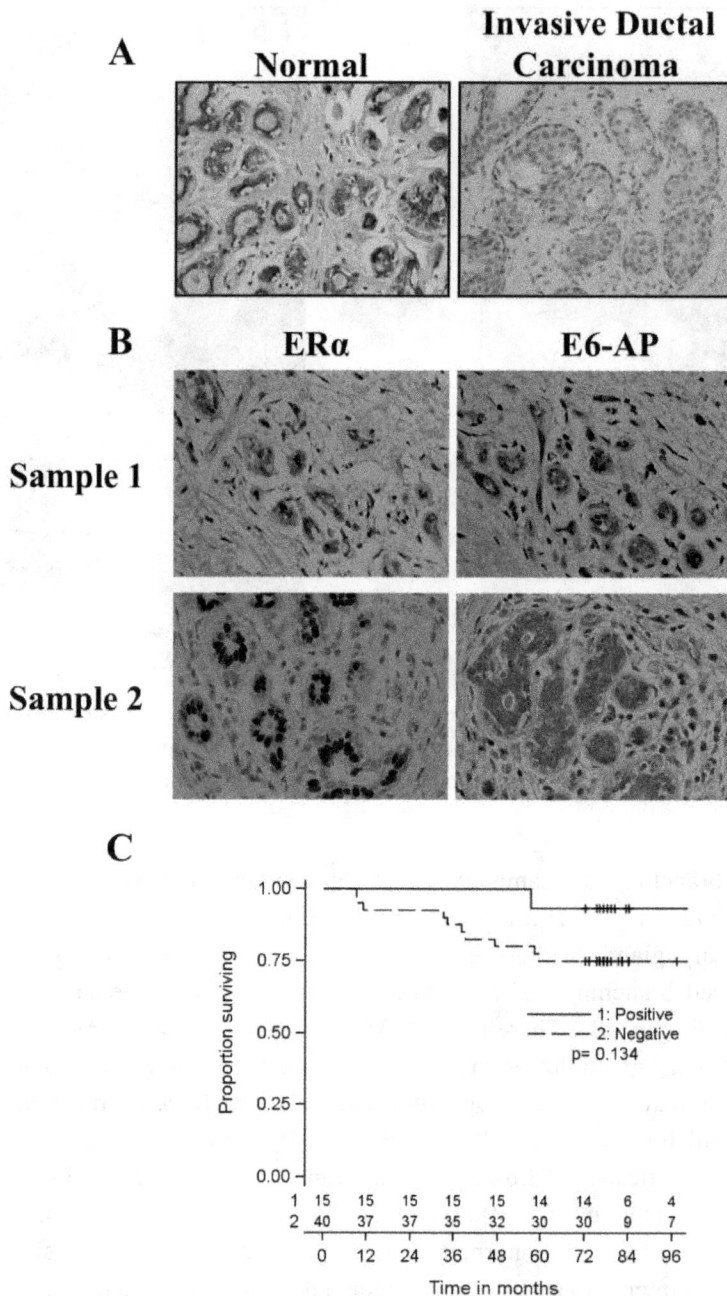

Figure 8: E6-AP expression in human carcinomas. A: Immunohistochemical analysis of E6-AP in normal and invasive ductal carcinomas. B: Immunohistochemical analysis of ERα and E6-AP in two different human breast carcinomas. C: Kaplan-Meier curve showing that E6-AP negative patients have worse survival pattern compared to E6-AP positive patients.

In conclusion, we found that E6-AP, a steroid hormone receptor coactivator, acts as a negative regulator of mammary gland development. This finding is somehow surprising. Because coactivators potentiate the transactivation function of steroid hormone receptors, and because these are positively involved in proliferation it would be expected that a coactivator induces or facilitates proliferation and mammary gland development. This is the case for other coactivators, like steroid receptor coactivator 3 (SRC3) and Cdc25 (Freedman, 1999). We believe this peculiarity is due to the fact that E6-AP is both a steroid hormone receptor coactivator and an E3 ubiquitin ligase. More specifically, we have evidence that, in the mammary gland, E6-AP acts mainly, if not exclusively, as an ubiquitin ligase, while its coactivation functions are, at least for this organ, negligible (Ramamoorthy et al., 2010).

6.1   Therapeutic Intervention

About 50-70 % of breast cancers are ERα positive and are therefore likely to respond well to endocrine therapy, which functions inhibiting estrogen production (aromatase inhibitors) or its action (tamoxifen and fulvestrant).

Approximately 25 % of all breast cancers are however ERα–negative. These tumors have a worst prognosis, and cannot be treated with hormonal therapy. Many laboratories, including ours, are exploiting the possibility of reversing the ERα–negative phenotype of breast cancers, in order to make them susceptible to hormonal therapies. We have evidence that at least in a subset of ERα–negative breast cancers, the messenger mRNA for ERα is actually expressed, even if the ERα protein is not detectable or low (Creighton et al., 2006; Iwao et al., 2000). This might indicate that some ERα–negative breast cancers appear so because of accelerated degradation of ERα. Furthermore, as discussed above, we have discovered that E6-AP is involved in the degradation of ERα through the proteasome.

If this is the case, E6-AP deregulation may play a role in ERα negativity by enhancing ERα degradation. Therefore, inhibition of the proteasome would lead to re-expression of ERα protein. The cancer, now ERα positive, can be targeted by hormonal therapies, such as tamoxifen. We are currently in the process of starting a clinical trial in which we plan to investigate the combined action of a proteasome inhibitor (bortezomib/Velcade) and of an antiestrogen (tamoxifen) in women with metastatic ERα negative breast cancer. Bortezomib is currently used for the treatment of several cancers, especially multiple myeloma. Clinical trials have investigated if bortezomib can also be effectively used in the treatment of metastatic breast cancer. However it seems this drug is not effective for breast cancer, at least if used as single agent (Yang, et al., 2006). We want to use bortezomib in combination with tamoxifen (Figure 9): we foresee that by allowing the conversion of breast cancers from ERα-negative to ERα-positive, we can effectively target them through conventional hormonal therapy. This would allow targeted therapeutic intervention in the treatment of, as of today, a very aggressive form of breast cancer, associated with poor prognosis.

Acknowledgments

The authors would like to acknowledge Jimmy El Hokayemfor critically reading the manuscript. This research was supported by the 1R01DK079217-01A2 grant from NIH to Zafar Nawaz.

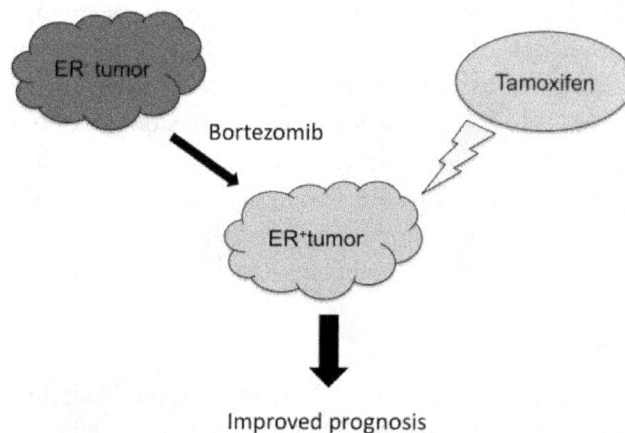

Figure 9: Schematic representation of the proposed clinical trial for woman with metastatic ERα negative breast cancer (see text for details).

References

Ahn, S. H., Kim, M., & Buratowski, S. (2004).Phosphorylation of serine 2 within the RNA polymerase II C-terminal domain couples transcription and 3' end processing. Mol Cell, 13(1), 67-76.

Bai, Z., & Gust, R. (2009).Breast cancer, estrogen receptor and ligands.Arch Pharm (Weinheim), 342(3), 133-149.

Barkhem, T., Haldosen, L. A., Gustafsson, J. A., & Nilsson, S. (2002). pS2 Gene expression in HepG2 cells: complex regulation through crosstalk between the estrogen receptor alpha, an estrogen-responsive element, and the activator protein 1 response element. Mol Pharmacol, 61(6), 1273-1283.

Bednarek, A. K., Laflin, K. J., Daniel, R. L., Liao, Q., Hawkins, K. A., & Aldaz, C. M. (2000). WWOX, a novel WW domain-containing protein mapping to human chromosome 16q23.3-24.1, a region frequently affected in breast cancer. Cancer Res, 60(8), 2140-2145.

Bell, O., Tiwari, V. K., Thoma, N. H., & Schubeler, D. (2011). Determinants and dynamics of genome accessibility. Nat Rev Genet, 12(8), 554-564.

Berger, S. L. (2007). The complex language of chromatin regulation during transcription. Nature, 447(7143), 407-412.

Bjornstrom, L., & Sjoberg, M. (2005). Mechanisms of estrogen receptor signaling: convergence of genomic and nongenomic actions on target genes. Mol Endocrinol, 19(4), 833-842.

Buffa, L., Saeed, A., & Nawaz, Z. (2012). Molecular mechanism of WW-domain Binding Protein 2 (WBP-2) coactivation function in estrogen receptor signaling. IUBMB Life, (In press).

Cabodi, S., Moro, L., Baj, G., Smeriglio, M., Di Stefano, P., Gippone, S., et al. (2004). p130Cas interacts with estrogen receptor alpha and modulates non-genomic estrogen signaling in breast cancer cells. J Cell Sci, 117(Pt 8), 1603-1611.

Carson-Jurica, M. A., Schrader, W. T., & O'Malley, B. W. (1990). Steroid receptor family: structure and functions. Endocr Rev, 11(2), 201-220.

Catoe, H. W., & Nawaz, Z. (2011). E6-AP facilitates efficient transcription at estrogen responsive promoters through recruitment of chromatin modifiers. Steroids, 76(9), 897-902.

Chen, H. I., & Sudol, M. (1995). The WW domain of Yes-associated protein binds a proline-rich ligand that differs from the consensus established for Src homology 3-binding modules, Proc Natl Acad Sci U S A92, 7819-7823.

Chen, J., & Li, Q. (2011). Life and death of transcriptional co-activator p300. Epigenetics, 6(8), 957-961.

Cohen, I., Poreba, E., Kamieniarz, K., & Schneider, R. (2011). Histone modifiers in cancer: friends or foes? Genes Cancer, 2(6), 631-647.

Creighton, C. J., Hilger, A. M., Murthy, S., Rae, J. M., Chinnaiyan, A. M., & El-Ashry, D. (2006). Activation of mitogen-activated protein kinase in estrogen receptor alpha-positive breast cancer cells in vitro induces an in vivo molecular phenotype of estrogen receptor alpha-negative human breast tumors. Cancer Res, 66(7), 3903-3911.

Dahlman-Wright, K., Cavailles, V., Fuqua, S. A., Jordan, V. C., Katzenellenbogen, J. A., Korach, K. S., et al. (2006). International Union of Pharmacology. LXIV. Estrogen receptors. Pharmacol Rev, 58(4), 773-781.

Del Mare, S., Kurek, K. C., Stein, G. S., Lian, J. B., & Aqeilan, R. I. (2011). Role of the WWOX tumor suppressor gene in bone homeostasis and the pathogenesis of osteosarcoma. Am J Cancer Res, 1(5), 585-594.

Dennis, A. P., Lonard, D. M., Nawaz, Z., & O'Malley, B. W. (2005). Inhibition of the 26S proteasome blocks progesterone receptor-dependent transcription through failed recruitment of RNA polymerase II. J Steroid Biochem Mol Biol, 94(4), 337-346.

Deroo, B. J., & Korach, K. S. (2006). Estrogen receptors and human disease. J Clin Invest, 116(3), 561-570.

Dhananjayan, S. C., Ramamoorthy, S., Khan, O. Y., Ismail, A., Sun, J., Slingerland, J., et al. (2006). WW domain binding protein-2, an E6-associated protein interacting protein, acts as a coactivator of estrogen and progesterone receptors. Mol Endocrinol, 20(10), 2343-2354.

Edwards, D. P. (2005). Regulation of signal transduction pathways by estrogen and progesterone. Annu Rev Physiol, 67, 335-376.

Forsberg, E. C., Johnson, K., Zaboikina, T. N., Mosser, E. A., & Bresnick, E. H. (1999). Requirement of an E1A-sensitive coactivator for long-range transactivation by the beta-globin locus control region. J Biol Chem, 274(38), 26850-26859.

Freedman, L. P. (1999). Increasing the complexity of coactivation in nuclear receptor signaling. Cell, 97(1), 5-8.

Fuda, N. J., Ardehali, M. B., & Lis, J. T. (2009). Defining mechanisms that regulate RNA polymerase II transcription in vivo. Nature, 461(7261), 186-192.

Gao, X., Loggie, B. W., & Nawaz, Z. (2002). The roles of sex steroid receptor coregulators in cancer. Mol Cancer, 1, 7.

Gao, X., Mohsin, S. K., Gatalica, Z., Fu, G., Sharma, P., & Nawaz, Z. (2005). Decreased expression of e6-associated protein in breast and prostate carcinomas. Endocrinology, 146(4), 1707-1712.

Greene, G. L., Sobel, N. B., King, W. J., & Jensen, E. V. (1984). Immunochemical studies of estrogen receptors. J Steroid Biochem, 20(1), 51-56.

Guenther, M. G., Levine, S. S., Boyer, L. A., Jaenisch, R., & Young, R. A. (2007). A chromatin landmark and transcription initiation at most promoters in human cells. Cell, 130(1), 77-88.

Harvey, K., & Tapon, N. (2007). The Salvador-Warts-Hippo pathway - an emerging tumour-suppressor network. Nat Rev Cancer, 7(3), 182-191.

Hatakeyama, S., Jensen, J. P., & Weissman, A. M. (1997). Subcellular localization and ubiquitin-conjugating enzyme (E2) interactions of mammalian HECT family ubiquitin protein ligases. J Biol Chem, 272(24), 15085-15092.

Huibregtse, J. M., Scheffner, M., & Howley, P. M. (1993). Cloning and expression of the cDNA for E6-AP, a protein that mediates the interaction of the human papillomavirus E6 oncoprotein with p53. Mol Cell Biol, 13(2), 775-784.

Iwao, K., Miyoshi, Y., Egawa, C., Ikeda, N., & Noguchi, S. (2000). Quantitative analysis of estrogen receptor-beta mRNA and its variants in human breast cancers. Int J Cancer, 88(5), 733-736.

Jenuwein, T., & Allis, C. D. (2001). Translating the histone code. Science, 293(5532), 1074-1080.

Jolliffe, C. N., Harvey, K. F., Haines, B. P., Parasivam, G., & Kumar, S. (2000). Identification of multiple proteins expressed in murine embryos as binding partners for the WW domains of the ubiquitin-protein ligase Nedd4. Biochem J, 351 Pt 3, 557-565.

Kim, M., Ahn, S. H., Krogan, N. J., Greenblatt, J. F., & Buratowski, S. (2004). Transitions in RNA polymerase II elongation complexes at the 3' ends of genes. EMBO J, 23(2), 354-364.

Kishino, T., Lalande, M., & Wagstaff, J. (1997). UBE3A/E6-AP mutations cause Angelman syndrome. Nat Genet, 15(1), 70-73.

Komuro, A., Nagai, M., Navin, N. E., & Sudol, M. (2003). WW domain-containing protein YAP associates with ErbB-4 and acts as a co-transcriptional activator for the carboxyl-terminal fragment of ErbB-4 that translocates to the nucleus. J Biol Chem, 278(35), 33334-33341.

Kouzarides, T. (2007). Chromatin modifications and their function. Cell, 128(4), 693-705.

Leader, J. E., Wang, C., Popov, V. M., Fu, M., & Pestell, R. G. (2006). Epigenetics and the estrogen receptor. Ann N Y Acad Sci, 1089, 73-87.

Levin, E. R. (2001). Cell localization, physiology, and nongenomic actions of estrogen receptors. J Appl Physiol, 91(4), 1860-1867.

Li, Q., Peterson, K. R., Fang, X., & Stamatoyannopoulos, G. (2002). Locus control regions. Blood, 100(9), 3077-3086.

Lonard, D. M., & O'Malley B, W. (2007). Nuclear receptor coregulators: judges, juries, and executioners of cellular regulation. Mol Cell, 27(5), 691-700.

Ludes-Meyers, J. H., Kil, H., Bednarek, A. K., Drake, J., Bedford, M. T., & Aldaz, C. M. (2004). WWOX binds the specific proline-rich ligand PPXY: identification of candidate interacting proteins. Oncogene, 23(29), 5049-5055.

Mangelsdorf, D. J., Thummel, C., Beato, M., Herrlich, P., Schutz, G., Umesono, K., et al. (1995). The nuclear receptor superfamily: the second decade. Cell, 83(6), 835-839.

McDonald, C. B., McIntosh, S. K., Mikles, D. C., Bhat, V., Deegan, B. J., Seldeen, K. L., et al. (2011). Biophysical analysis of binding of WW domains of the YAP2 transcriptional regulator to PPXY motifs within WBP1 and WBP2 adaptors. Biochemistry, 50(44), 9616-9627.

McKenna, N. J., Lanz, R. B., & O'Malley, B. W. (1999). Nuclear receptor coregulators: cellular and molecular biology. Endocr Rev, 20(3), 321-344.

McKenna, N. J., & O'Malley, B. W. (2002). Combinatorial control of gene expression by nuclear receptors and coregulators. Cell, 108(4), 465-474.

Mosselman, S., Polman, J., & Dijkema, R. (1996). ER beta: identification and characterization of a novel human estrogen receptor. FEBS Lett, 392(1), 49-53.

Naar, A. M., Lemon, B. D., & Tjian, R. (2001). Transcriptional coactivator complexes. Annu Rev Biochem, 70, 475-501.

Nawaz, Z., Lonard, D. M., Smith, C. L., Lev-Lehman, E., Tsai, S. Y., Tsai, M. J., et al. (1999). The Angelman syndrome-associated protein, E6-AP, is a coactivator for the nuclear hormone receptor superfamily. Mol Cell Biol, 19(2), 1182-1189.

Nawaz, Z., & O'Malley, B. W. (2004). Urban renewal in the nucleus: is protein turnover by proteasomes absolutely required for nuclear receptor-regulated transcription? Mol Endocrinol, 18(3), 493-499.

Nilsson, S., Makela, S., Treuter, E., Tujague, M., Thomsen, J., Andersson, G., et al. (2001). Mechanisms of estrogen action. Physiol Rev, 81(4), 1535-1565.

Nitsch, R., Di Palma, T., Mascia, A., & Zannini, M. (2004). WBP-2, a WW domain binding protein, interacts with the thyroid-specific transcription factor Pax8. Biochem J, 377(Pt 3), 553-560.

Novac, N., & Heinzel, T. (2004). Nuclear receptors: overview and classification. Curr Drug Targets Inflamm Allergy, 3(4), 335-346.

Overholtzer, M., Zhang, J., Smolen, G. A., Muir, B., Li, W., Sgroi, D. C., et al. (2006). Transforming properties of YAP, a candidate oncogene on the chromosome 11q22 amplicon. Proc Natl Acad Sci U S A, 103(33), 12405-12410.

Pan, Y., Tsai, C. J., Ma, B., & Nussinov, R. (2009). How do transcription factors select specific binding sites in the genome? Nat Struct Mol Biol, 16(11), 1118-1120.

Pan, Y., Tsai, C. J., Ma, B., & Nussinov, R. (2010). Mechanisms of transcription factor selectivity. Trends Genet, 26(2), 75-83.

Pedram, A., Razandi, M., Aitkenhead, M., Hughes, C. C., & Levin, E. R. (2002). Integration of the non-genomic and genomic actions of estrogen. Membrane-initiated signaling by steroid to transcription and cell biology. J Biol Chem, 277(52), 50768-50775.

Perissi, V., Aggarwal, A., Glass, C. K., Rose, D. W., & Rosenfeld, M. G. (2004). A corepressor/coactivator exchange complex required for transcriptional activation by nuclear receptors and other regulated transcription factors. Cell, 116(4), 511-526.

Pickart, C. M. (2001). Mechanisms underlying ubiquitination. Annu Rev Biochem, 70, 503-533.

Ramamoorthy, S., Dhananjayan, S. C., Demayo, F. J., & Nawaz, Z. (2010). Isoform-specific degradation of PR-B by E6-AP is critical for normal mammary gland development. Mol Endocrinol, 24(11), 2099-2113.

Ramamoorthy, S., Tufail, R., Hokayem, J. E., Jorda, M., Zhao, W., Reis, Z., et al. (2012). Overexpression of ligase defective E6-associated protein, E6-AP, results in mammary tumorigenesis. Breast Cancer Res Treat, 132(1), 97-108.

Rochette-Egly, C. (2005). Dynamic combinatorial networks in nuclear receptor-mediated transcription. J Biol Chem, 280(38), 32565-32568.

Sommer, S., & Fuqua, S. A. (2001). Estrogen receptor and breast cancer. Semin Cancer Biol, 11(5), 339-352.

Sudol, M. (1996). Structure and function of the WW domain. Prog Biophys Mol Biol, 65(1-2), 113-132.

Sudol, M., Chen, H. I., Bougeret, C., Einbond, A., & Bork, P. (1995). Characterization of a novel protein-binding module--the WW domain. FEBS Lett, 369(1), 67-71.

Sudol, M., & Hunter, T. (2000). NeW wrinkles for an old domain. Cell, 103(7), 1001-1004.

Wang, K., Degerny, C., Xu, M., & Yang, X. J. (2009). YAP, TAZ, and Yorkie: a conserved family of signal-responsive transcriptional coregulators in animal development and human disease. Biochem Cell Biol, 87(1), 77-91.

Yager, J. D. (2000). Endogenous estrogens as carcinogens through metabolic activation. J Natl Cancer Inst Monogr(27), 67-73.

Yang, C. H., Gonzalez-Angulo, A. M., Reuben, J. M., Booser, D. J., Pusztai, L., Krishnamurthy, S., et al. (2006). Bortezomib (VELCADE) in metastatic breast cancer: pharmacodynamics, biological effects, and prediction of clinical benefits. Ann Oncol, 17(5), 813-817.

York, B., & O'Malley, B. W. (2010). Steroid receptor coactivator (SRC) family: masters of systems biology. J Biol Chem, 285(50), 38743-38750.

Zaret, K. S., & Carroll, J. S. (2011). Pioneer transcription factors: establishing competence for gene expression. Genes Dev, 25(21), 2227-2241.

Angiotensin II in Breast Cancer Metastasis: Strategy, Tools and Models Towards New Cancer Therapies

Clara Nahmias
Inserm, U1016, Institut Cochin, Paris, France
Cnrs, UMR8104, Paris, France
Université Paris Descartes, Sorbonne Paris Cité, France
INSERM, U981, Gustave Roussy, Villejuif, France

Sylvie Rodrigues-Ferreira
Inserm, U1016, Institut Cochin, Paris, France
Cnrs, UMR8104, Paris, France
Université Paris Descartes, Sorbonne Paris Cité, France
INSERM, U981, Gustave Roussy, Villejuif, France

1   Introduction

Breast cancer is the most frequent cause of death by malignancy among women in developing countries, and the occurrence of distant metastasis is a critical event that limits the survival of patients with breast cancer. While targeted molecular therapies have considerably improved the management of primary breast tumors, these remain poorly effective for the treatment of distant metastases. The identification of molecular agents that may contribute to breast cancer cell dissemination and colonization is therefore essential for future development of new anti-metastatic therapeutic strategies.

In this chapter, we will describe the processes of breast cancer development and progression. We will next focus on Angiotensin II (AngII) as a novel interesting target against metastatic breast tumors. Finally we will present models and strategies to investigate AngII functions in experimental breast cancer metastasis.

1.1   Breast Cancer General Features

Breast cancer is the most common cancer among women affecting more than 1 million women worldwide. Each year, more than 450,000 patients die due to the disease (Jemal *et al.*, 2011). Breast cancer is not a single disease. There are indeed several types of breast tumors that have diverse histopathology, genetic and genomic variations, and clinical outcomes (Vargo-Gogola and Rosen, 2007).

Multiple subgroups of tumors with different molecular signatures, prognosis and response to therapies have been identified. Currently, breast tumors can be classified into three major molecular subtypes associated with differences in therapy and clinical outcome (Sorlie *et al.*, 2001; Higgins & Basselga, 2011):

- Luminal, or estrogen receptor positive tumors (ER+), are characterized by expression of estrogen receptor ER and progesterone receptor PR. This subtype concerns 70-80% of breast tumors and benefits from efficient hormonal therapy such as Tamoxifen or Aromatase inhibitors.

- HER2 (Human Epidermal growth factor Receptor 2) tumors are characterized by amplification of the ErbB2/HER2 oncogene and represent 10-15% of the tumors. Patients are treated with specific therapy targeting HER2 with monoclonal antibodies like Trastuzumab/Herceptin®.

- Triple negative tumors, that do express neither hormone receptors (ER, PR) nor HER2, belong to a heterogeneous molecular subtype which is the most aggressive, being highly proliferative and metastatic. Triple negative tumors represent only 10-15% of tumors but are responsible for 25% of deaths by breast cancer. Patients with triple negative breast tumors do not benefit from targeted therapy and remain of poor prognosis.

1.2   Breast Cancer Development and Progression

Breast cancer develops within epithelial cells of lobules and ducts of the breast. The transformation of breast epithelial cells is a combination of epigenetic and genetics changes. During this multistage process, control of proliferation and survival becomes deregulated allowing the emergence of breast tumors. As the tumor grows, the need in oxygen and nutrients increases and the center of the tumor becomes inaccessible to peripheral blood vessels, and thus hypoxic. Hypoxia activates neoangiogenesis necessary for tumor growth and progression. In highly aggressive tumors, some cells with metastatic properties initiate the metastatic program by detaching from the primary tumor, invading and migrating through the surrounding matrix stroma until reaching the blood flow by intravasation. This is quite an efficient step since most of the disseminated metastatic cells succeed in reaching the circulation. However, metastasis remains an inefficient process (Luzzi *et al.*, 1998). Among the large number of cancer cells that detach from the primary tumor and invade adjacent tissues to reach the bloodstream, most remain quiescent or die in the circulation. Few circulating tumor cells are able to cross the blood barrier and migrate toward distant organs to grow as a metastasis (Chambers *et al.*, 2002) (Figure 1). Metastasis is thus initiated by cancer cell dissemination, but extravasation and colonization remain the critical steps of the whole process.

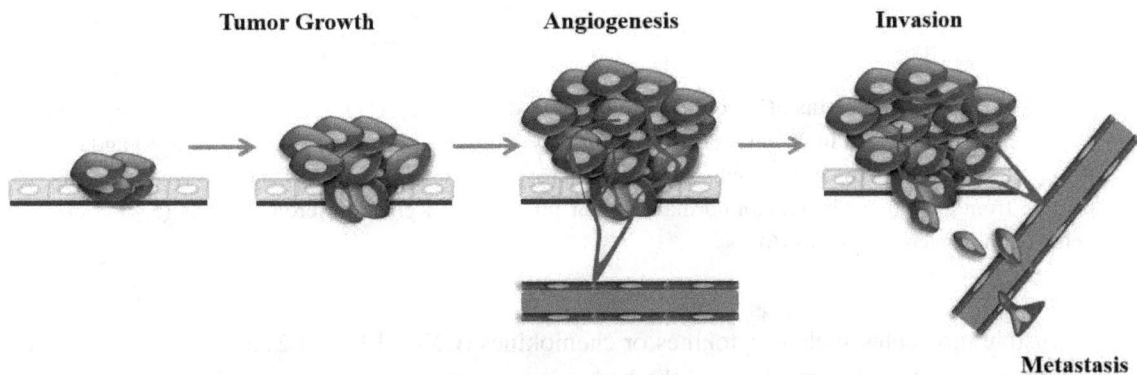

Figure 1: Scheme of tumor progression: Shown are the 4 majors steps of tumor progression namely growth, angiogenesis, invasion and metastasis. Blue cells represent epithelial cells over basement matrix (blue line); brown cells represent tumor cells; red cells are for endothelial cells.

1.3   Breast Cancer Metastasis: A Complex and Fatal Disease

Patients with metastatic breast cancer receive chemotherapy, but most of the time patients suffer from treatment resistance and recurrence of the disease. There is an urgent need to identify molecular factors of breast cancer cell dissemination and colonization in order to develop new anti-metastatic therapeutic options.

Networks of genes altered in primary tumors have been shown to contribute to the metastatic path, leading to the notion of "metastasis gene signatures" (Nguyen *et al.*, 2009). Among them, genes with pleiotropic effects that control both early and late stages of metastasis were classified as "metastasis progression genes" (Nguyen & Massagué, 2007) and are of high interest for novel efficient therapies against cancer metastasis. In addition to intrinsic metastasis gene signatures that predict the ability of tumor cells to colonize distant tissues, close interactions between circulating tumor cells and the host microenvironment are critical to the establishment of cancer cells at secondary sites (Fidler, 2003; Joyce & Pollard, 2009). Adaptative cancer cells can either proliferate to give rise to a micrometastasis, or remain latent in a dormant state. Reactivation of dormant cancer cells allows them to develop into a macrometastasis (Joyce & Pollard, 2009; Shibue & Weinberg, 2011). Breast cancer progression and metastasis strongly depend on the selection of adapted cancer cells and their close interactions with the stromal microenvironment (Figure 2).

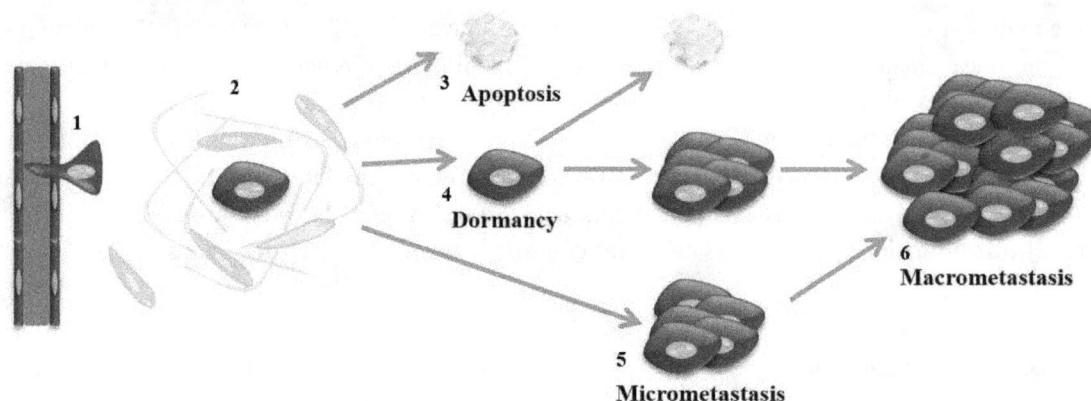

Figure 2: Scheme of metastatic colonization: After extravasation (1), metastatic cancer cells (in brown) migrate and seed in the target organ where they interact with stromal cells (in yellow) and extracellular matrix (yellow curves) present in the microenvironment (2). At this stage, metastatic cells can die from apoptosis (3), remain dormant (4), or proliferate to give a micrometastasis (5) that develops into a macrometastasis (6).

Diffusible molecules such as cytokines or chemokines (CXCL12, CCL2) are key factors in the interplay between metastatic tumor cells and the host microenvironment, and play a decisive role in breast cancer metastasis (Muller *et al.*, 2001; Qian *et al.*, 2011). We have hypothesized that other small molecules such as vasoactive peptides (Angiotensins, Endothelins or Bradykinins), either produced locally or released in the blood flow, may trigger activating signals contributing in an autocrine or paracrine way to cancer cell extravasation, colonization and metastasis (Rodrigues-Ferreira *et al.*, 2012a). In this review, we will present our recent studies investigating the effects of angiotensin II on breast cancer metastasis.

2   Angiotensin II as a New Potential Therapeutic Target

2.1   Angiotensin II and the Renin-angiotensin System

Angiotensin II (AngII) has been initially identified as the major biologically active peptide of the renin-angiotensin system (RAS), but it is now well established that other peptides derived from the RAS, namely Ang1-7, AngIII and AngIV, also display biological activities (Wright & Harding, 1997; Crowley & Coffman, 2012 ; *Santos et al.*, 2012). All angiotensin peptides derive from a unique precursor, angiotensinogen (AGT), synthesized and released from the liver. In response to blood changes (such as decrease in blood pressure or plasma sodium level), the kidneys produce and release the renin protease which cleaves AGT into a decapeptide designated Angiotensin I (AngI). AngI is in turn cleaved by Angiotensin Converting Enzyme (ACE) to produce the octapeptide AngII. AngII can then be processed by either the Angiotensin Converting Enzyme 2 (ACE2) to produce Ang1-7, or by aminopeptidase A and N to produce AngIII and AngIV, respectively (George *et al.*, 2010; Crowley & Coffman, 2012) (Figure 3). Angiotensin peptides, and in particular AngII, are produced in the plasma but also in several organs where a local RAS is active (Paul *et al.*, 2006). Interestingly, angiotensin peptides exert diverse biological effects, such as vasoconstriction/vasodilatation, inflammation, proliferation and apoptosis, through binding to different receptors, namely AT1R, AT2R, AT4R and MAS-R (Santos *et al.*, 2012; George *et al.*, 2010) (Figure 3).

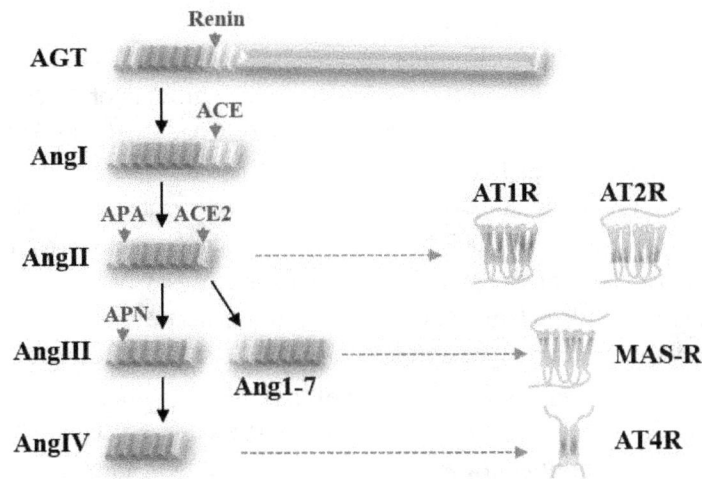

Figure 3: The Renin-Angiotensin system: Shown are the RAS peptides. Each enzyme is indicated in red and cleavage sites are indicated by an arrow head. Corresponding Angiotensin peptide receptors are indicated by dashed lines. AGT: Angiotensinogen; Ang: Angiotensin; ACE: Angiotensin converting enzyme, APA Aminopeptidase A, APN: Aminopeptidase N.

Both AngII and its cleavage product Ang1-7 have been shown to contribute to cancer processes, by different mechanisms. Studies reporting an effect of Ang1-7 acting though the MAS receptor have been recently reviewed (Santos *et al.*, 2012) and their role in cancer have first been described by Tallant's group (Gallagher *et al.*, 2004, 2011; Soto-Pantoja *et al.*, 2009). In this chapter, we will mainly focus on the effects of AngII in cancer progression.

2.2 AngII and Cancer

AngII is a major regulator of blood pressure and cardiovascular homeostasis, acting through activation of specific receptors AT1R and AT2R. These two subtypes of receptors belong to the superfamily of G-protein-coupled receptors, but have distinct distribution and intracellular signaling pathways (Nouet & Nahmias, 2000). Most of AngII actions involve the AT1R whereas AT2R often functions as a negative regulator of the AT1 subtype. Activation of the AT1 receptor triggers a large number of intracellular effectors leading to modulation of various cell processes, among which proliferation, migration, angiogenesis and inflammation, which are closely associated with tumor progression (Deshayes & Nahmias, 2005).

Strategies to investigate AngII functions in cancer include either blockade of AngII production with ACE inhibitors, or inhibition of AngII signaling pathways with Angiotensin receptor blockers (ARBs) (Deshayes & Nahmias, 2005). Of note, these drugs are widely used in the clinics to efficiently treat hypertensive patients. A retrospective cohort study performed by Lever and co-workers aimed to assess the risk of cancer in hypertensive patients receiving ACE inhibitors or other antihypertensive drugs. They showed that long-term use of ACE inhibitors may protect against cancer (Lever *et al.*, 1998). In an independent study of 1051 cases, users of ACE inhibitors or ARBs were shown to have significantly reduced risks in developing basal and squamous cell carcinomas (Christian *et al.*, 2008). These findings have been challenged by a recent meta-analysis that suggested that ARBs medication may be associated with a modest increase in cancer risk (Sipahi *et al.*, 2010). However, these results have not been further validated by other groups, which rather found no effect of ARBs related to the risk of cancer (Bangalore *et al.*, 2011; Connolly *et al.*, 2011). These results might reflect the heterogeneity of patient cases included in the studies. Regarding breast cancer, the use of ACE inhibitors or ARBs has not been associated with breast cancer risk (Li *et al.*, 2003; Fryzek *et al.*, 2006; Chae *et al.*, 2013; Sørensen *et al.*, 2013), but with significant reduction of breast cancer recurrence (Chae *et al.*, 2011). Furthermore, attempts to correlate RAS polymorphism with breast cancer risk have not been conclusive and require further investigation (Gonzalez-Zuloeta Ladd *et al.*, 2007; Xi *et al* 2011). Whether angiotensin receptors variation or blockade has beneficial effects in cancer patients still remains a matter of debate. This question needs to be better explored in distinct subpopulations of tumors classified according to histological, molecular and clinical characteristics, and according to the expression of different RAS components.

In breast tumors, most components of the classical RAS including angiotensinogen, angiotensin converting enzyme and angiotensin receptors are locally expressed (De Paepe *et al.*, 2001; Tahmasebi *et al.*, 2006; Herr *et al.*, 2008; Inwang *et al.*, 1997; George *et al.*, 2010). Interestingly, a large-scale meta-analysis performed on 31 breast cancer profiling datasets has revealed overexpression of AT1 receptor in 10-20% of invasive breast tumors (Rhodes *et al.*, 2009). Such studies highlight the potential use of ARBs as novel therapeutic agents against a subpopulation of breast cancer.

ARBs and ACE inhibitors have been assayed both in cancer cells and in mouse experimental models to characterize AngII functions in tumor growth, angiogenesis and metastasis. It is well established that AT1 receptor activation by AngII induces cell proliferation in several cell types including cancer cells (Deshayes & Nahmias, 2005). In agreement, ARBs such as losartan or candesartan were shown to inhibit cell proliferation *in vitro* and tumor growth in mice xenografts (Chen *et al.*, 2012). Tumor growth reduction in response to ARBs is associated with reduced tumor vascularization (Fujita *et al.*, 2002 and 2005), which is essential to the progression of primary tumors as well as initiation of metastasis.

Local production of AngII was shown to facilitate tumor progression and lymph node metastasis (Carl-McGrath *et al.*, 2007; Kinoshita *et al.*, 2009). Evidence for a role of AT1 receptor on cancer cell metastasis came from *in vivo* studies of lung models of metastasis. Cancer cells were injected into the tail vein of mice perfused with the ARB Candesartan. Inhibiting AngII signalling strongly reduced lung metastasis (Miyajima *et al.*, 2002; Fujita *et al.*, 2005), although it was not clear whether ARBs were acting on tumor cells or on the stromal microenvironment. The role of AT1R in the tumor microenvironment has been investigated by comparing the growth and the vascularization of tumors injected subcutaneously into wild type (WT) or AT1R knockout mice (Egami *et al.*, 2003; Fujita *et al.*, 2005; Imai *et al.*, 2007). Tumor growth and tumor-associated angiogenesis were strongly reduced in AT1R null mice indicating that the AT1R of host cells contributes to both tumor growth and angiogenesis. Of interest, the results show that AT1R-dependent tumor growth requires tumor angiogenesis that is promoted by AT1R-induced VEGF synthesis, a well known angiogenic factor. Furthermore, AT1R is highly expressed in the stromal tissue surrounding the tumors, in particular in tumor-associated macrophages TAMs. Macrophage infiltration, as well as levels of TAMs-released VEGF, was strongly reduced in AT1R null mice, supporting the hypothesis that host AT1R might also participate in inflammation-related tumor angiogenesis to maintain tumor growth (Egami *et al.*, 2003; Fujita *et al.*, 2005; Deshayes & Nahmias, 2005).

A remaining question is whether AngII produced locally may also directly act on tumor cells to promote tumor growth and metastasis.

3   Experimental Models to Study AngII and its Receptors in Breast Cancer Metastasis

3.1   Experimental Mouse Models of Metastasis

"Classical metastasis" experiments are performed by orthotopic injection of cancer cells that are allowed to grow and spontaneously form metastases. This model recapitulates all steps of cancer metastasis from primary tumor dissemination to distant organ colonization and constitutes the most relevant model of metastasis, but kinetics are very long and results are hardly reproducible due to variation of mouse response.

An alternative model of metastasis consists in injection of cancer cells directly in the blood flow. This model recapitulates the late rate-limiting steps of the metastatic process, i.e. extravasation and colonization. Cancer cells can be inoculated either by tail vein injection, in the case of lung metastasis experiments, or by intracardiac injection to promote the dissemination of cancer cells throughout the whole body including the lungs, bones and brain which are the major sites of breast metastases.

With no labelling of cancer cells, metastases can only be detected by histological or Polymerase Chain Reaction (PCR) analysis of selected tissues at the end of the experiment, which makes it difficult to monitor the establishment of metastatic foci in bones and soft organs. To follow and identify tumor cells in the whole organism, we used breast cancer cells stably expressing high levels of luciferase. Luciferase is an enzyme that reacts with its substrate luciferin to generate a photon. The number of photons released is proportional to the number of cancer cells. Bioluminescence is a powerful alternative to fluorescence labelling which is of weak sensitivity due to its high signal-to-noise ratio. Major limitation remains poor spatial resolution, light scattering and absorption by the tissue, although partially circumvent by three-dimensional imaging. Thus Bioluminescence Imaging (BLI) allows noninvasive real time follow up of tumor growth and metastasis formation at distant site in living mouse.

3.2   Model to Target AngII in Breast Cancer Cells Metastasis

To investigate the role of AngII on breast cancer metastasis, and address the question of whether locally produced AngII may act directly on tumor cells to promote tumor progression, we used the D3H2LN subline derived from the metastatic and triple negative breast cancer cells MDA-MB-231, expressing high levels of luciferase (Jenkins et al., 2005). D3H2LN cells are of particular interest for the study of breast cancer cell progression both *in vitro* and *in vivo* since they are highly invasive and metastatic. After intracardiac injection into nude mice, these cells rapidly disseminate and colonize distant organs including the brain, the lungs and the bones (Jenkins et al., 2005).

In our experiments, D3H2LN cells were exposed for 24 hrs to 100nM of AngII *in vitro*, before being injected intra-cardiacally into the bloodstream of nude mice (Rodrigues-Ferreira et al., 2012a). Such strategy allowed us to evaluate the effects of AngII on cancer cells while avoiding any direct effect of the peptide on the host microenvironment. Injection efficiency was monitored immediately after intra-cardiac injection by acquisition of luminescence in whole mice. Injection was considered successful when cancer cells propagated though the left ventricle reached the blood flow and labeled the whole animal (Figure 4). Only mice with successful injection were included in the study.

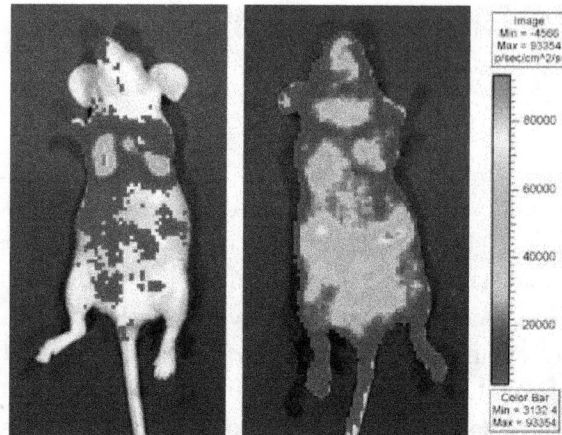

Figure 4: Bioluminescence imaging of nude mice at T0 after intracardiac injection of 100,000 D3H2LN cells. Left picture shows a failed injection where tumor cells achieve pulmonary artery instead of the systemic circulation and then remained in the lungs. Picture on the right shows a successful intracardiac injection with a widespread distribution of bioluminescent D3H2LN cells throughout the entire animal.

The establishment of tumor micrometastases in various organs was then evaluated by intravital bioluminescent imaging. Nineteen days after intracardiac injection all mice harbored metastases confirming high aggressiveness of the D3H2LN cell line. However, tumor cells exposed to AngII acquired a more aggressive behavior since at least one metastasis was already detectable in 86% of mice at day 9 as compared to only 40% for control mice, without any preferential tropism. Furthermore, AngII pre-treatment not only increased the percentage of mice with metastasis, but also increased the number of detectable metastatic foci per mouse (Figure 5) as well as the total number of tumor cells disseminated in the whole body, as assessed by quantification of bioluminescence (Rodrigues-Ferreira *et al.*, 2012a).

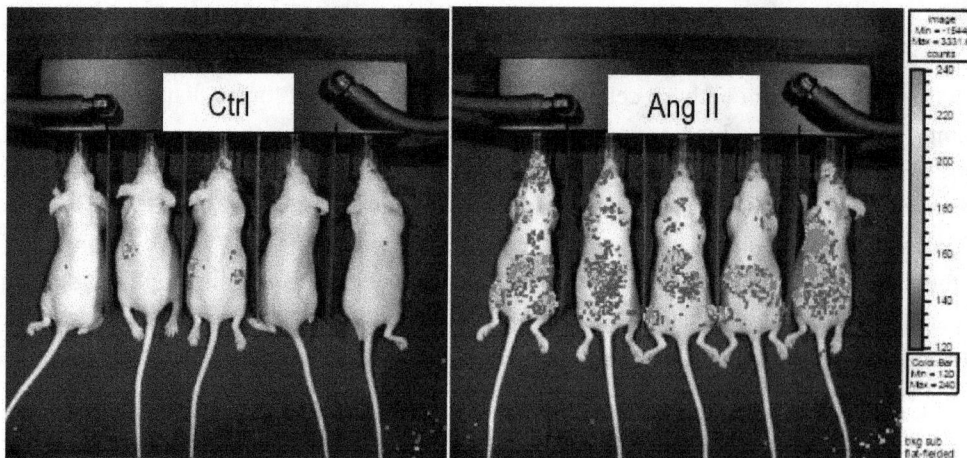

Figure 5: Intravital Imaging of mice taken 9 days after injection of control cells (Ctrl) or AngII-treated cells (AngII).

Our results indicate that D3H2LN breast cancer cells exposed to AngII show increased metastatic potential *in vivo* and are more prone to rapidly establish at distant organs. As AngII can be locally produced both in blood flow and cancer tissues, we hypothesize that this local production may accelerate the metastatic progression of breast cancer cells. Furthermore, we showed that direct exposure of breast cancer cells to AngII contributes to the metastasis process by increasing tumor-endothelial cell adhesion, trans-endothelial migration and motility (Rodrigues-Ferreira *et al.*, 2012a). Of interest, AngII concomitantly regulates a set of genes that ultimately influence the host microenvironment to facilitate cancer cell extravasation, adaptation to the soil and subsequent metastatic colonization. Among those genes, we have identified a set of genes related to MAP Kinase (MAPK1), a major effector of cell proliferation, and another one connected to matrix metalloproteases (MMP2/9), well-known mediators of cell invasion and matrix remodeling (Rodrigues-Ferreira *et al*, 2012a) (Figure 6). These results are in agreement with *in vitro* and *in vivo* effects of AngII and suggest that AngII may contribute to the cross-talk between tumor cells and their microenvironment to potentiate the metastatic colonization process. This model supports the notion that targeting AngII production or action using ACE inhibitors or ARBs, respectively, may represent an interesting therapeutic option to prevent metastatic progression of invasive breast tumors.

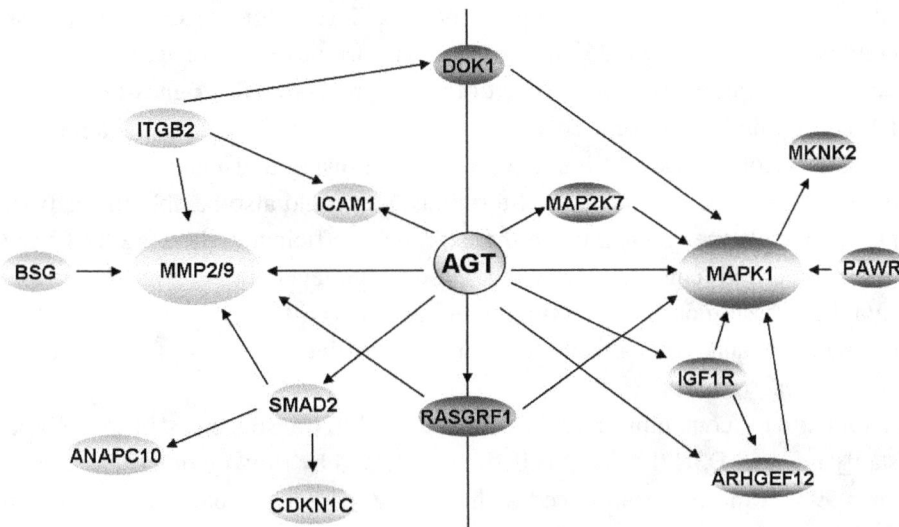

Figure 6: Networks of genes regulated by AngII centered around AngII precursor Angiotensinogen AGT. This network was obtained using the Ingenuity Pathway Analysis (IPA) software. Shown are the two main groups of connected genes associated to Metalloproteases 2 and 9 (MMP2/9 on the left) or to MAP-Kinase 1 (MAPK1 on the right).

3.3   Model to Target AT2 Effects on Breast Cancer Cells

It is generally admitted that AT1 receptor activation is responsible for most of the reported effects of AngII. Studies of AngII in cancer were mainly performed using AT1 receptor antagonists. But it is important to keep in mind that antagonizing the AT1 receptor by ARBs leaves the AT2 receptor fully available for activation by local AngII. As AT2 receptor levels have also been shown to be increased in ductal and invasive breast carcinomas (De Paepe *et al.*, 2002), it is essential to determine whether the AT2 receptor may antagonize, or mimic, the effects of the AT1 subtype on cancer cells. To date, results from the literature about AT2 receptor functions in cancer remain controversial. It has been shown that AT2 receptor expression or activation reduces growth of pheochromocytomas as well as pancreatic and lung carcinomas (Brown *et al.*, 2006; Doi *et al.*, 2010; Pickel *et al.*, 2010). In agreement, exogenous administration of AT2 receptor by nanoparticules significantly attenuates lung cancer growth in an orthotopic model of tumor grafts in syngenic mice (Kawabata *et al.*, 2012). In addition, activation of AT2 receptor with the agonist CGP42112A reduces colorectal liver metastasis (Ager *et al.*, 2010), suggesting that AT2 receptor activation might provide a novel strategy to inhibit tumor growth. However, in some other studies, AT2 receptor expression is rather correlated with poor prognosis and its blockade is associated with delayed tumor progression (Arrieta *et al.*, 2008; Clere *et al.*, 2010). As both subtypes of angiotensin receptors are concomitantly expressed in cancer cells and tissues, relative expression of each subtype in addition to their ability to dimerize may trigger different signalling and thus contradictory responses. Hence, establishment of a model to specifically address the function of AT2 receptor independently of the AT1 subtype is of particular interest.To study the implication of AT2 in breast cancer, we generated a human breast cancer cell line stably expressing high amounts of human AT2 receptors at the plasma membrane. We chose the previously described, breast cancer D3H2LN cell line (Jenkins *et al.*, 2005), and we first evaluated the expression level of the angiotensin receptors by RT-PCR (Reverse Transcription PCR) and their presence at the cell surface by radiolabelled AngII binding experiments. Our results indicate that D3H2LN cells express very low levels of endogenous AT2 receptor transcripts as assessed by RT-PCR and no detectable binding sites for I125-labeled AngII (Rodrigues-Ferreira *et al.*, 2012b).

We then designed an expression vector for the AT2 receptor (Rodrigues-Ferreira et al., 2012b). To facilitate AT2 receptor detection, we used a Flag-tagged human AT2 receptor (Flag-hAT2), which can be revealed by immunofluorescence and immunoprecipitation using anti-Flag antibodies. We reasoned that by tagging the receptor at the extracellular N-terminus, we would also be able to easily detect its expression at the plasma membrane. To maximize the expression efficiency, the Flag-hAT2 receptor sequence was cloned into a modified lentiviral vector that allows high levels of AT2 receptor expression, together with concomitant expression of the green fluorescent protein (GFP). GFP serves both as a positive control for infection efficiency, and as a valuable tool for the sensitive detection of the infected cells by FACS and immunofluorescence studies.

Lentiviral particles containing Flag-hAT2 were used to transduce D3H2LN cells. Transduction efficiency of stably infected D3H2LN-AT2 cells was evaluated by flow cytometry measuring GFP positive cells. More than 99% of the cells transduced with the AT2 lentiviral vector were positive for GFP expression, indicating that almost all infected cells had incorporated the construct (Figure 7 left).

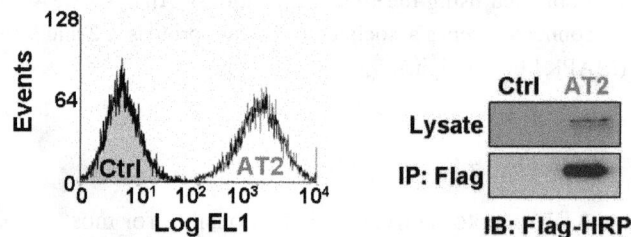

Figure 7: Left: FACS analysis of GFP positive cells. Grey filled area represents parental D3H2LN cells (Ctrl) and white area represents infected D3H2LN-AT2 (AT2) cells. Right: Biochemical validation of Flag-AT2 expression by western blot in total cell lysate (upper panel) or in anti-Flag immunoprecipitation fraction (lower panel) revealed by an anti-Flag-HRP antibody.

We then performed western blotting and immunoprecipitation analyses using anti-Flag antibodies to evaluate whether D3H2LN-AT2 cells also expressed detectable amounts of the AT2 receptor. As shown in Figure 7 (right), anti-Flag-HRP antibodies revealed the expression of Flag-hAT2 receptor in D3H2LN-AT2, but not in parental D3H2LN cells. To investigate whether the ectopically expressed Flag-hAT2 receptor was able to bind AngII with high affinity at the cell surface of D3H2LN-AT2, competition binding experiments were performed on intact cells using tritium labeled AngII (^{3}H-AngII) in the presence of increasing concentrations of unlabelled AngII. Results revealed a classical competition binding profile in D3H2LN-AT2 cells indicating the presence of a single population of receptors for AngII (Rodrigues-Ferreira et al., 2012b). In agreement, total binding of radiolabelled AngII to D3H2LN-AT2 cells could be displaced by 75% by adding an excess of the selective AT2 receptor antagonist PD123319, but not in the presence of an excess of the AT1 receptor antagonist losartan (Figure 8).

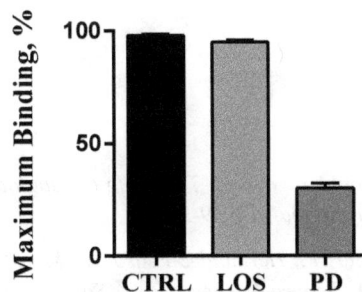

Figure 8: Maximum binding obtained in the presence of the AT1 receptor antagonist Losartan (LOS) or AT2 receptor antagonist PD123319 (PD), as compared to control (CTRL).

These results indicate that AT2 is the major AngII binding site in D3H2LN-AT2 cells and that ectopically expressed Flag-hAT2 receptors in D3H2LN breast cancer cells are correctly folded at the plasma membrane, and are able to bind the natural agonist.

We report the generation and characterization of a novel model of human invasive breast cancer cells (D3H2LN-AT2) that express high amounts of Flag-tagged human AT2 receptor at the plasma membrane. These cells also express GFP and luciferase, which makes them suitable for fluorescence and bioluminescence studies in vitro and in vivo. Of interest, D3H2LN-AT2 cells do not express detectable AT1 binding sites, as evaluated by radioligand binding assay, and overexpression of AT2 in breast cancer cells does not modulate levels of membrane AT1 receptors. This model allows the characterization of AT2 functions independently of those related to AT1 receptor activation, which is of great interest in the context of AT1 blockade by ARBs. The cellular model presented here offers a unique opportunity to evaluate the consequences of AT2 receptor activation and blockade on breast cancer proliferation, invasion and migration, as well as on tumor growth and metastasis formation. This model is of particular interest with the emergence of novel non-peptidic selective agonists of the AT2 receptor such as compound 21 (Wan et al., 2004; Unger & Dahlöf, 2010).

4   Conclusion

Data accumulated over the past two decades have highlighted important effects of the AngII vasoactive peptide in cancer, acting both on tumor cells and the host micro-environment. In this chapter, we summarize our recent studies indicating that AngII facilitates breast cancer metastasis by contributing to the cross-talk between cancer cells and the host stroma. While AT1 receptor blockade by ARBs is clearly beneficial in animal models, relevance to human cancer still remains to be evaluated and further studies should focus on selected populations of tumors overexpressing RAS components. Whether AT2 receptor activation may be beneficial or detrimental to cancer progression remains controversial; this question should benefit from a novel cellular model of breast cancer metastasis recently developed in our laboratory. Altogether, studies summarized here may translate into new therapeutic strategies against cancer, using blockers of the renin angiotensin system which are already used in the clinics as anti-hypertensive drugs with mild side effects.

References

Ager, E.I., Chong, W.W., Wen, S.W., & Christophi, C. (2010). Targeting the angiotensin II type 2 receptor (AT2R) in colorectal liver metastases. Cancer Cell International, 10, 19-30.

Arrieta, O., Pineda-Olvera, B., Guevara-Salazar, P., Hernández-Pedro, N., Morales-Espinosa, D., Cerón-Lizarraga, T.L., González-De la Rosa, C.H., Rembao., D., Segura-Pacheco, B., & Sotelo, J. (2008). Expression of AT1 and AT2 angiotensin receptors in astrocytomas is associated with poor prognosis. British Journal of Cancer, 99(1), 160-166.

Bangalore, S., Kumar, S., Kjeldsen, S.E., Makani, H., Grossman, E., Wetterslev, J., Gupta, A.K., Sever, P.S., Gluud, C., & Messerli, F.H. (2011). Antihypertensive drugs and risk of cancer: network meta-analyses and trial sequential analyses of 324,168 participants from randomised trials. Lancet Oncology, 12(1), 65-82.

Brown, M.J., Mackenzie, I.S., Ashby, M.J., Balan, K.K., & Appleton, D.S. (2006). AT2 receptor stimulation may halt progression of pheochromocytoma. Annals of the New York Academy of Sciences, 1073, 436-443.

Carl-McGrath, S., Ebert, M.P., Lendeckel, U., & Röcken, C. (2007). Expression of the Local Angiotensin II System in Gastric Cancer May Facilitate Lymphatic Invasion and Nodal Spread. Cancer Biology & Therapy, 6, 1218-1226.

Chae, Y.K., Valsecchi, M.E., Kim, J., Bianchi, A.L., Khemasuwan, D., Desai, A., & Tester, W. (2011). Reduced risk of breast cancer recurrence in patients using ACE inhibitors, ARBs, and/or statins. Cancer Investigation, 29(9), 585-593.

Chae, Y.K., Brown, E.N., Lei, X., Melhem-Bertrandt, A., Giordano, S.H., Litton, J.K., Hortobagyi, G.N., Gonzalez-Angulo, A.M., & Chavez-Macgregor, M. (2013). Use of ACE Inhibitors and Angiotensin Receptor Blockers and Primary Breast Cancer Outcomes. Journal of Cancer, 4(7), 549-556.

Chambers, A.F., Groom, A.C., & MacDonald, I.C. (2002). Dissemination and growth of cancer cells in metastatic sites. Nature Reviews Cancer, 2(8), 563-572.

Chen, X., Meng, Q., Zhao, Y., Liu, M., Li, D., Yang, Y., Sun, L., Sui, G., Cai, L., & Dong, X. (2012). Angiotensin II type 1 receptor antagonists inhibit cell proliferation and angiogenesis in breast cancer. Cancer Letter, in Press.

Christian, J.B., Lapane, K.L., Hume, A.L., Eaton, C.B., Weinstock, M.A., Marcolivio, K., Weinstock, M., Bingham, S., DiGiovanna, J.J., Hall, R., Naylor, M., Taylor, J.R., Vertrees, J., White, C., White ,CR. Jr., Piepkorn, M., Hall, R., Sidhu-Malik, N., Hannah, D., Eilers, D., Liang, T., Sakla, N., Kreuger, A., Cole, G., Jeffes, E., Labrador, T., Taylor, J.R., Kirsner, R., Kerri, J.E., Falabella, A.G., Givens, M., Naylor, M., Benson, M.B., Perry, L., Kalivas, J., Yanni, C., Targovnik, S., Austin, J., Collier, S., Point, P., Collins, J.F., Bingham, S., Calvert, B., Connor, P., Crigler, C., Davis, D., Grubb, P., Kelly, J., Kirk, G., Lawson, K., Linzy, L., Palmer, L., Rhoads, M., Sather, M., Copeland, E., Fye, C.,

Gagne, W., de Naranjo, P.G., Messick, C., Vertrees, J., Lew, R., Braverman, I., Cole, B., Kalish, R., McLean, D., & Thiers, B.H. (2008). Association of ACE inhibitors and angiotensin receptor blockers with keratinocyte cancer prevention in the randomized VATTC trial. Journal of the National Cancer Institute, 100(17), 1223-1232.

Clere, N., Corre, I., Faure, S., Guihot, A.L., Vessières, E., Chalopin, M., Morel, A., Coqueret, O., Hein, L., Delneste, Y., Paris, F., & Henrion, D. (2010). Deficiency or blockade of angiotensin II type 2 receptor delays tumorigenesis by inhibiting malignant cell proliferation and angiogenesis. International Journal of Cancer, 127(10), 2279-2291.

Connolly, S., Yusuf, S., Swedberg, K., Pfeffer, M.A., Granger, C.B., McMurray, J.J., Yusuf, S., Sjoelie, A.K., Massie, B.M., Carson, P., Lewis, J.B., Wachtell, K., Dahlöf, B., Devereux, R.B., Kjeldsen, S.E., Julius, S., Ibsen, H., Lindholm, L.H., Olsen, M.H., Okin, P.M., Califf, R., Holman, R.R., Haffner, S.M., Teo, K.K., Sleight, P., Gao, P., Schumacher, H., Dagenais, G., Probstfield, J., Anderson, C., Diaz, R., Dans, A., Levine, M., Unger, T., Fagard, R., Diener, H.C., Sacco, R.L., Zanchetti, A., Cohn, J.N., Solomon, S.D., Velazquez, E.J., & Weber, M. (2011). Effects of telmisartan, irbesartan, valsartan, candesartan, and losartan on cancers in 15 trials enrolling 138,769 individuals. Journal of Hypertension, 29(4), 623-635.

Crowley, S.D. & Coffman, T.M. (2012). Recent advances involving the renin-angiotensin system. Experimental Cell Research, 318(9):1049-1056.

De Paepe, B., Verstraeten, V.L., De Potter, C.R., Vakaet, L.A., & Bullock, G.R. (2001). Growth stimulatory angiotensin II type-1 receptor is upregulated in breast hyperplasia and in situ carcinoma but not in invasive carcinoma. Histochemistry and Cell Biology, 116, 247-254.

De Paepe, B., Verstraeten, V.M., De Potter, C.R., & Bullock, G.R. (2002). Increased angiotensin II type-2 receptor density in hyperplasia, DCIS and invasive carcinoma of the breast is paralleled with increased iNOS expression. Histochemistry and Cell Biology, 117(1), 13-19.

Deshayes, F. & Nahmias, C. (2005). Angiotensin II receptors: a new role in cancer ? Trends in Endocrinology and Metabolism, 16, 293-299.

Doi, C., Egashira, N., Kawabata, A., Maurya, D.K., Ohta, N., Uppalapati, D., Ayuzawa, R., Pickel, L., Isayama, Y., Troyer, D., Takekoshi, S., & Tamura, M. (2010). Angiotensin II type 2 receptor signaling significantly attenuates growth of murine pancreatic carcinoma grafts in syngeneic mice. BMC Cancer, 10, 67-79.

Egami, K., Murohara, T., Shimada, T., Sasaki, K., Shintani, S., Sugaya, T., Ishii, M., Akagi, T., Ikeda, H., Matsuishi, T., & Imaizumi, T. (2003). Role of host angiotensin II type 1 receptor in tumor angiogenesis and growth. Journal of Clinical Investigation, 112, 67-75.

Jemal, A., Bray, F., Center, M.M., Ferlay, J., Ward, E., & Forman, D. (2011). Global cancer statistics. CA:Cancer Journal for Clinicians. 61(2), 69-90.

Fidler, I.J. (2003). The pathogenesis of cancer metastasis: the 'seed and soil' hypothesis revisited. Nature Reviews Cancer, 3, 453-458.

Fryzek, J.P., Poulsen, A.H., Lipworth, L., Pedersen, L., Nørgaard, M., McLaughlin, J.K., & Friis, S. (2006). A cohort study of antihypertensive medication use and breast cancer among Danish women. Breast Cancer Research Treatment, 97(3), 231-236.

Fujita, M., Hayashi, I., Yamashina, S., Itoman, M., & Majima, M. (2002). Blockade of angiotensin AT1a receptor signaling reduces tumor growth, angiogenesis, and metastasis. Biochemical and Biophysical Research Communications, 294, 441-447.

Fujita, M., Hayashi, I., Yamashina, S., Fukamizu, A., Itoman, M., & Majima, M. (2005). Angiotensin type 1a receptor signaling-dependent induction of vascular endothelial growth factor in stroma is relevant to tumor-associated angiogenesis and tumor growth. Carcinogenesis, 26(2), 271-279.

Gallagher, P.E & Tallant, E.A. (2004). Inhibition of human lung cancer cell growth by angiotensin-(1-7). Carcinogenesis. 25(11), 2045-2052.

Gallagher, P.E., Cook, K., Soto-Pantoja, D., Menon, J., & Tallant, E.A. (2011). Angiotensin peptides and lung cancer. Current Cancer Drug Targets, 11(4), 394-404.

George, A.J., Thomas, W.G., & Hannan, R.D. (2010). *The renin-angiotensin system and cancer: old dog, new tricks. Nature Reviews Cancer, 10, 745-759.*

Gluz, O., Liedtke, C., Gottschalk, N., Pusztai, L., Nitz, U., & Harbeck, N. (2009). *Triple-negative breast cancer-current status and future directions. Annals of Oncology, 12, 1913-1927.*

González-Zuloeta Ladd, A.M., Arias Vásquez, A., Siemes, C., Yazdanpanah, M., Coebergh, J.W., Hofman, A., Stricker, B.H., & van Duijn, C.M. (2007). *Differential roles of Angiotensinogen and Angiotensin Receptor type 1 polymorphisms in breast cancer risk. Breast Cancer Research Treatment, 101(3), 299-304.*

Herr, D., Rodewald, M., Fraser, H.M., Hack, G., Konrad, R., Kreienberg, R., & Wulff, C. (2008). *Potential role of Renin-Angiotensin-system for tumor angiogenesis in receptor negative breast cancer. Gynecologic Oncology, 109(3), 418-425.*

Higgins, M.J. & Baselga, J. (2011). *Targeted therapies for breast cancer. Journal of Clinical Investigations, 121(10), 3797-3803.*

Imai, N., Hashimoto, T., Kihara, M., Yoshida, S., Kawana, I., Yazawa, T., Kitamura, H., & Umemura, S. (2007). *Roles for host and tumor angiotensin II type 1 receptor in tumor growth and tumor-associated angiogenesis. Laboratory Investigation, 87, 189-198.*

Inwang, E.R., Puddefoot, J.R., Brown, C.L., Goode, A.W., Marsigliante, S., Ho, M.M., Payne, J.G., & Vinson, G.P. (1997). *Angiotensin II type 1 receptor expression in human breast tissues. British Journal of Cancer, 75(9), 1279-1283.*

Jenkins, D.E., Hornig, Y.S., Oei, Y., Dusich, J., & Purchio, T. (2005). *Bioluminescent human breast cancer cell lines that permit rapid and sensitive in vivo detection of mammary tumors and multiple metastases in immune deficient mice. Breast Cancer Research, 7(4), R444-R454.*

Joyce, J.A. & Pollard, J.W. (2009). *Microenvironmental regulation of metastasis. Nature Reviews Cancer, 9(4), 239-252.*

Kawabata, A., Baoum, A., Ohta, N., Jacquez, S., Seo, G.M., Berkland, C., & Tamura, M. (2012). *Intratracheal administration of a nanoparticle-based therapy with the angiotensin II type 2 receptor gene attenuates lung cancer growth. Cancer Research, 72(8), 2057-2067.*

Kinoshita, J., Fushida, S., Harada, S., Yagi, Y., Fujita, H., Kinami, S., Ninomiya, I., Fujimura, T., Kayahara, M., Yashiro, M., Hirakawa, K., & Ohta, T. (2009). *Local angiotensin II-generation in human gastric cancer: correlation with tumor progression through the activation of ERK1/2, NF-kappaB and survivin. International Journal of Oncology, 34, 1573-1582.*

Lever, A.F., Hole, D.J., Gillis, C.R., McCallum, I.R., McInnes, G;T., MacKinnon, P.L., Meredith, P.A., Murray, L.S., Reid J.L., & Robertson, J.W. (1998). *Do inhibitors of angiotensin-I-converting enzyme protect against risk of cancer? Lancet, 352(9123), 179-184.*

Li, C.I., Malone, K.E., Weiss, N.S., Boudreau, D.M., Cushing-Haugen, K.L., & Daling, J.R. (2003). *Relation between use of antihypertensive medications and risk of breast carcinoma among women ages 65-79 years. Cancer, 98(7), 1504-1513.*

Luzzi, K.J., MacDonald, I.C., Schmidt, E.E., Kerkvliet, N., Morris, V.L., Chambers, A.F., & Groom, A.C. (1998). *Multistep nature of metastatic inefficiency: dormancy of solitary cells after successful extravasation and limited survival of early micrometastases. American Journal of Pathology, 153(3), 865-873.*

Miyajima, A., Kosaka, T., Asano, T., Asano, T., Seta, K., Kawai T., & Hayakawa, M. (2002) *Angiotensin II type I antagonist prevents pulmonary metastasis of murine renal cancer by inhibiting tumor angiogenesis. Cancer Research, 62, 4176-4179.*

Muller, A., Homey, B., Soto, H., Ge, N., Catron, D., Buchanan, M.E., McClanahan, T., Murphy, E., Yuan, W., Wagner, S.N., Barrera, J.L., Mohar, A., Verástegui, E., & Zlotnik, A. (2001). *Involvement of chemokine receptors in breast cancer metastasis. Nature 410, 50-56.*

Nguyen, D.X., Bos, P.D., & Massagué, J. (2009). *Metastasis: from dissemination to organ-specific colonization. Nature Reviews Cancer, 9, 274-284.*

Nguyen, D.X. & Massagué, J. (2007). Genetic determinants of cancer metastasis. Nature Reviews Genetics, 8, 341-352.

Nouet, S. & Nahmias, C. (2000). Signal transduction from the angiotensin II AT2 receptor. Trends in Endocrinology Metabolism, 11(1), 1-6.

Paul, M., Poyan Mehr, A., & Kreutz, R. (2006). Physiology of local renin-angiotensin systems. Physiological Reviews, 86(3), 747-803.

Pickel, L., Matsuzuka, T., Doi, C., Ayuzawa, R., Maurya, D.K., Xie, S.X., Berkland, C., & Tamura, M. (2010). Overexpression of angiotensin II type 2 receptor gene induces cell death in lung adenocarcinoma cells. Cancer Biology & Therapy, 9(4), 277-285.

Qian, B.Z., Li, J., Zhang, H., Kitamura, T., Zhang, J., Campion, L.R., Kaiser, E.A., Snyder, L.A., & Pollard, J.W. (2011). CCL2 recruits inflammatory monocytes to facilitate breast-tumour metastasis. Nature, 475, 222-225.

Rhodes, D.R., Ateeq, B., Cao, Q., Tomlins, S.A., Mehra, R., Laxman, B., Kalyana-Sundaram, S., Lonigro, R.J., Helgeson, B.E., Bhojani, M.S., Rehemtulla, A., Kleer, C.G., Hayes, D.F., Lucas, P.C., Varambally, S., & Chinnaiyan, A.M. (2009). AGTR1 overexpression defines a subset of breast cancer and confers sensitivity to losartan, an AGTR1 antagonist. Proceedings of the National Academy of Sciences of the United States of America, 106, 10284-10289.

Rodrigues-Ferreira, S., Abdelkarim, M., Dillenburg-Pilla, P., Luissint, A.C., di-Tommaso, A., Deshayes, F., Pontes, C.L., Molina, A., Cagnard, N., Letourneur, F., Morel, M., Reis, R.I., Casarini, D.E., Terris B., Couraud, P.O., Costa-Neto, C.M., Di Benedetto, M., & Nahmias, C. (2012a). Angiotensin II facilitates breast cancer cell migration and metastasis. PLoS One, 7(4), e35667- e35674.

Rodrigues-Ferreira, S., Morel, M., Reis, R.I., Cormier, F., Baud, V., Costa-Neto, C.M., & Nahmias, C. (2012b). A Novel Cellular Model to Study Angiotensin II AT2 Receptor Function in Breast Cancer Cells. International Journal of Peptides, 2012, doi:10.1155/2012/745027.

Santos, R.A., Ferreira, A.J., Verano-Braga, T., & Bader, M. (2013). Angiotensin-converting enzyme 2, Angiotensin-(1-7) and Mas: new players of the Renin Angiotensin System. Journal of Endocrinology, 216(2), R1-R17.

Sørensen, G.V., Ganz, P.A., Cole, S.W., Pedersen, L.A., Sørensen, H.T., Cronin-Fenton, D.P., Garne, J.P., Christiansen, P.M., Lash, T.L., & Ahern, T.P. (2013). Use of β-blockers, angiotensin-converting enzyme inhibitors, angiotensin II receptor blockers, and risk of breast cancer recurrence: a Danish nationwide prospective cohort study. Journal of Clinical Oncology, 31(18):2265-2272.

Soto-Pantoja, D.R., Menon, J., Gallagher, P.E., & Tallant, E.A. 2009 Angiotensin-(1-7) inhibits tumor angiogenesis in human lung cancer xenografts with a reduction in vascular endothelial growth factor. Molecular Cancer Therapeutics, 8(6), 1676-1683.

Shibue, T. & Weinberg, R.A. (2011). Metastatic colonization: settlement, adaptation and propagation of tumor cells in a foreign tissue environment. Seminars in Cancer Biology, 21(2), 99-106.

Sipahi, I., Debanne, S.M., Rowland, D.Y., Simon, D.I., & Fang, F.C. (2010). Angiotensin-receptor blockade and risk of cancer: meta-analysis of randomised controlled trials. Lancet Oncology, 11(7), 627-636.

Sørlie, T., Perou, C.M., Tibshirani, R., Aas, T., Geisler, S., Johnsen, H., Hastie, T., Eisen, M.B., van de Rijn, M., Jeffrey, S.S., Thorsen, T., Quist, H., Matese, J.C., Brown, P.O., Botstein, D., Lønning, P.E., & Børresen-Dale, A.L. (2001). Gene expression patterns of breast carcinomas distinguish tumor subclasses with clinical implications. Proceedings of the National Academy of Sciences of the United States of America, 98(19), 10869-10874.

Tahmasebi, M., Barker, S., Puddefoot, J.R, & Vinson, G.P. (2006). Localisation of renin-angiotensin system (RAS) components in breast. British Journal of Cancer, 95, 67-74.

Unger, T. & Dahlöf, B. (2010). Compound 21, the first orally active, selective agonist of the angiotensin type 2 receptor (AT2): implications for AT2 receptor research and therapeutic potential. Journal of the Renin-Angiotensin-Aldosterone System, 11(1), 75-77.

Vargo-Gogola, T. & Rosen, J.M. (2007). Modelling breast cancer: one size does not fit all. Nature Reviews Cancer, 7, 659-672.

Wan, Y., Wallinder, C., Plouffe, B., Beaudry, H., Mahalingam, A.K., Wu, X., Johansson, B., Holm, M., Botoros, M., Karlén, A., Pettersson, A., Nyberg, F., Fändriks, L., Gallo-Payet, N., Hallberg, A., & Alterman, M. (2004). Design, synthesis, and biological evaluation of the first selective nonpeptide AT2 receptor agonist. Journal of Medicinal Chemistry, 47(24), 5995-6008.

Wright, J.W. & Harding, J.W. (1997). Important role for angiotensin III and IV in the brain renin-angiotensin system. Brain Research Reviews. 25(1), 96-124.

Xi, B., Zeng, T., Liu, L., Liang, Y., Liu, W., Hu, Y., & Li, J. (2011). Association between polymorphisms of the renin-angiotensin system genes and breast cancer risk: a meta-analysis. Breast Cancer Research Treatment, 130(2), 561-568.

Innovative Strategies for Breast Cancer Therapy: Concepts and Applications

Lorena González
Institute of Biochemistry and Biophysics (IQUIFIB)
University of Buenos Aires, Argentina

Ezequiel Monteagudo
Department of Pharmaceutical Technology
University of Buenos Aires, Argentina

Sebastián E. Pérez
Department of Pharmaceutical Technology
University of Buenos Aires, Argentina

Yamila Gándola
Institute of Biochemistry and Biophysics (IQUIFIB)
University of Buenos Aires, Argentina

Adriana Mónica Carlucci
Department of Pharmaceutical Technology
University of Buenos Aires, Argentina

1   Introduction

1.1   Breast Cancer: Statistics and State of Art

Breast cancer (BC) is by far the most frequent cancer among women with an estimated 1.38 million new cancer cases diagnosed in 2008 (23% of all cancers), and ranks second overall (10.9% of all cancers). The range of mortality rates is much less (6-19 per 100,000) because of the more favorable survival in (high-incidence) developed regions, but it is still the most frequent cause of cancer death in women in both developing and developed regions (Kamangar *et al.*, 2006).

Other unfortunate statistics indicate that less than 10% of all patients diagnosed with BC have metastatic disease at the time of presentation; and approximately one-third of the patients with early-stage disease would eventually relapse (Higa, 2009). There is still uncertainty about many issues regarding BC treatment, including the choice of the appropriate therapies for different cases and stages of the illness. This situation arises in spite of the recent advances in the understanding of biological mechanisms involved in tumor promotion and progression.

Nowadays, the overall prognosis of patients with operable BC differs depending on a number of tumor-specific characteristics including: size; expression of the estrogen (ER), progesterone receptors (PR), HER2/neu (Her2), and proteins linked to cell division such as Ki-67; as well as to nuclear grade, S-phase fraction, and ploidy (Viale, 2008). However, the single most important prognostic factor associated with disease-free survival and overall survival is the extent of axillaries node involvement.

In spite of the careful assessment of tumor characteristics that has been instrumental in the management of the disease, it is clear that cure has not been achieved in all patients with early BC. Basic research must continue to enhance the probability that novel principles will translate into clinical benefits (Simon, 2010).

1.2   Currently Used Therapy

Some of the local therapies for BC had substantially different effects on the rates of local recurrence — such as the reduced recurrence with the addition of radiotherapy to surgery — but there were no definite differences in overall survival at 10 years (Fisher *et al.*, 1985). Because of that, the addition of systemic therapy was included in the therapy protocol after some clinical trials' evidence (Fisher *et al.*, 1990; Fisher *et al.*, 1989; Mansour *et al.*, 1989).

Nowadays, it is considered that as the mainstay of aggressive forms of BC will continue to rely heavily on cytotoxic therapies for the foreseeable future, agents without these characteristics will be particularly valuable in combination trials (Place *et al.*, 2011). Cytotoxic chemotherapy is the only option currently available for patients with "triple-negative" (ER-negative, PR-negative, and HER2-negative) BCs. However, preoperative (neo-adjuvant) systemic therapy is currently preferable for patients with inoperable inflammatory or locally advanced BC. A favorable clinical response to neo-adjuvant therapy can convert many patients with inoperable cancers into candidates for surgical resection. Combined modality postsurgical treatment has resulted in an interesting improvement in survival compared to those who do not receive any form of systemic therapy (Liu, 2010; Pierga *et al.*, 2003).

The use of systemic therapy in the adjuvant has demonstrated to reduce the risk of relapse and death for both hormonal therapy and chemotherapy. Allocation to about 6 months of anthracycline-based polychemotherapy reduces the annual BC death rate by about 38% for women younger than 50 years of age when diagnosed and by about 20% for those of age 50—69 years when diagnosed. Such regimens are significantly more effective than CMF (cyclophosphamide, methotrexate, fluorouracil) chemotherapy (EBCTC group 2005). However, the single most important prognostic factor associated with disease-free survival and overall survival is the extent of axillaries node involvement (Lane & Esserman, 2004). The last report of the EBCTC group updated meta-analyses of 20 trials of 5 years of adjuvant TMX in early BC versus no adjuvant TMX, with about 80% compliance. This protocol safely reduces 15-year risks of BC recurrence and death. ER status was the only recorded factor importantly predictive of the proportional reductions (EBCTCGroup, 2011).

Because of the risks of systemic therapy, investigators have been searching for ways to identify patients who will benefit most from chemotherapy, while enabling others to avoid cytotoxic agents without altering their prognoses. In agree with this position is the fact that histological similar BC cells often display a distinct array of gene-expression patterns (Van de Vijver *et al.*, 2002).

Although TMX is still the endocrine therapy of choice for premenopausal women with ER (+), clinical trials are evaluating whether addition of ovarian ablation or ovarian ablation plus an aromatase inhibitor is more effective than TMX alone. Other unresolved question is if longer duration of therapy may be beneficial and with which cost. Moreover, the currently used protocol has also demonstrated clinical benefits regardless of menopausal status, nodal status, or administration of chemotherapy (Higa, 2009).

A number of caveats are noted with regard to the choice of systemic therapy. First, the presence of the (ER) in the primary tumor does not necessarily indicate endocrine-responsiveness (Goldhirsch *et al.*, 2003). Second, the timing of endocrine therapy may depend on the sites and burden of metastatic disease, as well as on patient symptoms, performance status, and personal preferences. Third, nearly all patients with hormone-responsive tumors will, inevitably, develop hormone refractory disease (Pinder *et al.*, 2008). Consequently and in spite of the uncertainty that still exists about the most appropriate therapy for each case, there is a general agreement in searching for more effective protocols using well-known agents.

The currently recommendations for postmenopausal women with early-stage, ER (+) BC is the use of TMX as a dyuvant. At the current stage, many experts in the field recommend a switch to an aromatase inhibitor (anastrozole, for instance) following 2–3 years on TMX as standard adjuvant treatment for postmenopausal women. However, aromatase inhibitors may also be used as first-line adjuvant treatment for 5 years, in particular when patients with a known risk for trombo-embolic events and/or HER-2 overexpressing patients are considered (Geisler *et al.*, 2006, PEBC Canada, 2011).

Tamoxifen citrate (TMX-C) is an anti-estrogen, non-steroidal derivative of triphenylethylene with poor water solubility (Gao & Singh, 1998). Even though TMX-C mechanism of action has not been completely elicited, it was reported that it acts primarily through (ER) by modulation of gene expression that finally leads to cell cycle arrest. However, it has been informed that at higher concentrations could induce BC cell apoptosis (Dhiman *et al.*, 2005; Jones *et al.*, 2002; Sutherland *et al.*, 1983; Tagne *et al.*, 2008). It is an estradiol competitive inhibitor for the ER. Currently, two different ERs have been identified; ERα and Erβ; while isolation of the ER was crucial for understanding the hormone's molecular mechanism of action, the discovery also became the most tangible guide for appreciating how hormone receptors could mediate tumor dependence on estrogens. Intra-nuclear binding of the estrogen–ER complex to a portion of DNA known as the estrogen- response-elements results in several biologic effects including stimulation of mammary gland duct growth (Heldring, 2007; Marino *et al.*, 2006).

It is also thought to induce a tumoricidal effect on ER(-) cells by increasing the secretion of inhibitory growth factors. This is an ER independent and nongenomic effect; it was found in ER(-) BC cells and other cell types such as malignant gliomas, pancreatic carcinomas and melanomas (Gelmann, 1997). More recently it has been demonstrated that TMX-C may possess anti-angiogenic activity through its anti-estrogenic effects (Chawla & Amiji, 2003). On the other hand, estradiol has an anti-apoptotic influence in both, ER (+) and ER (-) cells, in addition to its proliferative effect on ER (+) cells; the anti-apoptotic effect has also been reported in MCF-7 BC cell line (Zheng et al., 2006).

Estrogen deprivation is believed to be the operative mode of all hormonal therapies in the treatment of BC. Hence, pharmacologic agents that directly or indirectly deprive tumor cells of estrogens have significantly improved tumor and health-related quality of life outcomes in patients with early and advanced BC.

TMX-C is still the systemic hormonal therapy of choice in premenopausal women and an appropriate alternative in postmenopausal women intolerant to, or with disease progressing on, aromatase inhibitors. It was also described as an useful anti-hormone agent in inflammatory breast cancer (Chang et al, 1998) and also as a prevention therapy for recurrence in patients who have undergone surgery (Fisher et al., 2005).

TMX-C is administered by oral route in dose ranges from 20 to 40 mg a day, but up to 200 mg a day has been reported (Hardman et al., 2006). Regarding pharmacokinetics, its oral bioavailability is affected by the first pass effect and is a substrate for some protein families that mediate toxic compounds efflux outside the organism (Shin et al., 2006). It also presents vulnerability to enzymatic degradation in both intestine and liver. Following long-term therapy, TMX-C has some major side effects, including higher incidence of endometrial cancer, liver cancer, thromboembolic disorders and development of drug resistance (Chawla & Amiji, 2003).

1.3   General Concepts of Nanotechnology Applied to Breast Cancer Therapy

Nanoparticulate drug delivery has become an area of extensive research as these systems enable bioavailability improvement of poorly water-soluble compounds as well as targeted delivery of active pharmaceutical ingredients to various tissues and organs. Generally, nanoparticles in drug delivery are defined as submicron colloidal particles ranging from 10 to 1000 nm3. The US Patent and Trademark Office, however, define nanotechnology using a scale from only 1 to 100 nm and slightly larger (Bosselmann & Williams, 2012).

As one of the more important challenges to overcome in cancer therapy is the administration of the required therapeutic active compound concentration at the tumor site for a convenient period of time nanotechnology arises as a promising tool. Targeted drug delivery to solid tumors is necessary in order to achieve optimum therapeutic outcomes. It would, therefore, be desirable to develop chemotherapeutics that can either passively or actively target cancerous cells (Peer et al., 2007). Because of this, scientific research is focused towards the development of novel drug delivery strategies like drug targeting which would enhance the therapeutic efficacy of drugs while reducing their side toxicity (Basile et al., 2012). Additionally, nanoparticles show increased uptake and interaction with biological tissues (Bosselmann & Williams, 2012).

The tumor vasculature is highly heterogeneous in distribution and more permeable in some places, however, large areas of tumors may be poorly perfused. Impaired lymphatic drainage in tumors contributes to increased interstitial fluid pressure (IFP) adding another barrier to drug delivery. The elevated IFP has been described to be one of the main factors contributing to limited extravasation and trans-vascular transport of macromolecules despite the leaky tumor microvasculature, and it inhibits the transport of molecules in tumor interstitial space. High tumor cell density and dense tumor stroma can further hamper the movement of drugs within tumors (Barenholz, 2012).

The high permeability of tumor vasculature and the lack of proper lymphatic drainage result in the so called enhanced permeability and retention effect (EPR) in the tumor microenvironment, which has been suggested to improve tumor drug delivery for nanoparticles and macromolecules that have the ability to circulate with a long half life (Barenholz, 2012).

Passive targeting exploits this effect (Chawla & Amiji, 2003); whereas free drugs may diffuse nonspecifically, a nanocarrier can extra vasate into the tumor tissues via the leaky vessels by the EPR effect. The preferential localization of nanoparticles at the site of interest is beneficial in that it reduces the occurrence of adverse side effects associated with nonspecific drug distribution (Bosselmann & Williams, 2012). The dysfunctional lymphatic drainage in tumors retains the accumulated nanocarriers (Peer *et al.,* 2007; Cuckierman& Khan, 2010). The tumor vasculature is known to be leaky with junctions between the epithelial cells ranging from 100 to 600 nm depending on the type of tumor. Therefore, the optimal size of nanoparticles was thought to be between 10 and 100 nm (Bosselmann & Williams, 2012) but nanoparticle size does have an effect on particle clearance and circulation times and should be considered in BC targeting studies. The optimal size of a nanoparticle for active targeting to tumor cells *in vivo* remains an unanswered question. Host and tumor factors including tumor size, tumor stage, and tumor location may also impact the efficacy of targeted nanoparticles for anti-cancer applications and should be more carefully considered as well (Grobmyera *et al.*, 2012).

Targeting molecules, such as antibodies, small molecular weight ligands, or aptamers, attached to the surface of nanocarriers contribute to drug delivery to the tumors, thus allowing specific binding to tumoral cells by the nanocarriers. However, its *stealth effect*, which is necessary for the selective tumor distribution, and the *targeting effect* is hard to achieve simultaneously (Gullotti & Yeo, 2009). The three most studied types of nanoparticles for active targeting in cancer treatment are liposomes, lipid and polymer nanoparticles, and micelles (Basile *et al.*, 2012). The advantage of actively (cancer cell-) targeted nanomedicines over passively targeted formulations is that they are taken up by cancer cells much more efficiently, but it is necessary to remark that they need to penetrate several cell layers before being able to bind to cancer cells. Despite the significant progress that has been made with regard to better understanding the (patho-) physiological principles of drug targeting to tumors, several important pitfalls has been identified, such as insufficient incorporation of nanomedicine formulations in clinically relevant combination regimens. Another pitfall is related to the fact that medical need relates to metastasis and not to solid tumor treatment. It is well-known that patients with locally confined tumors can often be curatively treated with surgery and/or radiotherapy, and chemotherapy is only given in an adjuvant setting, to prevent and treat metastasis (Lammers *et al.*, 2012).

It is currently asked for a rational formulation design, based on standard criteria for acceptable safety and efficacy, and desirable pharmaceutical characteristics (*e.g.*, stability, ease of administration, *etc.*); a detailed physicochemical characterization as well as functional tests in order to support highly reproducible manufacturing processes are also recommendable. The minimum set of nanoparticle characteristics that should be measured and reported include size, morphology, state of dispersion, physical and chemical properties, surface area, and surface chemistry as they significantly contribute to the biologic activity of ligand targeted nanoparticles *in vivo* (Grobmyera *et al.*, 2012).

According to Barenholz and col, the ideal nanomedicine may embody the following features: 1) detailed understanding of critical components and their interactions; 2) identification of key characteristics and their relation to performance; 3) ability to replicate key characteristics under manufacturing conditions; 4) easy to produce in a sterile form; 5) ability to target or accumulate in the desired site of action by overcoming the restrictive biological barriers; 6) good in-use stability, easy to store and to administer (Barenholz, 2012).

Proper formulation design is critically important to achieve antitumor efficacy *in vivo* and in patients. As opposed to in animal models, in patients, nanomedicine formulations often fail to demonstrate significant therapeutic benefit. They are generally much better tolerated, and tend to have less (and other) side effects, but their ability to improve response rates and survival times is limited. It is considered that more time and effort should be invested in selecting and generating animal models which are physiologically and clinically more relevant and able to more confidently predict treatment efficacy in patients (Lammers *et al.*, 2012).

1.4   Nanocarriers Currently Tested for Breast Cancer Therapy

Abraxane® is an approved nanoparticulate paclitaxel (PTX) formulation composed of a hydrophobic drug core surrounded by a hydrophilic albumin coating rendered nanoparticles of mean diameters of 130 nm (Bosselmann & Williams, 2012). It can leave the circulation through leaky tumor microvasculature and accumulate in the interstitium. In addition, the albumin shell facilitates interaction with receptors on endothelial cells (gp60) and in the tumor interstitium secreted protein acidic rich in cysteine (SPARC). Specifically, albumin gp60 binding leads to endothelial transcytosis of the nanocarrier into the extravascular space, where SPARC, which is overexpressed in many types of cancer, entraps the albumin in tumor cells resulting in high intratumoral accumulation (Bosselmann & Williams, 2012; Barenholz, 2012; Ernsting *et al.*, 2012).

Doxil®, the first FDA-approved nano-drug (1995), has shown prolonged drug circulation time and avoidance of reticuloendothelial system (RES) due to the use of PEGylated nano-liposomes and high and stable remote loading of doxorubicin. Due to the EPR effect, Doxil is "passively targeted" to tumors and shows superiority to free doxorubicin clinical performance in a variety of neoplastic conditions reducing side effects, this explains why it has the most extensive clinical use. Eventhough Doxil® is an excellent example to demonstrate the essential and obligatory role of lipid physical chemistry, lipid biophysics, and nano-technology in the success of liposome-based drugs delivery (Barenholz, 2012) its use in metastatic breast cancer could only reduce the incidence and/or intensity of side effects (Lammers *et al.*, 2012).

The new generation of doxorubicin-loaded liposomes is thermo sensitive; Termodox®, for example, releases their encapsulated drugs in regions where local tissue temperatures are elevated where it undergoes a gel-to-liquid crystalline phase change when heated that renders the liposomes more permeable, releasing the drug (Yarmolenko *et al.*, 2012).

Genexol-PM ® is a polymeric micelle formulated PTX composed of block copolymers which include poly-(ethylene glycol) (PEG) used as non-immunogenic carriers and biodegradable core-forming poly-(D,L-lactic acid) to solubilize hydrophobic drug. Based on results from Phase I and II trials in Korea/US, the therapeutic dose recommended is $300mg/m^2$, much higher than Taxol (Cremophor EL-based formulation) ($175 mg/m^2$) (Oerlemans *et al.*, 2010).

One of the synthetic polymers that have been used to bind many anticancer agents is poly-N-(2-hydroxypropyl) methacrylamide (pHPMA). It was initially developed as a plasma expander but proved to show all the characteristics required for a polymer used for targeting purposes. Antitumor agents have been bound to pHPMA copolymers via peptidyl spacers designed to limit drug release in plasma and serum, but to degrade enzymatically by the lyosomal proteases particularly cathepsins B, H, and L. It is currently in Phase II trials for Doxorubicin delivery (PK1®), an active-targeted nanomedicine for which the recommended doses were 280 mg/m2 instead of 50-75 mg/m2 conventionally administered of the free drug (Lammers *et al.*, 2012).

An important issue that must be considered is the fact that several factors may simultaneously affect biodistribution and targeting. Systemic therapies using nanocarriers require methods that can overcome non-specific uptake by mononuclear phagocytic cells and by non-targeted cells. It is also necessary to remark once more that the particular complexity and multicomponent nature of nanomedicines introduce large number of additional variables that may substantially increase the level of difficulty in controlling processes and predictability of behavior in a biological system (Barenholz, 2012).

Through the large number of clinical trials performed up to date, formulations have been combined with other treatment modalities, such as standard chemotherapy and/or radiotherapy, becoming clear that tumor-targeted nanomedicines – as do standard chemotherapeutic drugs – perform particularly well when integrated in combined modality anticancer therapy. Therefore, in the years to come efforts should also focus on establishing rational combination regimens, in order to better exploit the biocompatibility and the beneficial biodistribution of nanomedicines (Lammers *et al.*, 2012; Bosselmann, 2012; Hrkach *et al.*, (2012).

2   Microemulsions as Tamoxifen Delivery Systems

2.1   Microemulsions, an Extensively Studied Nanocarrier

Microemulsions (MEs) are extensively studied nanocarriers; they are defined as a system of water, oil and amphiphile which is a single optically isotropic and thermodynamically stable liquid solution. Their structure consists in micro-domains of lipids or water stabilized by an interfacial film of surfactant and co-surfactant molecules. They can be classified as oil in water (o/w) or water in oil (w/o) and the droplet size is lower than 150 nanometers. They present a number of advantages as drug delivery system, such as the ability to solubilize hydrophobic drugs, spontaneous assembly, long term physical stability and ease in manufacturing (Lawrence & Rees, 2000). They presented successful results for all administration routes. There has also been increasing interest for their administration via the parenteral route (Strickley, 2004; Tagne *et al.*, 2008) due to the number of acceptable excipients available nowadays (Date & Nagarsenker, 2008; Gupta & Moulik, 2007). Because of this, TMX represents a promising lipophilic model drug either for oral or parenteral administration using MEs as passive targeting drug delivery system. It is well-known that the oncology community awaits another wave of conceptual discoveries that could translate into ground-breaking clinical trials and new treatment paradigms (Higa, 2009). Therefore, an alternative protocol for oral, IM or IV administration in BC or in ER (-) tumors would be evaluated taking advantage of ME properties.

The aim of the work published by our group was to design and characterize o/w MEs composed by pharmaceutically accepted excipients for TMX-C delivery. They would be further proposed for alternative protocols with oral or parenteral administration. The biological behavior of the selected compositions for passive targeting drug delivery was also evaluated in MCF-7 human breast cancer cell line.

In the following paragraphs the main steps carried out during the work are presented as an alternative proposal for a rationale formulation design of an useful nanomedicine for BC (Monteagudo *et al.*, 2012).

2.2   Preliminary Solubility Evaluation

First of all, the solubility of TMX in a number of excipients was estimated. The oily phases were Isopropyl myristate (IPM), Mygliol 840, Captex 355, Oleic acid, Imwitor 408, phosphatidylcholine (PC) and Capmul MCM L. PC is solid at room temperature, so a suspension was prepared (being 16% m/v the maximum concentration tested). These oils are widely used as no polar phases for ME formulation (Pouton, 2006; Kale &Patravale, 2008). It is remarkable that PC has also been used for the formulation of parenteral MEs (Spernath *et al.*, 2006). Five Co-surfactants were tested; Ethanol, Polyethilenglycol 400 (PEG 400), Transcutol P® (TC P), Labrafil 1944 CS ®, and Propylenglycol (PG). All of them are included in the FDA inactive ingredients guide. Polysorbate 80 (PS 80) was selected as surfactant model because it is listed as a Generally Recognized as safe (GRAS) excipient. In addition, it is extensively used for different ways of administration, including the parenteral route (Rowe *et al.*, 2010; Gupta & Moulik, 2008).

TMX-C resulted almost insoluble in IPM, Mygliol 840, Captex 355, Oleic acid and Imwitor 408, and showed solubility near 20 mg/g in the PC suspension and in Capmul MCM L (Figure 1a). Therefore, only PC and Capmul MCM L were selected for the forthcoming screening. The selection of the oily phase is very important because the drug solubility in the formulation depends mainly on it (Palamakula & Khan, 2004; Porter *et al.*, 2008). So, this property results fundamental in the search for high solubilizing capacity systems. Lipid solubility values found in this work are in accordance with the most effective ones published to date (Elnaggar *et al.*, 2009) and they also were significantly higher than TMX-C solubility in water (≈20 mg/mL and ≈0.4 µg/mL, respectively).

Solubility of TMX-C in the five co-surfactants and in PS 80 is depicted in figure 1b. The highest solubilizing capacity was achieved with PG and ethanol; therefore, both compounds were selected to act as co-emulsifiers in the forthcoming ME screening. Solubility of TMX-C in PS 80 was around 5 mg/g; however, it is expected that these results slightly impact on the final therapeutic agent solubilization. The most important factor that contributes to the final ME solubilizing capacity in poorly water soluble drugs is the solubility in the lipid internal phase (Sznitowska *et al.*, 2002b).

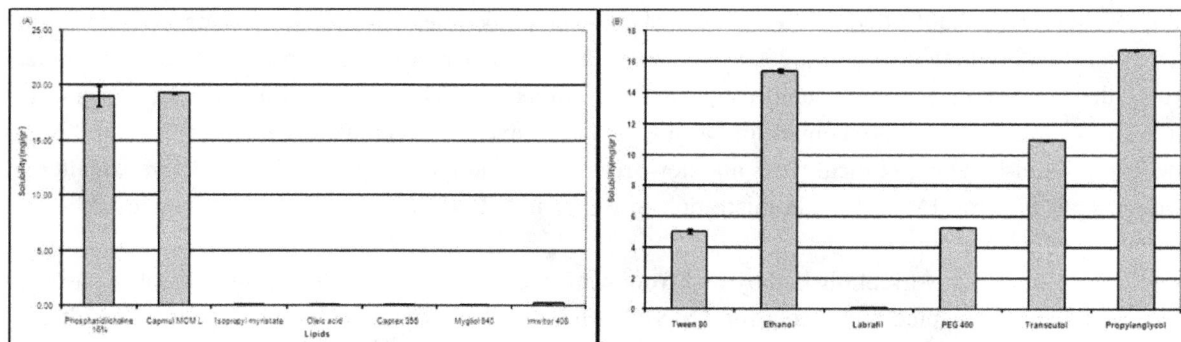

Figure 1: a) Solubility of Tamoxifen citrate in oil phases; b) Solubility of Tamoxifen Citrate in Polysorbate 80 and co-surfactants. Solubility is expressed in mg/g). Each bar represents the mean of three samples ± SD.

2.3   Preliminary Cytotoxicity Study

In order to avoid interference when testing selected vehiclesfor *in vitro* performance, a preliminary cyto-toxicity experiment on the MCF-7 cancer cell line was performed. As it can be observed in Figure 2a, only samples containing 5% m/v of PS 80 exhibited low cytotoxicity. As a result of the preliminary sur-factant cytotoxicity experiments and, in order to avoid excipient related effects on the cells, final formula-tions have been diluted prior to their *in vitro* performance evaluation. Oleic acid was the only no polar phase associated with cytotoxicity effect at both assayed concentrations (Figure 2b). Labrafil CS was the only cosurfactant which showed that inconvenient.

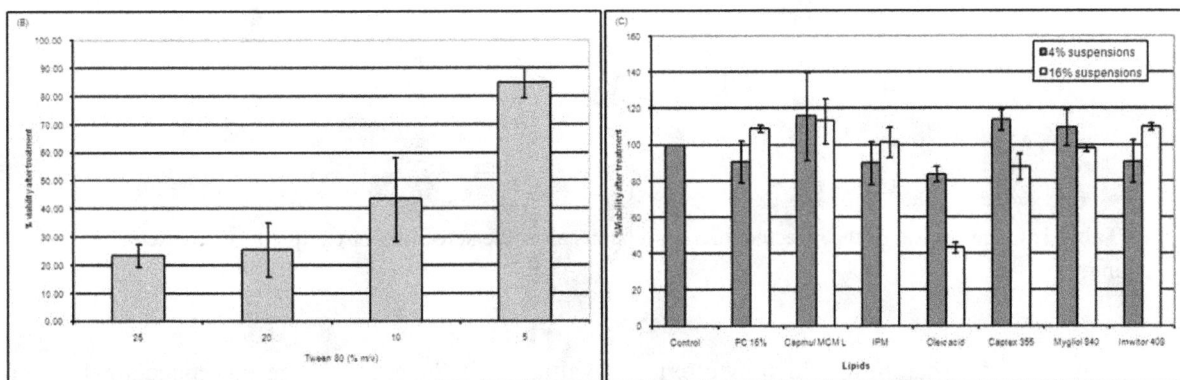

Figure 2: a) Cell viability shown by Polysorbate 80 at 25, 20, 10 and 5 % m/v, respectively. **b)** Cell viability exhibited with suspensions of 4% and 16% of each one of the selected lipids. Cell viability was evaluated using MCF-7 breast cancer cells at 37°C for 48 hs. Each bar represents the mean of three samples ± SD.

2.4   Screening and Optimization of Microemulsions

Based on solubility and cytotoxicity results, the following excipients were selected to perform the prelim-inary ME screening: PS 80 as surfactant, ethanol and PG as co-surfactants and PC and Capmul MCM L as the oil phases. Once the screening and the Ternary Phase Diagram were finished, a number of compo-sitions which resulted to be isotropic were selected. The selection included compositions with a relative proportion of PS 80 lower than 20%, relative concentrations of each one of the oil phases between 8 and 16%; the level of the co-surfactants were fixed in 25 %.

None of these compositions containing PG as co-surfactant, matched the adopted criterion for con-sidering ME system and they were discarded for the next step of selection. In relation to Capmul MCM L, promising results were observed in agreement with other authors; as it has been recorded medium chain mono-glycerides are known for their ease of emulsification when compared to fixed oils or long chain fatty acids (Stricley, 2004; Kale & Patravale, 2008). They also exhibit good solubilizing capacity. How-ever, this oil phase could not be forthcoming evaluated in MEs´ selection because of the high cytotoxicity exhibited in cell cultures (Data not shown). At this stage of the work, only MEs containing PC, ethanol and PS 80 were selected (Table 1).

Formula	Polysorbate 80	PC	Capmul MCM L	Propylene glycol	Ethanol	Water
1	20	8			25	47
2	20	12			25	43
3	20	16			25	39
4	15	8			25	52
5	15	12			25	48
6	20		8		25	47
7	20		12		25	43
8	20		16		25	39
9	15		8		25	52
10	15		12		25	48
11	20		8	25		47
12	20		12	25		43
13	20		16	25		39
14	15		8	25		52
15	15		12	25		48

Table 1: Composition of the selected microemulsions after the screening of excipients expressed as % m/m.

This way of research, in which cytotoxicity evaluation is done during the pharmaceutical development process, may result at last, in biological findings more representative; and additionally in a shorter period of time. This idea is based on the widespread opinion that asks for a formulation design that must be done along with the interpretation of biological representative parameters. It is also remarkable that Cavalli et al. (2011) have recently reported that sometimes the results are partially affected by the conditions of culture medium, as the use of Dimethyl sulfoxide (DMSO) in cytotoxicity assays, for example.

2.5   Preparation and Solubility Evaluation of Selected MEs Containing Tamoxifen

Results are shown in Figure 3 and as it can be observed, there is a synergic effect regarding drug solubility in the MEs compared to the solubility in the isolated excipients. This means that, in some cases, the difference observed for solubilizing capacity is ten-fold higher. The determination of solubilizing capacity shown by formulations was carried out at the same conditions used for isolated excipients. Considering TMX-C water solubility ($\approx$0.4 µg/mL) (De Lima et al., 2003; Cavallaro et al., 2004; Hu et al., 2006), these systems represent an improvement of around 150000 fold for vehicle 4, which exhibited a solubility of 60 mg/g.

2.6   Physicochemical Characterization

A significant lowering effect of approximately 1.5 points in pH values was observed when TMX-C was added. Conductivity values obtained for the selected compositions correspond to those of o/w MEs (Boonme et al., 2006; Zhu et al., 2008). The low viscosity values are representative for MEs (Table 2). The differences observed for viscosity values might be the result of the interaction between ME droplets in oil/water systems. It is expected that PS 80 hydrophilic chains are strongly hydrated and connected with hydrogen bonds; this allows the interaction between the droplets, thus raising the viscosity values (Podlogar et al., 2004).

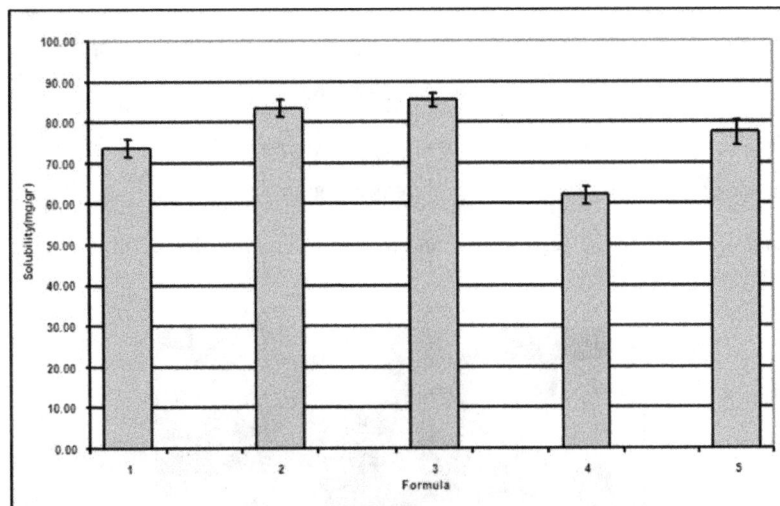

Figure 3: Solubility of Tamoxifen citrate in the selected vehicles. Each bar represents the mean of three samples ±SD (standard deviation for n=3).

Formula	Viscosity (mPa.s) Empty-ME	pH (Empty ME)	pH (Loaded ME)	Conductivity (uS/cm) Empty-ME	Density (g/mL) Empty-ME
1	45.7 ± 1.8	6.11 ± 0.02	4.62 ± 0.02	71.1 ± 0.9	1.00 ± 0.01
2	59.4 ± 4.3	6.09 ± 0.01	4.62 ± 0.02	40.7 ± 1.1	0.98 ± 0.01
3	79.3 ± 7.7	5.96 ± 0.02	4.67 ± 0.01	65.2 ± 1.6	0.99 ± 0.01
4	21.2 ± 2.3	6.15 ± 0.02	4.54 ± 0.01	42.6 ± 0.8	0.99 ± 0.01
5	29.9 ± 2.2	6.00 ± 0.05	4.61 ± 0.02	40.2 ± 1.1	0.97 ± 0.01

Table 2: Physicochemical parameters measured in the selected microemulsions. Data are expressed as mean ± SD (n = 3).

It is also to remark that the higher PC concentrations in the compositions, the higher viscosity was observed. All selected formulations were non-birefringent when analyzed with the polarized microscope, confirming their isotropy. It was concluded that MEs were not electrically charged (z potential equal to 0 mV) due to their ionic characteristics and dipolar attributes.

Since ME formation process is generally a random stirring process; the resulting delivery system may result in a polydispersed system in which different droplet sizes can coexist. This information is extremely valuable in practice because both stability and viscosity depend on the drop size distribution (Charman *et al.*, 1992). The later *in vivo* or *in vitro* behavior depends on this property as well (Tarr & Yalkowski, 1989). Results shown in Table 3 are in the typical range for a ME composition with a narrow range of polydispersion as the Polydispersity index (PDI) shown (Date & Nagarsenker, 2008). TEM images also confirmed this size distribution (Figure 4) for blank-ME N° 2. The addition of TMX-C did not significantly change droplet size of formulations comparing with empty ones, even at the highest TMX-C concentration (20 mM). This is an interesting advantage for the selected compositions, because the loading of a lipophilic active compound could result in an increase in the droplet size and, eventually, could compromise the system physical stability (Tarr & Yalkowski, 1989).

Formula	Droplet size(nm) Empty- ME	pdI	Droplet size (nm)-Loaded ME	pdI
1	5.72	0.344	6.04	0.407
2	5.37	0.237	6.04	0.297
3	5.41	0.256	4.97	0.174
4	9.54	0.365	9.62	0.368
5	8.43	0.389	8.33	0.210

Table 3: Mean droplet size for selected empty and loaded-microemulsions. PdI: Polydispersity index.

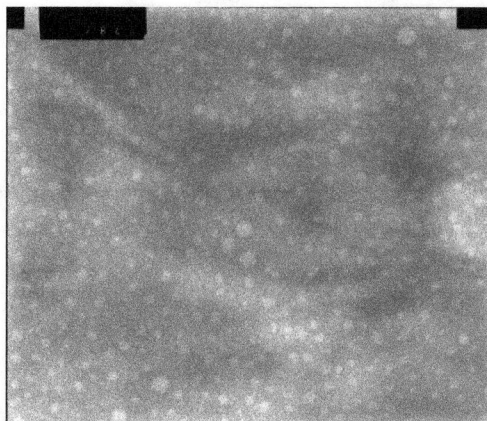

Figure 4: TEM photograph of Formulation 2 (x 100000; dilution 1:40).

A short stability testing was carried out with selected formulations. For this purpose, TMX-C 10 mM was loaded in order to achieve a final concentration of approximately 5.10^{-4} M in the culture media as the higher dose, according to literature data (Dhiman *et al.*, 2005). Results demonstrated that all formulations showed a $100 \pm 2\%$ of the initial content after a month of observation. Obtained values confirm the total solubilization of the drug and absence of rapid degradation (Data not shown).

Regarding physicochemical values no significant changes in the values measured at the beginning of the study were obtained after the studied period. No precipitation or change in appearance was observed by direct visual observation. None of the fifteen ME formulations have shown any sign of instabilization during the Thermodynamic stability tests carried out.

2.7   *In vitro* Performance of Selected Microemulsions

As a preliminary experiment, the five empty selected MEs were assayed in cultured cells to assess if they had any effect on cell proliferation in presence of 10 nM of estradiol. Two controls were also included: one adding estradiol (10 nM) to the cells in order to determine its proliferation effect and the other containing only the cells. As it is shown in Figure 5, none of the empty-ME showed effects *per se* over the MCF-7 cell line; it can be observed, instead, the proliferative effect of estradiol on MCF-7 cell line. Results confirmed that the dilution adopted was not cytotoxic.

The five selected formulations were loaded with the following TMX-C concentrations: 11 mg/g (20 mM), 5.5 mg/g (10 mM) and 2.2 mg/g (4 mM); it is important to remark that the *in vitro* performance of selected MEs was carried out in a culture media containing estradiol 10 nM.

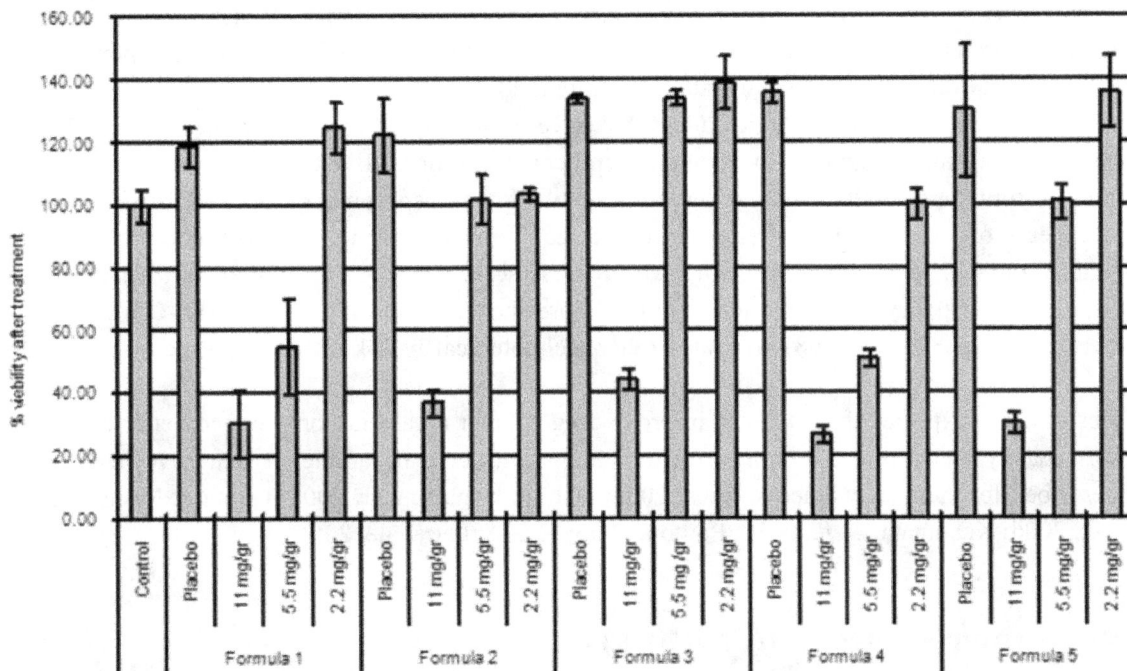

Figure 5: Cell viability of MCF-7 breast cancer cells incubated with empty-microemulsions and formulations containing Tamoxifen citrate in the following concentrations: 11 mg/g (20 mM), 5.5 mg/g (10 mM), 2.2 mg/g (4 mM). Each bar represents the mean of three samples ± SD.

The percentage of cellular viability of MCF-7 cells following inoculation of the above mentioned TMX-C concentrations is illustrated in Figure 5. There was a significant decrease in cell growth for all formulations containing the highest concentration of TMX. The viable cell percentages after treatment were around 30 to 40 % in all cases, that is, at least 90% less of viable cells than the empty compositions; ME N° 4 was the one which showed the highest cytotoxic effect. The same behavior was shown by the formulations 1 and 4 with the intermediate concentration of drug; in these cases the differences shown were 75% and 90%, respectively.

Even though TMX mechanism of action has not been completely elucidated, it was reported that it acts primarily through (ER) by modulating gene expression that finally leads to cell cycle arrest. However, it has been informed that at higher concentrations it could induce BC cell apoptosis (Dhiman *et al.,* 2005). This ER independent and nongenomic effect was found in ER (-) BC and other cell types (malignant gliomas, pancreatic carcinomas and melanomas). On the other hand, estradiol has an anti-apoptotic influence in both, ER positive and negative cells, in addition to its proliferative effect on ER (+) cells; the anti-apoptotic effect has also been reported in MCF-7 breast cancer cell line (Zheng *et al.,* 2006). Thus and taking into consideration the obtained results in cell cultures, it might be concluded that all the compositions containing 20mM of TMX-C showed an important cytotoxic effect. This phenomenon would be related to the induction of cellular apoptosis described above; the effect was also observed in ME N° 1 and 4 containing 10 mM TMX-C. The percentage of viable cells observed would indicate that seven of the fifteen assayed compositions were able to solubilize enough amount of TMX-C capable to show a modification in apoptosis cellular induction. It is also interesting to remark that this phenomenon is observed in presence of the above demonstrated proliferative effect of estradiol. It can be concluded that formulations 1 and 4 had the best *in vitro* performance because they were able to show an important anti-proliferative effect even when they were loading the intermediate dose.

Regarding other nanotechnological tools that have been reported for BC treatment using TMX as hormone-therapy agent, we can point out some general considerations. MEs designed in this work did not show signs of limited transport indicating that no saturable drug transport was involved (Chawla & Amiji, 2003); their ease of preparation is a frequently asked requirement for nanomedicines, nor High pressure Homogenization (Al Haj *et al.*, 2008) neither electrospray were necessary to be used in their formation (Cavalli *et al.*, 2011); they were able to solubilize more than 100-fold higher of TMX-C reported for nanoemulsions (Tagne *et al.*, 2008) with also other technological well-known differences (Shah *et al.*, 2010).

Besides, it is expected that MEs can improve drug cellular uptake not only due to better drug solubilization capacity but also to the improvement in biopharmaceutical parameters that have been extensively described for them (Lawrence & Rees, 2000; Date & Nagarsenker, 2008; Gupta & Moulik, 2007; Shin *et al.*, 2006; Kakumanu *et al.*, 2011; Pouton, 2006; Kale & Patravale, 2008)

3   Small Interference RNA (siRNA)

3.1   siRNA: aPromising Tool for Innovative Therapy

The silencing of genes by interference with RNA (iRNA) is a natural biological process in which small fragments of RNA (siRNA) can knock-down their cognate targets specifically and effectively based on direct homology dependent post-transcriptional gene silencing (Fire *et al.*, 1998; Hannon *et al.*, 2002; Caplen *et al.*, 2003). Common features of RNA silencing are production of small (21–23 nucleotide) RNAs (siRNA). Double-stranded RNA produced by transposons, replicating viruses or regulatory non coding micro-RNAs are recognized by the endonuclease Dicer, and cleaved into fragments called siRNA. A multi-enzyme complex, which includes Argonaute 2 (AGO 2) and the RNA-induced silencing complex (RISC), binds to siRNA duplex and discards the sense strand to form an activated complex containing the antisense strand. The AGO2-RISC complex then targets an mRNA strand sharing a complementary sequence and leads to its degradation, shutting down protein expression (Matranga *et al.*, 2005).

After iRNA demonstration in mammalian cells in 2001, it was quickly realized that this highly specific mechanism of sequence-specific gene silencing might be harnessed to develop a new class of drugs that inhibit the expression of pathologically relevant genes, which show aberrant (over-)expression, *e.g.*, in tumors or other pathologies (de Fougerolles *et al.*, 2007; Güntherm *et al*, 2011). One of the most important advantages of using siRNA is that, compared to antisense oligonucleotides, siRNA is 10–100-fold more potent for gene silencing (Ozpolat *et al.*, 2009). In contrast to the tangible and obvious effectiveness of RNAi *in vitro*, silencing target gene expression *in vivo* has been a very challenging task due to multiscale barriers, including rapid excretion, low stability in blood serum, nonspecific accumulation in tissues, poor cellular uptake and inefficient intracellular release (Shim, 2010; Katas, 2006; Wu, 2010; Schroeder, 2009).

To date, the production of effective gene delivery vectors is the bottleneck limiting the success of gene-based drugs in clinical trials. Because of this situation, most of the siRNA based therapies that have entered into clinical trials imply local delivery such as the intravitreal or intranasal routes. On the other hand, it is currently recognized that systemic delivery of siRNA for anti-cancer therapies, for example, depends on the development of effective nanocarriers for siRNA systemic administration, as they offer great advantages to fulfill the requirements (Ozpolat *et al.*, 2009, Nishikawa & Huang, 2001; Anderson *et al.*, 1998; Khurana *et al.*, 2010). The ideal *in vivo* delivery system for siRNA is expected to provide robust gene silencing, be biocompatible, biodegradable and nonimmunogenic, and bypass rapid hepatic or renal clearance.

Nonselective systemic delivery approaches result in the nonspecific distribution of siRNAs throughout the body, requiring consequently large amounts of siRNA for gene silencing *in vivo* which can also potentially affect cellular miRNA activity by saturating the RISC. It is also necessary to consider that siRNAs can also induce toxicities such as the activation of innate immunity through the induction of interferon responses as well as off-target gene silencing. Some of these toxicities can be minimized by better design of siRNAs to avoid the immune stimulatory motifs and to reduce the amounts required by restricting the delivery to only the desired tissue and/or specific cell types (Kim *et al.*, 2012). Furthermore, an ideal delivery system should be able to target siRNA specifically into the tumor by interacting with tumor-specific receptors (Ozpolat *et al.*, 2009).

Regarding potential molecular targets in breast cancer, Murrow *et al.* performed a synthetic siRNA-mediated RNAi screen of the human tyrosine kinome. A primary RNAi screen conducted in the triple-negative/basal-like breast cancer cell line MDA-MB231 followed by secondary RNAi screens and further studies in this cell line and two additional triple-negative/basal-like BC cell lines, BT20 and HCC1937, identified the G2/M checkpoint protein, WEE1, as a potential therapeutic target. Similar sensitivity to WEE1 inhibition was observed in cell lines from all subtypes of breast cancer. WEE1-inhibited cells underwent apoptosis, increased sub-G1 DNA content, apoptotic morphology. In contrast, the nontransformed mammary epithelial cell line, MCF10A, did not exhibit any of these downstream effects following WEE1 silencing (Murrow *et al.*, 2010).

Due to the reasons mentioned above, latest advances have focused on achieving targeted siRNA delivery restricted to relevant tissues and cell types *in vivo*; thereby advancing the field of siRNA therapy towards clinical use (Kim *et al.*, 2012).

In the following paragraphs successfully siRNA-based delivery systems are described based on recently published advances.

3.2   SiRNA Delivery Systems

3.2.1   Lipid-based Delivery Systems

Nanoparticles such as liposomes, emulsions and solid lipid nanoparticles, have been used for siRNA delivery. Cationic lipids have been traditionally the most popular and widely used delivery systems. Liposomes are uni- or multilamellar vehicles consisting of a phospholipid bilayer with hydrophilic and / or aqueous inner compartment (Weyermanna *et al.*, 2004). DNA/cationic lipid (lipoplexes), DNA/cationic polymer (polyplexes) and DNA/cationic polymer/cationic lipid (lipopolyplexes) electrostatic complexes were proposed as non-viral nucleic acids delivery systems (Midoux *et al.*, 2009). Lipoplexes containing siRNA resulted in acceptable *in vitro* transfection efficiency. Nevertheless, they have had limited success for *in vivo* gene down regulation, they have also exhibited a dose-dependent toxicity, and a low colloidal stability under physiological conditions with poor intracellular release of the oligonucleotides (Li & Szoka, 2007). Cationic lipids can also activate the complement system and cause their rapid clearance by macrophages of the reticuloendothelial system (RES) (Lemke, 2008); potential for lung and other toxicities may require alternative preparations for safety (Dokka *et al.*, 2000; Spagnou *et al.*, 2004, Lv *et al.*,

2006). Therefore, careful selection of lipids and formulation strategies may help reduce or eliminate toxicity and potential adverse effects (Ozpolat *et al.*, 2009).

These effects can also be minimized or avoided by altering the chemical composition of the lipids or the use of complex mixture of different types of lipids. SNALP, stable nucleic-acid–lipid particle, is a class of lipid nanoparticles and is one of the leading liposomal formulations for siRNA delivery. The key components; cationic lipid and helper lipid coated with polyethylene glycol (PEG) ensure efficient binding to siRNA, endosomal escape and sufficient nanoparticle stability in circulation. The lipid bilayer surfaces of these particles consist of cationic and helper lipid molecules that facilitate the cellular internalization of the nucleic acid payload. The inclusion of PEG–lipids into the bilayer provides a neutral, hydrophilic exterior that enhances particle stability and helps to overcome systemic barriers to delivery such as rapid clearance upon systemic administration. The PEG–lipid dissociates from the particle at a defined rate, yielding a transfection-competent agent. The cationic lipid component governs cellular internalization of the particle while the helper lipid component aids in endosomal escape (Lammers *et al.*, 2012).

SNALP-mediated delivery of siRNAs targeting hepatitis B virus (HBV) sequences suppressed HBV replication in mouse hepatocytes. Similar results were seen for the delivery of siRNA targeting ApoB in both mice and rhesus macaques with a corresponding decrease in serum cholesterol levels (Lammers *et al.*, 2012; Manjunath, 2010).

One of the most important advances in the siRNA delivery field has been the development of neutral 1,2-dioleoyl-sn-glycero-3-phosphatidylcholine (DOPC) based nanoliposomes (Landen *et al.*, 2005; Halder *et al.*, 2006; Gray *et al.*, 2008; Merritt *et al.*, 2008). These nanoliposomes can deliver siRNA *in vivo* into tumour cells 10- and 30-fold more effectively than cationic liposomes (DOTAP) and naked siRNA, respectively (Gewirtz *et al.*, 2007). However, the preparation technique involves the use of organic solvents and addition of surfactants of limited biocompatibility.

Natural lipids are currently preferred because they are biocompatible, biodegradable and non immunogenic. 1,2-Dioleoyl-sn-glycero-3-phosphoethanolamine (DOPE) is a fusogenic lipid which has proved to facilitate the endosomal release of siRNA (Heyes J, 2005; Hassani Z, 2005). Hatakeyama and col modified a multifunctional envelope-type nano device (MEND) for efficient *in vivo* delivery of siRNA using PEG. However, PEGylation also inhibits both uptake and endosomal escape of MENDs; in order to overcome these limitations, they developed a PEG-peptide-DOPE (PPD) and modified the system with a pH-sensitive fusogenic GALA peptide (GALA/PPD-MEND). They demonstrated that introduction of the pH-sensitive fusogenic peptide facilitates nanoparticle endosomal escape, thereby enhancing the efficiency of siRNA delivery and gene silencing after topical *in vivo* administration (Hatakeyama H., 2009).

3.2.2   Polymer-based Delivery Systems

To prevent deactivation in extracellular circumstances, nucleic acid drugs were traditionally condensed with cationic polymers or encapsulated with hydrophobic polymers. The condensed or encapsulated complexes are often cross linked to enhance the physicochemical stability and coated with biocompatible polymers for safety. Delivery of the nucleic acid drugs to a specific site and subsequent intracellular entry can be partially accomplished by passive targeting based on the enhanced permeability and retention (EPR) effect or nonspecific endocytosis, but more effectively by receptor-mediated endocytosis (Lee & Kataokoa, 2012).

One widely studied cationic polymer for siRNA delivery is polyethylene imine (PEI); however, PEI has failed to progress clinically primarily owing to its poor toxicity profile and *in vivo* instability especially during systemic administration (Lammers *et al.*, 2012). Polypeptides, such as poly-L-lysine and protamine, have also commonly been used to deliver siRNA, but undesirable biological effects, such as necrosis and apoptosis have appeared in a number of cell lines (Kim *et al.*, 2008).

Because of the disadvantages often related to polymers use, natural cationic polymers which have demonstrated to be biocompatible, biodegradable and non toxic, are currently more desirable for *in vivo* release siRNA. Chitosan-based carriers are one of the synthetic vectors which have gained increasing interest because of its safety along with its cost-effective balance. Their comparative advantages include low toxicity, low immunogenicity, excellent biodegradability, biocompatibility and a high positive charge (Katas, 2006; Rudzinski, 2010; Shim, 2010). Howard and col reported chitosan-based nanoparticles for *in vitro* and *in vivo* siRNA delivery; rapid cellular uptake followed by accumulation during 24 hours and protein silencing around 80% were the most significant results (Howard, 2006). Katas *et al.* have prepared optimized chitosan-based delivery systems which have shown a promising siRNA loading efficiency (Katas,2006). It has also been demonstrated that physicochemical properties (mean droplet size, z potential, morphology and complex stability) and *in vitro* silencing efficiency are strongly dependent on the chitosan characteristics and on the polymer/siRNA ratio (Rudinski, 2010). Howard reported successfully *in vivo* silencing for α tumoral necrosis factor in macrophages by optimization of the formulation (Howard, 2008).

More recently, CDP a cyclodextrin-based cationic polymer delivery system was developed; it is comprised of three delivery components CDP, adamantane–PEG (AD–PEG) and adamantane–PEG–Transferrin (AD– PEG–Tf), each playing a specific but complimentary role in overcoming numerous *in vivo* barriers for siRNA delivery. The first two components are required for efficient binding to siRNA, endosomal escape and nanoparticle stability in circulation. The last component enhances cell specific uptake and increases specificity and potency (Alabi *et al.*, 2012).

3.2.3   Alternatively Studied SiRNA Delivery Systems

The use of chemically modified siRNA with greater serum stability and nuclease resistance has lead to the development of new delivery platforms with promising pre-clinical results. One of these emerging platforms is the siRNA Dynamic Poly Conjugate which was able to mask the lytic activity of the membrane active polymer before reaching the endosomal compartment via a pH sensitive carboxylated dimethyl maleic acid chemistry (Alabi *et al.*, 2012).

Dendrimers are synthetic, highly branched, spherical, and monodisperse macromolecules with three-dimensional nanometric structure, which are obtained by an iterative sequence of reaction steps producing a precise, unique branching structure. Structure of dendrimers with controllable molecular weight, large number of readily accessible terminal functional groups, and ability to encapsulate guest molecules within internal cavities makes them interesting scaffolds for gene delivery (Kesharwani *et al.*, 2012), eventhough silencing efficiency and toxicity would be improved. Dendrosomes are supramolecular entities wherein the dendrimer-nucleic acid complex is encapsulated within a lipophilic shell. An optimized dendrosome containing siRNA against E6 and E7 oncogenes in cervical cancer was found to knock down the genes considerably when evaluated in HeLa cells; no significant toxic effect was observed (Dutta *et al.*, 2010).

Carbon nanotubes based siRNA delivery (CNTs) are currently under scrutiny as new tools for biomedical applications. CNTs are cylindrical molecules composed of carbon atoms, exclusively in a series of hexagonal lattice structure formed from a graphite sheet. CNTs ends resemble hemispherical bucky balls connected by a graphene cylinder. Generally the diameter of a nanotube is in the order of a few nanometers. They have been proposed to easily cross the plasma membrane and to translocate directly into the cytoplasm of target cells because of their nano-needle structure, utilizing an endocytosis independent mechanism without inducing cell death. This property makes them very suitable as siRNA delivery system (Kesharwani *et al.*, 2012).

3.2.4   New Trends in SiRNA-based Therapy

As it has been mentioned before most of the siRNA- based therapies that have entered into clinical trials imply local delivery such as the intravitreal or intranasal routes. One of them is ALN-RSV01 for the treatment of the respiratory syncytial virus in lung transplant patients; it is in Phase IIb clinical trials. Administered via inhalation once daily for five consecutive days the treatment was associated with a clinically meaningful treatment effect, with a reduction of over 50% in the incidence of day 180 Bronchiolitis Obliterans Syndrome (Zamora *et al.*, 2011).

Another siRNA-based drug undergoing Phase II clinical trials is PF-655 for the treatment of age-related macular degeneration and diabetic macular edema (DME). The target gene, RTP801, is rapidly up regulated in response to ischemia, hypoxia and/or oxidative stress. Intravitreal injection of PF-655 in preclinical animal models of laser-induced choroidal neovascularization (CNV) led to inhibition of RTP801 expression, induction of expression of anti-angiogenic and neurotrophic factors, and subsequent reduction of CNV volume, vessel leakage and infiltration of inflammatory cells into the choroid (Gooding *et al.*, 2012).

TKM-08031(R) is a SNALP developed as anti-tumor drug that suppresses the polo-like kinase 1 (PLK1) protein; its efficacy has been demonstrated for an orthotopic bladder cancer model via intravesical instillation (Seth *et al.,* 2011). Another promising SNALP-formulated siRNA sunder clinical trial was able to target vascular endothelial growth factor (VEGF) and kinesin spindle protein (KSP) for treatment of hepato-cellular carcinoma; VEGF is critical to tumor angiogenesis while KSP is an essential protein for cellular proliferation (Judge *et al.*, 2009). AtuPLEX (R) is a SNALP which was proposed to be responsible for the effective condensation of siRNA because of the small amount of lipid required, being able in consequence to reduce the potential for lipid-associated toxicity. It is used in repeated systemic administration for antiangiogenic therapeutic interventions (Nguyen *et al.*, 2008).

It was recently recommended the co-delivery of siRNA and therapeutic agents using nanocarriers, one of the most interesting benefits for this combination is the possibility to overcome cancer resistance. It seems that the use of both the siRNA and drug is most effective when delivered in the same device. Additionally it could also prevent healthy cells from protecting themselves from antineoplastic agents, increasing the toxicity of the drug (Creixell & Peppas, 2012). Zao have reported that simultaneous delivery of PTX and P-gp-targeted siRNAs with liposomes or nanoparticles shown satisfactory results for multiple drug resistance (MDR) cancer therapy. In other protocol, PTX was administered after 24 h of MDR-1 gene silencing to provide sufficient time for substantial down-regulation of P-gp expression. The results showed that MDR-1 gene silencing by siRNA significantly enhanced the chemotherapeutic effects in drug-resistant tumor cells. The former approach is easier because it uses a single dosage protocol and can ensure that both cargos are delivered into the same MDR cancer cell. However, more studies are needed to compare the effect of co-delivery versus sequential treatment for drug-resistant tumor therapy (Gao *et al.*, 2012).

Although the recent description of multiple targeted delivery systems heralds future therapeutic applications, there are still a number of concerns and scope for improvement. These include the efficacy levels of *in vivo* delivery and possible competition with endogenous cellular RNAi components. In addition, the possibility of toxicities and immune responses to the vehicle component as well as to the targeting component needs better evaluation. Many current delivery vehicles require many components and multiple, laborious assembly steps to complex siRNA to the vehicle (Kim *et al.*, 2012).

This statement underlines the importance of I) realizing that biological systems are inherently very complex and variable, that II) carrier materials should be versatile, flexible, biocompatible, well-characterized and reproducible (*i.e.*, low batch-to-batch variability) and that III) pharmaceutical products should be as simple and straightforward as possible with relatively easy and cost-effective to prepare. It has also been agreed that the future will also see advances in the development of nontoxic liposomal and other forms of nanoparticle-based approaches because the vehicle allows relatively large amounts of siRNAs to be packaged (Lammers *et al.*, 2012).

3.3   Preliminary Studies Carried Out with Lecithin-based Nanoparticles for SiRNA Delivery

Lecithin is a mixture of phospholipids with phosphatidylcholine (PC) as a main component (up to 98% w/w) with extensively uses for pharmaceutical purposes as components of liposomes, mixed micelles and submicron emulsions. Water lecithin dispersion (WLD) is a system that has been reported for drug delivery and which is obtained by dispersing lecithin in water or in an isotonic aqueous solution (*e.g.*, mixture of glycerol and water) with means of extensive mixing at temperature 40 – 60 °C in order to obtain good hydration of lecithin. Neither special manufacturing procedure nor additional lipids and surfactants are used (Sznitowska *et al.*, 2002).

Cui *et al.* (2006) have proposed the use of lecithin for the design of nucleic acid delivery systems; they have achieved a significant improvement in the stability of a previously reported nanoparticle-based DNA delivery. A plasmid was adsorbed onto the surface of the lecithin nanoparticles and was successfully transfected to cultured cells; however, this formulation resulted very toxic because of the cationic tensioactive CTAB (Cetyltrimethylammonium bromide) added for improvement electrostatic interactions with the plasmid.

The idea of our recently published work was to take advantage of lecithin's biocompatibility along with its physicochemical properties for the preparation of WLD using different isotonic solutions; these dispersions would be used then as carriers for siRNA delivery (Pérez *et al.*, 2012).

Dispersions of soybean lecithin (Phospholipon® 90G, 90% w/w of PC) from 25mM to 100mM in different diluents (distilled water, isotonic solution of glycerol 2.76% w/w, 66mM isotonic phosphate buffer pH 7.0 and 50mM isotonic acetate buffer pH 5.0) were prepared. Buffers were isotonized by adding sodium chloride when necessary according to Sörensen and White-Vincent methods. Lecithin was first dispersed in the appropriate diluent with means of extensive mixing at 60°C by use of a thermostated magnetic stirrer in order to obtain good hydratation. Next, the dispersion was stirred for 2 minutes at the same temperature with a high-shear mixer (Ultra-Turrax T25 basic, IKA Werke, Staufen, Germany) at 13,000 rpm and sonicated at 20 kHz for 10 minutes. Lecithin dispersed in different concentrations in water, glycerol, pH 7.0 and pH 5.0 buffers were combined with 10 pmol of RNAi and allowed to stay at room temperature for 20 minutes for dsRNA binding.

The sizes of the resulting lecithin-based nanoparticles determined by Photon Correlation Spectroscopy (PCS) showed particles in the range of 180-250 nm. Lecithin bound the oligonucleotide when dispersed in pH 5.0 and pH 7.0 buffers, but was unable to assemble when dispersed in water or glycerol. The same results were obtained for all the different lecithin concentrations tested.

Lecithin-based nanoparticles obtained at pH 5.0 buffer containing 25mM PC exhibited nanometric size and irregular shape; when loaded with siRNA, the particles changed to a spherical shape of a smaller diameter. Probably, this change in shape is due to the change in the electrostatic interactions present in the polar head of PC when the oligonucleotide is added, allowing a structural reorganization. While at pH 5.0, small, spherical, isolated particles are presented (Figure 6a and 6 b), at pH 7.0 more elongated, locally cylindrical structures are observed (Figure 6c and 6 d).

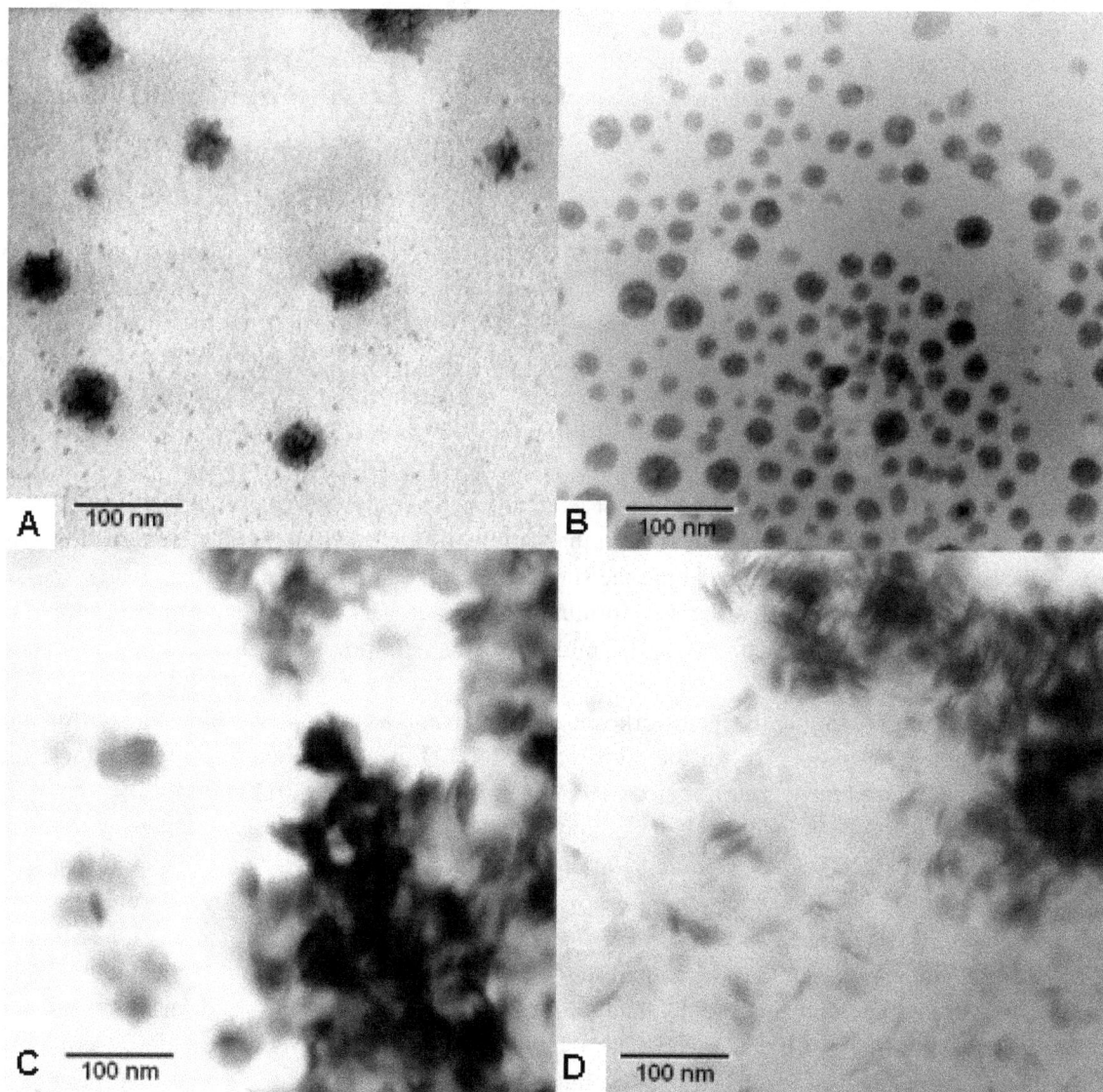

Figure 6: Transmission electron micrographs of the lecithin-based nanoparticles. Lecithin-based dispersions containing 25mM phosphatidylcholine, alone in pH 5.0 (A) and pH 7.0 (C) buffers are shown. The same dispersions were then loaded with siRNA at N/P=8000 and incubated, and the siRNA-loaded nanoparticles were observed (B and D respectively).

The phosphocholine polar head is zwitterionic at pH between 3 and 11; this means that in this pH range the phosphate group of the polar head has a net negative charge and the choline group has an equal positive charge with a spatial separation. In aqueous solution, 3–5 water molecules are bound to the phosphate group while none is bound to the choline group. When salts are added to the solution, anions are attracted by the choline group and cations are bound to the phosphate group (Huang, 1997); it can be supposed, then, that nanometric spherical particles are formed at pH 5.0 because of the interaction between siRNA and PC, more specifically because of the interaction between the positively charged amine group of PC and the phosphate groups of siRNA. Meanwhile, at pH 7.0 these interactions could be less relevant as a result of the decrease in the proportion of the positively charged forms of the zwitterionic phosphocholine polar head of the amphiphile, that is in agreement with the z potential values obtained which was positive when using pH 5.0 buffer as diluent and negative in pH 7.0 buffer.

Results demonstrated that lecithin assembled with siRNA in a broad range of N/P (Nitrogen/Phosphate) ratios, especially above 1000. Meanwhile, it is to remark that only lecithin-based nanoparticles obtained at pH 5.0 buffer was able to at least weakly associate at much lower ratios, whereas at pH 7.0 binding was not observed below N/P 100. This fact can be related to the higher proportion of the positively charged form of the phosphocholine polar head at lower pH values, supported by the zeta potential as well.

Regarding citotoxicity effects, no significant differences were observed for the different formulations when compared with untreated control cells (Figure 7). A preliminary stability study demonstrated flocculation tendency of nanoparticles. Though, it is to remark that redispersion and macroscopic reconstitution was easily achieved by gentle shaking.

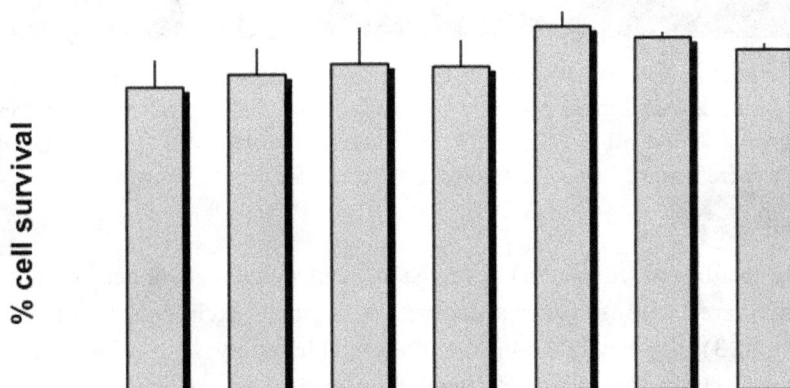

Figure 7: Cytotoxicity assay in MCF-7 cells of WLDs (25mM, 50mM and 100mM phosphatidylcholine) prepared in pH 5.0 and pH 7.0 buffers. No significant differences in cytotoxicity were observed for the different formulations when compared with untreated control cells (Dunnet Test; P > 0.05). Data shown are mean ± SD (n=3).

Proper internalization of the delivered siRNA was tested on MCF-7 cells transfected with the vehicle. Both lecithin dispersions at pH 5.0 and pH 7.0 were able to efficiently deliver a fluorescent-labeled double stranded RNA (BLOCK-iTTMAlexa Fluor® Red Fluorescent Oligo, Invitrogen) in MCF-7 cells. Fluorescent siRNA mainly located in the cytoplasm of the cells near the nucleus (Figure 8).

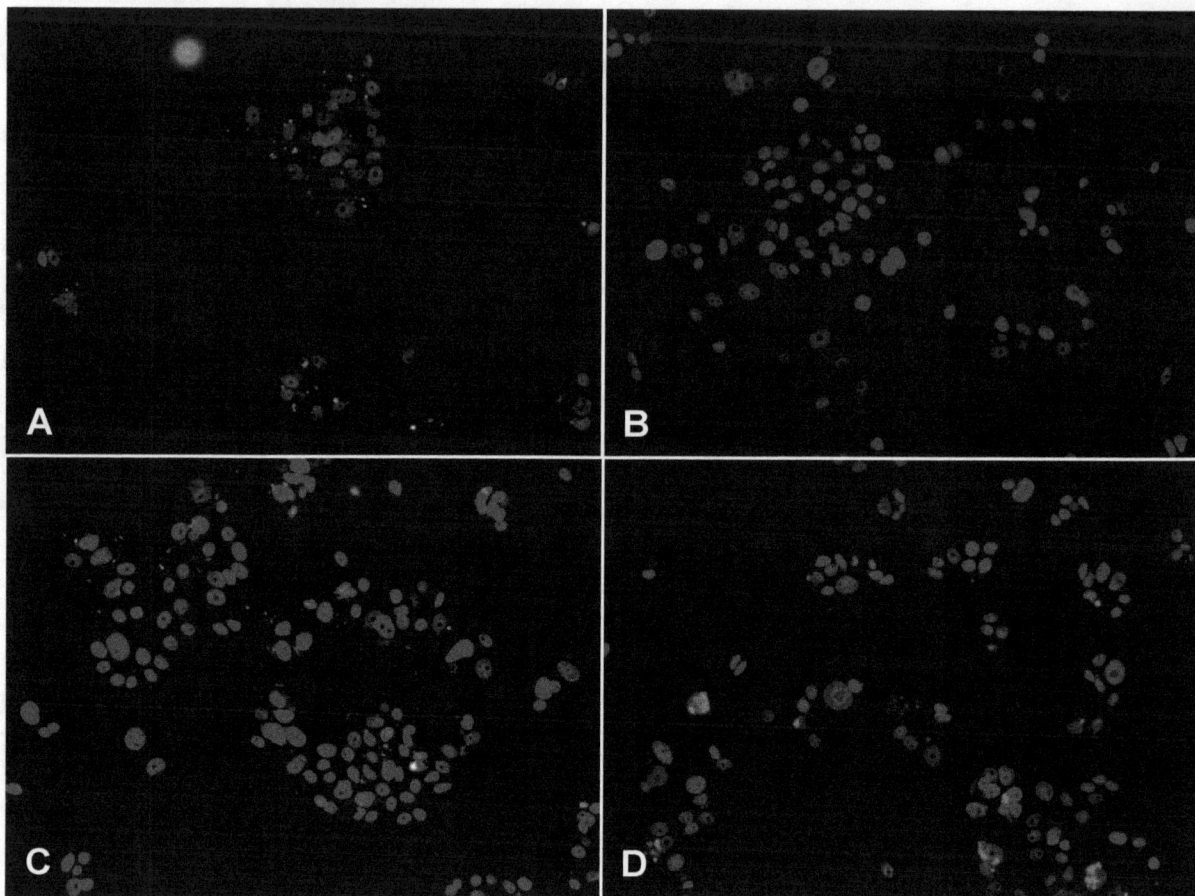

Figure 8: FluosiRNA uptake by MCF-7 cells transfected with lecithin dispersions in pH 5.0 and pH 7.0 buffers. Control dsRNA:Lipofectamin® (A), dsRNA alone (B), dsRNA: lecithin 25mM pH 5.0 (C), dsRNA:lecithin 25mM pH 7.0 (D) at N/P 8000 were incubated with the MCF-7 cells for 18 h. Afterwards cells were washed, fixed and fluorescent signal was visualized by microscopy

Finally, these lecithin-based nanoparticles have been developed under some currently required considerations: 1) they are based on pharmaceutically acceptable excipients; 2) they can be easily produced in a sterile form; 3) they have demonstrated acceptable safety; 4) a minimum set of nanoparticle characteristics has been studied; 5) an understanding of critical components and their interactions has been proposed. Furthermore the intracellular delivery of dsRNA was successfully achieved, because of these results, the present oligo delivery system represents a promising one for further investigation for the silencing of proteins over-expressed in BC.

4   Conclusions

There are many areas where uncertainty still exists concerning currently used therapies for different cases and stages of BC. This situation arises in spite of the recent advances in the biology fields. The diversity of clinical presentations of the illness, along with the absence of an appropriate understanding of definite factors that can certainly improve clinical outcomes drives the oncology community to ask for new therapy protocols. Literature has also well-stated the high potentiality of nanotechnological drug delivery systems for improving the current situation in this area of knowledge.

In this work, a novel interdisciplinary rational screening for a ME composition, its optimization and the corresponding *in vitro* performance evaluation, were proposed. The experimental design began with the selection of acceptable excipients for all the routes of administration. Then, they were evaluated for their solubilizing capacity and *in vitro* cytotoxic behavior; those which had shown acceptable parameters were selected by their ability to form MEs. It is our opinion that this design layout allows a faster optimization of MEs composition.

The results obtained after the *in vitro* inhibition of estradiol-induced proliferation in MCF-7 BC cells, demonstrated a significant effect in cell growth. A decreasing of at least 90% in viable cells was shown after the incubation with selected MEs containing 20 mM of TMX. It is also necessary to remark that the cell culture experiments were carried out with no reagent addition. In summary, most of the currently asked considerations for a rationale nanocarrier formulation design along with a detailed understanding of critical components, their interactions and the consequently biological effects on BC cells were considered.

Non-adherence to oral medication is an increasingly recognized concern in the care of cancer patients and considering that every year, hundreds of thousands of women worldwide are recommended to take TMX for 5 years; a different protocol of treatment would be evaluated. Moreover, the present would be an interesting alternative in the searching for more effective protocols using a well-known hormonal-therapy agent which is an important claim of the oncology community. Not other oral administration protocol but even an IM or IV formulation would eventually be proposed after *in vivo* experiments; these MEs would be also particularly valuable in combination trials not only for patients with metastasic disease but also for the ones who presented early BC.

On the other hand, a siRNA lecithin-based delivery system capable to improve some of the disadvantages that non-viral carriers normally present, like poor cellular uptake or high cytotoxicity, was readily obtained. It was not necessary to add other components like cationic lipids or cationic surfactants, of recognized toxicity, so as to improve siRNA loading capacity. In this case, the efficiency in loading was reached by means of the optimization of the critical parameters in the elaboration, such as pH and ionic strength. It has also been agreed that the future will also see advances in the development of non toxic-nanoliposomes and other forms of nanoparticle based approaches because the vehicle allows relatively large amount of siRNAs to be packaged. Eventhough it is necessary to remark that physical stability is an important technological issue that must be improved before further investigations.

Both systems, MEs and lecithin-based nanoparticles result in promising alternatives for further *in vivo* and ex vivo evaluation respectively. It is currently well-established that for rapid and effective clinical translation, the nanocarriers should present some characteristics that these ones do exhibit. They are made with biocompatible, well-characterized and easily functionalized excipients; they are both soluble and colloidal dosage forms under aqueous conditions which are related to increased effectiveness. MEs have also shown a low rate of aggregation and a long shelf-life, and they would also exhibit differential uptake efficiency in the target cells over normal cells because of passive targeting.

In conclusion, our proposal involves a work focused on well-established principles of pharmaceutical technology along with a better understanding of the biological responses in order to accelerate the incorporation of nanocarriers in the therapeutical progress of BC, improving in this way the transfer from concepts towards applications.

Acknowledgments

Support for these studies was provided by the National Agency of Scientific and Technological Promotion (ANPCyT); Ministry of Science, Technology and Productive Innovation, Argentina, the University of Buenos Aires and the National Science Research Council (CONICET). The authors have no relevant financial involvement with any organization or entity with a financial interest in or financial conflict with the subject matter or materials discussed in the manuscript. No writing assistance was utilized in the production of this manuscript.

References

Alabi C., Vegas A., Anderson D. (2012).Attacking the genome: emerging siRNAnanocarriers from concept to clinic.Current Opinion in Pharmacology, 12, 427–433.

Al Haj N.A., Abdullah R., Ibrahim S., Bustamam A. (2008). Tamoxifen drug loading solid lipid nanoparticles prepared by hot high pressure homogenization techniques.American Journal of Pharmacology and Toxicology, 3, 219-224.

Anderson W.F. (1998).Human gene therapy.Nature, 392, 25-30.

Barenholz Y. (2012). Doxil® — The first FDA-approved nano-drug: Lessons learned. Journal of controlled release, 160, 117-134.

Basile L, Pignatello R, Passirani C. (2012). Activetargeting strategies for anticancer drug nanocarriers. Current Drug Delivery, 9, 255-268.

Boonme P., Krauel K., Graf A., Rades T., Junyaprasert V.B. (2006). Characterization of Microemulsion Structures in the Pseudoternary Phase Diagram of Isopropyl Palmitate/Water/Brij 97:1-Butanol. AAPS PharmSciTech, 7 (2): Article 45. DOI: 10.1208/pt 070245.

Bosselmann S., Williams R.O. (2012). Has nanotechnology led to improved therapeutic outcomes? Drug Development and Industrial Pharmacy, 38, 158–170.

Caplen N.J. (2003). RNAi as a gene therapy approach.Expert Opinion in Biological Therapy, 3, 575-586.

Cavallaro G., Maniscalo L., Licciardi M., Giammona G. (2004). Tamoxifen loaded polymeric micelles: preparation, physico-chemical characterization and in vitro evaluation studies. Macromolecular Bioscience, 4, 1028–1038.

Cavalli R., Bisazza A., Bussano R., Trotta M., Criva A., Lembo D., Ranucci E., Ferrutti P. (2011). Poly(amidoamine)-Cholesterol Conjugate Nanoparticles Obtained by Electrospraying as Novel Tamoxifen Delivery System. Journal of Drug Delivery, Article ID 587604, 9 pages doi:10.1155/2011/587604.

Chang S., Parker S.L., Pham T., et al. (1998). Inflammatory breast carcinoma incidence and survival: the surveillance, epidemiology, and end results program of the National Cancer Institute, 1975-1992. Cancer, 82, 2366-2372.

Charman S.A., Charman W.N., Rogge M.C., Wilson T.D., Dutko F.J., Pouton C.W. (1992). Self-emulsifying drug delivery systems: formulation and biopharmaceutic evaluation of an investigational lipophilic compound. Pharmaceutical Research, 9, 87-93.

Chawla J.S., Amiji M.M. (2003). Cellular Uptake and Concentrations of Tamoxifen Upon Administration in Poly(-caprolactone) Nanoparticles. AAPS PharmSci, 5, Article 3. Avalaiblefrom http://www.aapsj.org/articles/ps0501/ps050103/ps050103.pdf

Creixell M., Peppas N.A. (2012).Co-delivery of siRNA and therapeutic agents using nanocarriers to overcome cancer resistance Nano Today , 7, 367-379.

Cui Z., Qiu F., Sloat B.R. (2006). Lecithin-based cationic nanoparticles as a potential DNA delivery system.International Journal of Pharmaceutics, 313, 206-213.

Cukierman E., Khan D.R. (2010). The benefits and challenges associated with the use of drug delivery systems in cancer therapy. Biochemical pharmacology, 80, 762-770.

Date AA.,Nagarsenker M.S. (2008). Parenteral microemulsions: An overview. International Journal of Pharmaceutics, 355, 19-30.

deFougerolles A., Vornlocher H.P., Maraganore J., Lieberman J. (2007). Interfering with disease: a progress report on siRNA-based therapeutics.Nature Reviews Drug Discovery, 6, 443-453.

De Lima G.R., Facina G., Shida J.Y., Chein M.B.C., Tanaka P., Dardes R.C. (2003). Effects of low dose tamoxifen on normal breast tissue from premenopausal women.European Journal of Cancer, 39, 891–898.

Dhiman H.K., A.R.Ray A.R., Panda A.K. (2005). Three-dimensional chitosan scaffold-based MCF-7 cell culture for the determination of the cytotoxicity of tamoxifen.Biomaterials, 26, 979–986.

Dokka S., Toledo D., Shi X., Castranova V., Rojanasakul Y. (2000).Oxygen radical-mediated pulmonary toxicity induced by some cationic liposomes.Pharmaceutical Research, 17: 521.

Dutta T., Burgess M., McMillan N.A.J., Parekh H.S. (2010).Dendrosome-based delivery of siRNA against E6 and E7 oncogenes in cervical cancer.Nanomedicine: Nanotechnology, Biology and Medicine, 6, 463-470.

Early Breast Cancer Trialists' Collaborative Group (2005). Effects of chemotherapy and hormonal therapy for early breast cancer on recurrence and 15-year survival: an overview of the randomised trials. Lancet, 365, 9472, 1687-1717.

Early Breast Cancer Trialists´Collaborative Group. Relevance of breast cancer hormone receptors and other factors to the efficacy of adjuvant tamoxifen: patient-level meta-analysis of randomised trials. Lancet.2011 27, 378 (9793), 771-84.

Elnaggar Y.S.R., El-Massik M.A., Abdallah O.Y. (2009). Self-nanoemulsifying drug delivery systems of tamoxifen citrate: Design and optimization. International Journal of Pharmaceutics, 380, 133-141.

Ernsting M.K., Murakami M., Undzys E., Aman A., Press B., Li S-D (2012). A docetaxel-carboxymethylcellulose nanoparticle outperforms the approved taxanenanoformulation, Abraxane, in mouse tumor models with significant control of metastases. Journal of Controlled Release 162, 575–581.

Fire A, Xu S, Montgomery MK, Kostas SA, Driver SE, Mello CC. (1998) Potent and specific genetic interference by double-stranded RNA in Caenorhabditiselegans. Nature, 391, 806-811.

Fisher B, Redmond C, Fisher ER, et al. (1985). Ten-year results of a randomized clinical trial comparing radical mastectomy and total mastectomy with or without radiation. New England ofJournal Medicine, 312, 674-681.

Fisher B. et al. (2005). Tamoxifen for the prevention of breast cancer: current status of the National Surgical Adjuvant Breast and Bowel Project P-1 study. Journal of the National Cancer Institute., 16, 1652-1662.

Fisher B., Brown A.M., Dimitrov N.V., et al. (1990) Two months of doxorubicin-cyclophosphamide with and without interval reinduction therapy compared with 6 months of cyclophosphamide, methotrexate, and fluorouracil in positive-node breast cancer patients with tamoxifen-nonresponsive tumors: results from the national surgical adjuvant breast and bowel project B-15. Journal of Clinical Oncology, 8, 1483-1496.

Fisher B., Redmond C., Dimitrov N.V., et al. (1989) A randomized clinical trial evaluating sequential methotrexate and fluorouracil in the treatment of patients with node-negative breast cancer who have estrogen receptor-negative tumors.New England Journal of Medicine, 320, 479-484.

Gao S., Singh J. (1998). In vitro percutaneous absorption enhancement of a lipophilic drug tamoxifen by terpenes.Journal of Controlled Release, 51, 193–199.

Gao Z., Zhang L., Yongjun Sun Y. (2012). Nanotechnology applied to overcome tumor drug resistance. Journal of Controlled Release, 162, 45–55.

Geisler J., Lonning P.E. (2006) Aromatase inhibitors as adjuvant treatment of breast cancer J¨urgenGeisler, Per E. Lønning. Critical Reviews in Oncology/Hemaology, 57, 53–61.

Gelmann EP. (1997). Tamoxifen for the treatment of malignancies other than breast and endometrial carcinoma.Seminars in Oncology.24, S1-65-S1-70.

Gewirtz A.M. (2007). On future's doorstep: RNA interference and the pharmacopeia of tomorrow. Journal of Clinical Investigation, 117, 3612–3614.

Goldhirsch A., Wood W.C., Gelber R.D., Coates A. S., Thürlimann B., Senn H-J. (2003). Meeting Highlights: Updated International Expert Consensus on the Primary Therapy of Early Breast Cancer. Journal of clinical oncoloty, 21, 357-365.

Gooding M., Browne L.P., Quinteiro F.M., Selwood D.L. (2012). siRNA Delivery: From Lipids to Cell-penetrating Peptides and Their Mimics.Chemical Biology & Drug Design, 80, 787–809.

Gray M.J., Van Buren G., Dallas N.A. (2008). Therapeutic targeting of neuropilin-2 on colorectal carcinoma cells implanted in the murine liver. Journal of National Cancer Insitute, 100, 109–120.

Grobmyera S.R., Zhoua G., Gutweina L.G., Iwakumab N., Sharmac P., Hochwald S.N. (2012). Nanoparticle delivery for metastatic breast cancer. Nanomedicine: Nanotechnology, Biology, and Medicine 8, S21–S30.

Gullotti E., Yeo Y. (2009) Extracellularly activated nanocarriers: A new paradigm of tumor targeted drug delivery. Molecular Pharmacology, 6, 1041–1051.

Gunther M., Lipka J., Malek A., Gutsch D., Kreyling W., et al. (2011).Polyethylenimines for RNAi-mediated gene targeting in vivo and siRNA delivery to the lung.European Journal of Pharmaceutics and Biopharmaceutics, 77: 438–449.

Gupta S., Moulik S.P. (2007). Biocompatible Microemulsions and Their prospective Uses in Drug Delivery.Journal of Pharmaceutical Sciences, 97, 22-46.

Halder J., Kamat A.A., Landen C.N. (2006). Focal adhesion kinase targeting using in vivo short interfering RNA delivery in neutral liposomes for ovarian carcinoma therapy.Clinical Cancer Research, 12, 4916–4924.

Hannon GJ. (2002). RNA interference.Nature, 418, 244-51.

Hardman J.G., Limbird L.E., A.G. Gilman A.G. (2006). The Pharmacological Basis of Therapeutics, New York:,McGraw-Hill.

Hassani Z., Lemkine G.F., Erbacher P., Palmier K., Alfama G. (2005). Lipid-mediated siRNA delivery down-regulates exogenous   gene expression in the mouse brain at picomolar levels. The Journal of Gene Medicine, 7, 198–207.

Hatakeyama H., Itoa E., Akitaa H., Oishib M., Nagasakib Y., Futakid S., Harashimaa H. (2009). A pH-sensitive fusogenic peptide facilitates endosomal escape and greatly enhances the gene silencing of siRNA-containing nanoparticles in vitro and in vivo. Journal of Controlled Release139, 2, 127–132.

Heldring N. (2007). Estrogen Receptors: How Do They Signal and What Are Their Target. Physiological Reviews, 87, 905-931.

Heyes J., Palmer L., Bremner K., MacLachlan I. (2005). Cationic lipid saturation influences intracellular delivery of encapsulated nucleic acids. Journal of Controlled Release, 107: 276–287.

Higa G.M. (2009). Breast cancer: beyond the cutting edge (2009). Expert opinion in Pharmacotherapy, 10, 2479-2498.

Howard, K.A., Paludan, S.R., Behlke, M.A., Besenbacher, F., Deleuran, B., Kjems, J (2009).Chitosan/siRNA nanoparticle-mediated TNF-alpha knockdown in peritoneal macrophages for anti-inflammatory treatment in a murine arthritis model.Molecular Therapy, 17, 162–168.

Howard K.A., Rahbek U.L., Liu X., Damgaard C.K., et al. (2006). RNA Interference in Vitro and in Vivo Using a Novel Chitosan/siRNA Nanoparticle System. Molecular Therapy, 14, 476–484.

Hrkach J. et al. (2012) Preclinical Development and Clinical Translation of a PSMA-Targeted Docetaxel Nanoparticle with a Differentiated Pharmacological Profile. Science Translational Medicine, 4, 128-139.

Hu F.X., Neoh K.G., Kang E.T. (2006). Synthesis and in vitro anti-cancer evaluation of tamoxifen-loaded magnetite/PLLA composite nanoparticles.Biomaterials, 27, 5725–5733.

Huang Y.X. (1997). Laser light scattering studies on thermodynamics of C8-lecithin and monovalent salt solutions.Journal of Chemical Physics, 107, 9141-9145.

Jones J.L., Daley B.J., Enderson L., Zho J.R., Karlstad M.D. (2002).Genistein inhibits tamoxifen effects on cell proliferation and cell cycle arrest in T47D breast cancer cells. American Surgeon, 68, 575-577.

Judge A.D., Robbins M., Tavakoli I., Levi J., Hu L., et al. (2009). Confirming the RNAi-mediated mechanism of action of siRNA-based cancer therapeutics in mice.The Journal of Clinical Investigation, 119, 3, 661–673.

Kakumanu S., Tagne J.B., Wilson T.A., Nicolosi R.J. (2011). A nanoemulsion formulation of dacarbazine reduces tumor size in a xenograft mouse epidermoid carcinoma model compared to dacarbazine suspension. Nanomedicine, 7, 277-283.

Kale A., Patravale V. (2008).Development and Evaluation of Lorazepam Microemulsions for Parenteral Delivery.AAPS PharmSciTech, 9, 966-971.

Kamangar F., Dores G.M. & Anderson W.F. (2006). Patterns of Cancer Incidence, Mortality, and Prevalence Across Five Continents: Defining Priorities to Reduce Cancer Disparities in Different Geographic Regions of the World. Journal of clinical oncology, 24, 2137-2150.

Katas H., OyaAlpar H. (2006). Development and characterization of chitosan nanoparticles for siRNA delivery. Journal of Controlled release, 115, 2, 216-225.

Kesharwani P., Gajbhiye V., Jain N.K. (2012). A review of nanocarriers for the delivery of small interfering RNA.Biomaterials 33, 7138-7150.

Khurana B., Goyal A.K., Budhiraja A., Arora D., Vyas S.P. (2010).siRNA delivery using nanocarriers - an efficient tool for gene silencing. Current Gene Therapy, 10, 139-155.

Kim S-S., Garg H., Joshi A., Manjunath N. (2009). Strategies for targeted nonviral delivery of siRNAs in vivo Trends.Molecular Medicine,15,11, 491-501.

Kim S.H., Jeong J.H., Lee S.H., Kim S.W., Park T.G. (2008). Local and systemic delivery of VEGF siRNA using polyelectrolyte   complex micelles for effective treatment of cancer.Journal of Controlled Release, 129,107–116.

Lammers T., Kiessling F. ,Hennink W.E., Storm G. (2012). Drug targeting to tumors: Principles, pitfalls and (pre-) clinical progress. Journal of Controlled Release 161, 175–187.

Landen C.N., Chavez-Reyes A., Bucana C. (2005).Therapeutic EphA2 gene targeting in vivo using neutral liposomal small interfering RNA delivery.Cancer Research, 65, 6910–6918.

Lane K.T., Esserman L.J. (2004). Sentinel lymph node dissection in early-stage breast cancer. Standards, controversies and future considerations.Oncology Exchange, 3 6-13.

Lawrence M.J., Rees G.D. (2000).Microemulsion-based media as novel drug delivery systems. Advanced Drug Delivery Reviews, 45, 89-121.

Lee Y., Kataoka K. (2012). Delivery of nucleic acid drugs.Advances in Polymer Science 249, 95-134.

Lemke, T.L. (2008). Foye´s Principles of Medicinal Chemistry. Philadelphia: Lippincott Williams & Wilkins.

Li W., Szoka F.C. (2007). Lipid-based Nanoparticles for Nucleic Acid Delivery.Pharmaceutical Research, 24, 438-449.

Liu S.V., Melstrom L., Yao K., Russell C.A., Sener S.F. (2010).Neoadjuvant Therapy for Breast Cancer.Journal of Surgical Oncology, 101, 283–291.

Lv H., Zhang S., Wang B., Cui S., Yan J. (2006). Toxicity of cationic lipids and cationic polymers in gene delivery.Journal of Controlled Release, 114, 100–109.

Manjunath N. (2010). Advances in synthetic siRNA delivery.Discovery medicine available from http://www.discoverymedicine.com/N-Manjunath/2010/05/07/advances-in-synthetic-sirna-delivery/.

Mansour E.G., Gray R., Shatila A.H., et al. (1989) Efficacy of adjuvant chemotherapy in high-risk node-negative breast cancer An intergroup study. New England Journal of Medicine, 320, 485-490.

Marino M., Galluzzo P., Ascenzi P. (2006).EstrogenSignaling Multiple Pathways to Impact Gene Transcription.Current Genomics, 7, 497–508.

Matranga C., Tomari Y., Shin C., Bartel D.P., Zamora P.D. (2005). *Passenger-strand cleavage facilitates assembly of siRNA into Ago2-containing RNAi enzyme complexes. Cell, 123, 607-620.*

Merritt W.M., Lin Y.G., Spannuth W.A. (2008). *Effect of interleukin-8 gene silencing with liposome-encapsulated small interfering RNA on ovarian cancer cell growth.Journal of National Cancer Institute, 100, 359–372.*

Midoux P., Pichon C., Yaouanc J.J., Jaffrès P.A. (2009). *Chemical vectors for gene delivery: A current review on polymers, peptides and lipids containing histidine or imidazole as nucleic acids carriers. British Journal of Pharmacology, 157, 166-178.*

Monteagudo E., Gándola Y, González L, Bregni C., Carlucci A.(2012). *Development, characterization and in vitro evaluation of tamoxifenmicroemulsions.Journal of Drug delivery.Article ID 236713, 11 pages. doi:10.1155/2012/236713.*

Murrow L.M., Garimella S.V., Jones T.L., Caplen N.J., Lipkowitz S. (2010). *Identification of WEE1 as a potential molecular target in cancer cells by RNAi screening of the human tyrosine kinome. Breast Cancer Research and Treatment, 122, 347-357.*

Nguyen T., Menocal E.M., Harborth J., Fruehauf J.H. (2008). *RNAi therapeutics: An update on delivery. Current Opinion in Molecular Therapeutics, 10, 2, 158-167.*

Nishikawa M., Huang L. (2001). *Non viral vectors in the new Millenium: delivery barriers in gene therapy. Human Gene Therapy, 12, 861-870.*

Oerlemans C., Bos M., Storm G., Nijsen F W., Hennink W.E. (2010). *Polymeric Micelles in Anticancer Therapy: Targeting, Imaging and Triggered Release. Pharmaceutical Research, 27, 12, 2569–2589.*

Ozpolat B, Sood AK, Lopez-Berestein G. (2009).*Nanomedicine based approaches for the delivery of siRNA in cancer. Journal of Internal Medicine, 267, 44-53.*

Palamakula A., Khan M.A. (2004).*Evaluation of cytotoxicity of oils used in coenzyme Q10 Self-emulsifying Drug Delivery Systems (SEDDS).International Journal of Pharmaceutics, 273, 63-73.*

PEBC, A Quality Initiative of the Program in Evidence-based Care). *The Role of Aromatase Inhibitors in Adjuvant Therapy for Postmenopausal Women with Hormone Receptor-positive Breast Cancer. (2011).Technical Report, Members of the Breast Cancer Disease Site Group - Cancer Care Ontario.*

Peer D., Karp J.M., Hong S., Farokhzad O.C., Margalit R., Langer R. (2007). *Nanocarriers as an emerging platform for cancer therapy.Nature nanotechnology, 2, 751-760.*

Pérez S.E., Gándola Y., Carlucci A.M., González L., Turyn D., Bregni C. (2012). *Formulation Strategies, Characterization, and In Vitro Evaluation of Lecithin-Based Nanoparticles for siRNA Delivery.Journal of Drug Delivery.Article ID 986265, 9 pages, doi:10.1155/2012/986265.*

Pierga J.Y., Mouret E., Laurence V. et al. (2003). *Prognostic factors for survival after neoadjuvant chemotherapy in operable breast cancer: the role of clinical response. European Journal of Cancer, 39, 1089-1096.*

Pinder M.C., Buzdar A.U., Anderson M.D. (2008).*Cancer Care Series. New York: Springer Science + Business Media, LLC.*

Place AE, et al. (2011) *The microenvironment in breast cancer progression: biology and implications for treatment. Breast Cancer Research, 13:227.*

Podlogar F., Gasperlin M., Tomsic M., Jamnik A., Rogac M.B. (2004). *Structural characterisation of water-Tween 40/Imwitor 308-isopropyl myristatemicroemulsions using different experimental methods. International Journal of Pharmaceutics, 276, 115-128.*

Porter C.J.H., Pouton C.W., Cuine J.F., Charman W.N. (2008). *Enhancing intestinal drug solubilisation using lipid-based delivery systems.Advanced Drug Delivery Reviews, 60, 673–691.*

Pouton C.W. (2006). *Formulation of poorly water-soluble drugs for oral administration: physicochemical and physiological issues and the lipid formulation classification system. European Journal of Pharmaceutical Sciences, 29, 278-287.*

Rowe R., Sheskey P., Quinn M. (2010).*Handbook of pharmaceutical excipients.London: Pharmaceutical Press.*

Rudzinski W.E., Aminabhavi T.M. (2010). Chitosan as a carrier for targeted delivery of small interfering RNA.   International. Journal of Pharmaceutics, 399, 31, 1-11.

Schroeder A., Levins C.G., Cortez C., Langer R., Anderson D.G. (2010).Lipid-based nanotherapeutics for siRNA delivery. Journal of Internal Medicine, 267, 1, 9-21.

Seth S., Matsui Y., Fosnaugh K., Liu Y., Vaish, N., et al. (2011). RNAi-based Therapeutics Targeting Survivin and PLK1 for Treatment of Bladder.Cancer Molecular Therapy, 19, 5, 928–935.

Shah P., Bhalodia D., Shelat P. (2010).Nanoemulsion: a pharmaceutical review. Systematic Reviews in Pharmacy, 1, 24-32.

Shim M.S., Kwon Y.J., (2010). Efficient and targeted delivery of siRNA in vivo.FEBS Journal 277, 23, 4814–4827.

Shin S., Choi J., Li X. (2006). Enhanced bioavailability of tamoxifen after oral administration of tamoxifen with quercetin in rats.International Journal of Pharmaceutics, 313, 144–149.

Simon R. (2010). Translational research in oncology: key bottlenecks and new paradigms. [Serial in internet] Expert Reviews inMolecular Medicine., 12, e32. doi:10.1017/S1462399410001638.

Spagnou S., Miller A.D., Keller M. (2004). Lipid carriers of siRNA: differences in the formulation, cellular uptake, and delivery with plasmid DNA. Biochemistry-US, 43, 13348–13356.

Spernath A., Aserin A., Garti N. (2006). Fully dilutablemicroemulsions embedded with phospholipids and stabilized by short-chain organic acids and polyols. Journal of Colloid and Interface Science, 299, 900–909.

Strickley R. (2004). Solubilizing Excipients in Oral and Injectable Formulations. Pharmaceutical research, 21, 201-230.

Sutherland R.L., Hall R.E., Taylor I.W. (1983). Cell Proliferation Kinetics of MCF-7 Human Mammary Carcinoma Cells in Culture and Effects of Tamoxifen on Exponentially Growing and Plateau-Phase Cells.Cancer Research, 43, 3998-4006.

Sznitowska M., Dabrowska E.A., Janicki S. (2002). Solubilizing potential of submicron emulsions and aqueous dispersions of lecithin.International Journal of Pharmaceutics, 246, 203-206.

Sznitowska M., Dabrowska E.A., Janicki S. (2002). Solubilizing potential of submicron emulsions and aqueous dispersions of lecithin.International Journal of Pharmaceutics, 246, 203-206.

Sznitowska M., Klunder M., Placzek M. (2008). Paclitaxel solubility in aqueous dispersions and mixed micellar solutions of lecithin.Chemical & Pharmaceutical Bulletin, 56, 70-74.

Tagne J.B., Kakumanu S., Ortiz D., Shea T., Nicolosi R.J. (2008). A nanoemulsion formulation of tamoxifen increases its efficacy in a breast cancer cell line. Molecular Pharmaceutics, 5, 280–286.

Tarr B.D., Yalkowski S.H. (1989). Enhanced intestinal absorption of cyclosporine in rats through the reduction of emulsion droplet size.Pharmaceutical Research, 6, 40-43.

Van de Vijver M.J., He Y.D., van't Veer L., et al. (2002) A gene-expression signature as a predictor of survival in breast cancer. NewEngland Journal of Medicine, 347, 1999-2009.

Viale G. (2008). Predictive Value of Tumor Ki-67 Expression in Two Randomized Trials of Adjuvant Chemoendocrine Therapy for Node-Negative Breast Cancer.Journal of National Cancer Institute, 100, 207-212.

Walter A., Kuehl G., Barnes K., VanderWaerdt G. (2000). The vesicle-to-micelle transition of phosphatidylcholine vesicles induced by nonionic detergents: effects of sodium chloride, sucrose and urea. BBA-Biomembranes, 1508, 20-33.

Weyermanna J., Lochmanna D., Zimmerb A. (2004).Comparison of antisense oligonucleotide drug delivery systems.Journal of Controlled Release, 100, 411-423.

Wu S.Y., Singhania A., Burgess M. et al. (2011). Systemic delivery of E6/7 siRNA using novel lipidic particles and its application with cisplatin in cervical cancer mouse models. Gene Therapy, . 18, 1, 14–22.

Yarmolenko P.S., Zhao Y., Landon C., Spasojevic I., Yuan F., Needham D., Viglianti B., Dewhirst M.W. (2010). Comparative effects of thermosensitive doxorubicin-containing liposomes and hyperthermia in human and murine tumours.International Journal ofJ Hyperthermia, 26, 5, 485–498.

Zamora M.R., Budev M., Rolfe M., Gottlieb J, Humar A. et al. (2011). RNA Interference Therapy in Lung Transplant Patients Infected with Respiratory Syncytial Virus. American Journal of respiratory and critical care medicine,183, 531-538.

Zheng A., Kalli A., Härkönen P. (2006). Tamoxifen-Induced Rapid Death of MCF-7 Breast Cancer Cells Is Mediated via Extracellularly Signal-Regulated Kinase Signaling and Can Be Abrogated by Estrogen. Endocrinology, 148, 2764-2777.

Zheng A., Kalli A., Härkönen P. (2006). Tamoxifen-Induced Rapid Death of MCF-7 Breast Cancer Cells Is Mediated via Extracellularly Signal-Regulated Kinase Signaling and Can Be Abrogated by Estrogen. Endocrinology, 148, 2764-2777.

Zhu W., Yu A., Wang W., Dong R., Wu J., Zhai G. (2008). Formulation design of microemulsion for dermal delivery of penciclovir.International Journal ofPharmaceutics, 360, 184-190.

mTOR Signaling in Endocrine Resistance Growth Control

Euphemia Leung
Auckland Cancer Society Research Centre
University of Auckland, New Zealand

Bruce C. Baguley
Auckland Cancer Society Research Centre
University of Auckland, New Zealand

1   Introduction

Breast cancer is the most common malignancy in women. After surgery, treatments with anti-estrogens and/or with aromatase inhibitors are the treatment of choice for patients with estrogen receptor positive (ER+) tumors. Aromatase inhibitors are effective in post-menopausal patients, as they do not inhibit estrogen synthesis from the ovary. Tamoxifen is also currently prescribed for the prevention of breast cancer in women who are at high risk (Jordan, 2008). Despite the efficacy of these two treatments, a proportion of patients relapse with recurrent, aggressive disease, which may be associated with a loss of ER and resistance to the above treatments. It has been found that up-regulation of the mTOR pathway occurs in a proportion of hormone-resistant breast cancers (Perez-Tenorio & Stal, 2002), as happens in a number of other tumour types including prostate cancer and hepatocellular cancer (Schenone *et al.*, 2011).

The clinical development of hormone resistance can also be studied using breast cancer cell lines. MCF-7, a commonly used breast cancer cell line, has been propagated for many years by multiple groups and it might be expected that propagation of cells from the original tumour specimen would select a single phenotype that had the highest growth rate. However, tamoxifen-resistant MCF-7 sub-lines that we and others generated appear to be derived not from metabolic adaptation but from outgrowth of pre-existing sub-populations (Baguley & Leung, 2012; Coser *et al.*, 2009; Leung *et al.*, 2010). These results suggest that MCF-7 lines are heterogeneous and contain sub-populations that are generated, possibly continuously, as a consequence of genetic or epigenetic changes. Some of the variant sub-lines generated by deprivation of estrogen or addition of tamoxifen show up-regulation of the mTOR pathway (Leung *et al.*, 2010). Such heterogeneity (Coser *et al.*, 2009) in culture may parallel processes occurring in clinical breast cancer and even in normal breast epithelium (Visvader, 2009). Thus, the in vivo appearance of tumors with up-regulated mTOR may reflect, as it does in vitro, the outgrowth of pre-existing sub-populations.

There is currently considerable interest in the use of mTOR inhibitors in the treatment of breast cancer (Baselga *et al.*, 2012) and attention has focused on mTOR both as a biomarker and as a target for mTOR inhibitors. The aim of this review is firstly to summarize both the pathways and the clinical results. We present results for the ER+ MCF-7 line and in phenotypic ER+ sub-lines that are resistant to the anti-estrogen tamoxifen. While the parental line and three tamoxifen-resistant sub-lines are sensitive to the mTOR inhibitors rapamycin and everolimus, two sub-lines are resistant to that show a low degree of mTOR pathway utilization and are resistant to mTOR inhibitors (Leung *et al.*, 2010).

2   The PI3K/Akt/mTOR Pathway

The mTOR pathway is a key regulator of multiple cell signaling pathways, integrating growth factors, nutrients, energy and stress (Zoncu *et al.*, 2011). In breast cancer, mitochondrial respiration is usually restricted (Warburg effect) and cells derive most energy from glycolysis, As shown in Figure 1, estrogen regulates glycolysis through pyruvate kinase M2 (Cai *et al.*, 2012), but in the absence of estrogen, mTOR may act on the same pathway (Q. Sun *et al.*, 2011). mTOR signaling in breast cancer is in turn stimulated by phosphatidylinositol 3-kinase (PI3K) and Akt (Vivanco & Sawyers, 2002), which are linked to signaling from external cellular receptors such as EGFR. This pathway may also control distinct regulatory motifs in mRNA that promote a pro-invasion translational program (Hsieh *et al.*, 2012; Thoreen *et al.*, 2012). Aberrant signaling through the PI3K/Akt/mTOR has emerged as the principal mechanism for endocrine resistance (Johnston, 2006). Inhibition of mTOR activity restores responsiveness to tamoxifen in

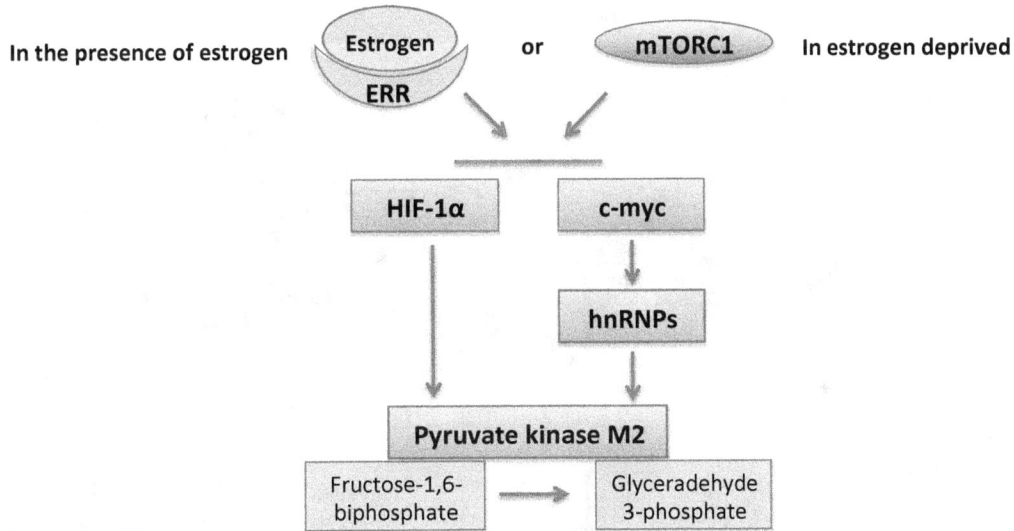

Figure 1: Roles of the estrogen and mTORC1 pathways in cellular energy production. The details of coupling to HIF-1α and c-myc are still unclear, but both seem to be utilized in regulating the activity of pyruvate kinase M2.

A pre-clinical xenograft model using MCF-7 breast cancer cells in which Akt is constitutively active (deGraffenried *et al.*, 2004). mTOR is the catalytic subunit of two distinct cell signaling complexes, mTORC1 and mTORC2 (Figure 2). RAPTOR and RICTOR are unique accessory proteins that distinguish mTORC1 and mTORC2, respectively. mTORC1 and mTORC2 also contain mLST8, which function as scaffolds and bind substrates and regulators. DEPTOR, and PRAS40) are specific for mTORC1 while mSIN1 is unique to mTORC2 (Laplante & Sabatini, 2012).

Recent research has revealed the complexity of the mTOR signaling network (Laplante & Sabatini, 2012; Zoncu *et al.*, 2011). mTORC1 regulates several growth-related process such as protein translation, ribosome biogenesis, metabolism including lipid synthesis, nutrient import, autophagy and cell cycle progression. The mTORC1 controls protein synthesis through mTOR substrates S6 kinase and 4E-BP1 associations with mRNAs and regulates mRNA translation initiation and progression. It appears that mTORC2, in contrast to mTORC1, is insensitive to energy and amino acid levels but sensitive to regulation by growth factors. mTORC2 is activated by association with the ribosome, and this mechanism ensures that mTORC2 is active only in growing cells (Zinzalla *et al.*, 2011). mTORC2 regulates the actin cytoskeleton and other processes via phosphorylation of AGC kinase family members including Akt, SGK1 and PKC (Laplante & Sabatini, 2012).

Cell cycle progression from the G1 to S phase is regulated through mTOR effectors S6K1 and 4E-BP1/eIF4E (Fingar *et al.*, 2004). mTORC1 directly phosphorylates the translational regulators 4E-BP1 and S6K1, which promote protein synthesis (Dowling *et al.*, 2010). Phosphorylation of 4E-BP1 prevents its association with eIF4E, thus promoting assembly of the eIF4F complex that is required for the initiation of cap-dependent translation. On activation, mTORC1 and S6K1 associate with mRNAs and facilitate the efficient assembly of the translation pre-initiation complex (Ma & Blenis, 2009). Hence, mTORC1 activation increases the translation of messenger RNAs that encode proteins involved in cell cycle progression and proliferation. In addition, mTORC2 is involved in cell cycle progression as RICTOR depletion reduced Akt phosphorylation and accumulated cells in G1 phase (Hietakangas & Cohen, 2008).

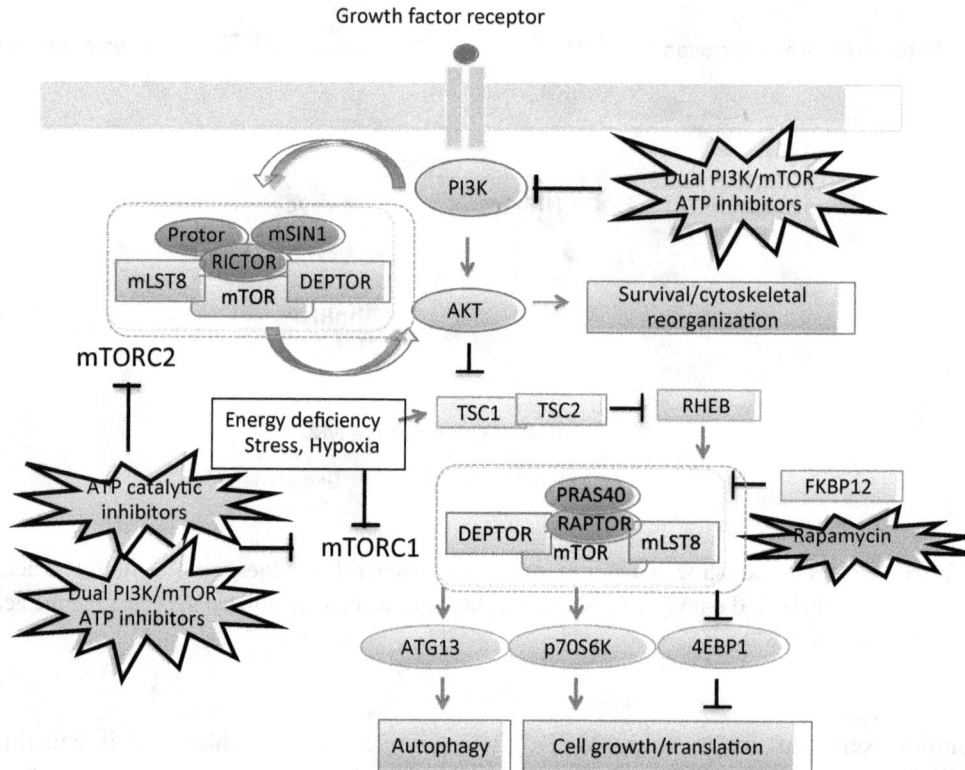

Figure 2: A network of mTOR complex signaling and function. Blue arrows and black lines represent activating and inhibitory connections, respectively.

Growth factors block TSC1–TSC2 activity and activate mTORC1 whereas stress, energy deficiency, and hypoxia promote TSC1–TSC2 action and inhibit mTORC1. mTORC1 mediates Akt-induced senescence in tumors with activated PI3K/Akt signaling (Astle *et al.*, 2012) and regulates the growth factor signaling by controlling the feedback loop to PI3K/Akt (Hsu *et al.*, 2011). mTORC1 negatively regulates the expression of DEPTOR, which suppresses S6K1, Akt and SGK1 (Peterson *et al.*, 2009). Partial mTOR inhibition leads to an inhibition of the feedback mechanism, subsequently activating the PI3K/Akt pathway that depends on the activity of an IGF-1R substrate (Wan *et al.*, 2007).

3   The mTOR Inhibitors

The mTOR inhibitors (Benjamin *et al.*, 2011) can be classified in two groups: allosteric inhibitors, which target mTORC1 but not mTORC2, and ATP-competitive inhibitors, which target the kinase domain of mTOR on both (Schenone *et al.*, 2011) (Table 2 and Figure 3) .

4   Allosteric mTOR inhibitors

Rapamycin and its analogues (rapalogs) are the most well-studied mTOR inhibitors and change the conformation and substrate specificity of mTORC1 by an allosteric mechanism (Ballou & Lin, 2008). Inter-

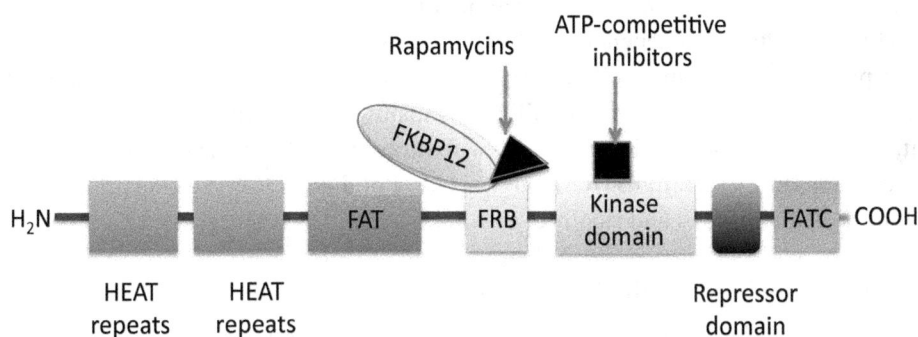

Figure 3: Structure of mTOR, showing tandem HEAT repeats, FAT domain, FRB domain, a catalytic kinase domain, repressor domain and FATC domain.

mTOR allosteric inhibitors in Clinical Trial		
Everolimus (RAD-001)	Phase III, oral dosing	Novartis Pharmaceuticals
Temsirolimus (CCI 779)	Phase II, i.v. infusion	Pfizer
Sirolimus (Rapamycin)	Phase II, oral dosing	Pfizer
Ridaforolimus (Deforolimus)	Phase II, oral dosing	Merck
ATP Competitive (TORC1/2) mTOR Kinase Inhibitors in Clinical Trial		
OSI-027	Phase I, oral dosing	Astellas Pharma Inc
AZD8055	Phase I/II, oral dosing	AstraZeneca
AZD2014	Phase I, oral dosing	AstraZeneca
INK128	Phase I, oral dosing	Intellikine
Palomid 529	Phase I, i.v. infusion	Paloma Pharmaceuticals, Inc.
CC-223	Phase I, oral dosing	Celgene Corporation
GDC-0349	Phase I, oral dosing	Genentech
DS-3078	Phase I, oral dosing	Daiichi Sankyo Inc.
Dual PI3K/mTOR Inhibitors in Clinical Trial		
NVP-BEZ235	Phase I/II, oral dosing	Novartis Pharmaceuticals
SF1126	Phase I, i.v. infusion	Semafore Pharmaceuticals
XL765	Phase I/II, oral dosing	Sanofi-Aventis
NVP-BGT226	Phase I/II, oral dosing	Novartis Pharmaceuticals
GSK1059615	Phase I, oral dosing	GlaxoSmithKline
GDC-0980	Phase I, oral dosing	Genentech
GSK2126458	Phase I, oral dosing	GlaxoSmithKline
PF-04691502	Phase I, oral dosing	Pfizer
GDC-0941	Phase II, oral dosing	Genentech
PKI-587	Phase I, i.v. infusion	Pfizer

Table 2: mTOR inhibitors in clinical trial. Data from http:/clinicaltrials.gov. Phase I clinical trials were assumed to include breast cancer.

action between ER signaling and mTOR pathway involves mTORC1 substrate, S6 kinase 1, which phosphorylates and triggers ligand-independent ER activation (Yamnik & Holz, 2010). Rapamycin and rapalogs form complexes with the intracellular receptor FKBP12 to inhibit mTORC1 signaling (Figure 3). Since the poor aqueous solubility and instability of rapamycin have limited its development as an anti-cancer agent, several analogues (called rapalogs) with more favorable pharmaceutical characteristics have been developed, including everolimus (RAD001), a U.S. Food and Drug Administration-approved mTOR allosteric inhibitor, temsirolimus and ridaforolimus.

4.1   Cell Culture Models for Evaluation of Allosteric Inhibitors

The anti-estrogen tamoxifen is commonly used in front-line treatment of women whose breast cancer biopsies show elevated levels of ER, regardless of menopausal status. The role of ovarian ablation in addition to tamoxifen in premenopausal breast cancer patients is still being investigated in ongoing clinical trials. Many women with early-stage breast cancers who initially respond to tamoxifen become resistant to the drug over time and develop recurrent tumors. Regardless of menopausal status, the continued expression of ER in many patients with tumor progression on tamoxifen indicates that mechanisms for resistance other than ER loss are common in breast cancer (Encarnacion et al., 1993). Sequential biopsies from breast cancer patients who relapsed on tamoxifen show that functional ER expression is retained in more than 50% of cases (Johnston, 2010). Cell culture models provide a method to investigate the onset of drug resistance. Tamoxifen resistance was associated with an activated PI3K pathway in some MCF-7 cell lines (Fox et al., 2011; Leary et al., 2010), either through IGF-1 receptor pathway or HER2/ER cross-talk. We have previously developed a series of sub-lines of the MCF-7 breast cancer cell line using conditions that mimic, in vitro, those conditions that appear in vivo lead to the development clinical resistance to anti-estrogens (Leung et al., 2010). Firstly, MCF-7 cells were cultured continuously in standard growth medium in the presence of increasing amounts of tamoxifen to produce the TamR7 sub-line in the presence of estrogen (which is present in fetal bovine serum), thus mimicking clinical anti-estrogen therapy. Secondly, cells were grown continuously in culture medium in the absence of both estrogen and phenol red (which has estrogenic properties) to produce the TamC3 and TamC6 sub-lines. The fetal bovine serum, used as a source of growth factors, had been previously absorbed with charcoal to remove estrogen, thus mimicking the clinical effects of either oophorectomy or treatment with aromatase inhibitors such as letrozole. Thirdly, cells were cultured continuously as above in the absence of estrogen but with the addition of tamoxifen to produce the TamR3 and TamR6 sub-lines, thus mimicking the effect of combined therapy with anti-estrogens plus aromatase inhibitors. Cell lines were then characterized by cellular DNA content (ploidy), modal cell volume and cell cycle time (Table 3) (Leung et al., 2010). Furthermore, these sub-lines still maintain their heterogeneity, as shown by cytogenetic analysis (data not shown). In accordance with the recent finding that intratumor heterogeneity leads to underestimation of the tumor genomic and transcriptional diversity (Gerlinger et al., 2012), human breast cancers may therefore contain pre-existing minor tamoxifen-resistant populations that expand during treatment.

4.2   Effects of Rapamycin and Everolimus on Cell Growth

Our previous study showed that the tamoxifen-resistant lines emerging following prolonged culture of MCF-7 cells in the presence of tamoxifen or in the absence of estrogen showed differential response to rapamycin (Leung et al., 2010). The TamC6 and TamR6 sub-lines, show high phosphorylation level of p70S6K and ERK (Figure 4). We have identified sub-lines, TamC3 and TamR3, that are highly resistant to both rapamycin and everolimus in growth inhibition (Figure 5), exhibit low levels of Akt and p70S6K phosphorylation, suggesting low utilization of PI3K pathway (Leung et al., 2010).

	Parental	TamR7	TamC3	TamR3	TamC6	TamR6
DNA content (ploidy)	1.5	1.9	1.4	1.4	2	2.1
Modal cell volume (pL)	2.4	2.6	1.6	1.2	2.2	2
Cell cycle time (hours)	31	31	27	27	36	37

Table 3: Characteristics of the MCF-7 line and its sub-lines, reproduced with permission from previously published data (Leung *et al.*, 2010).

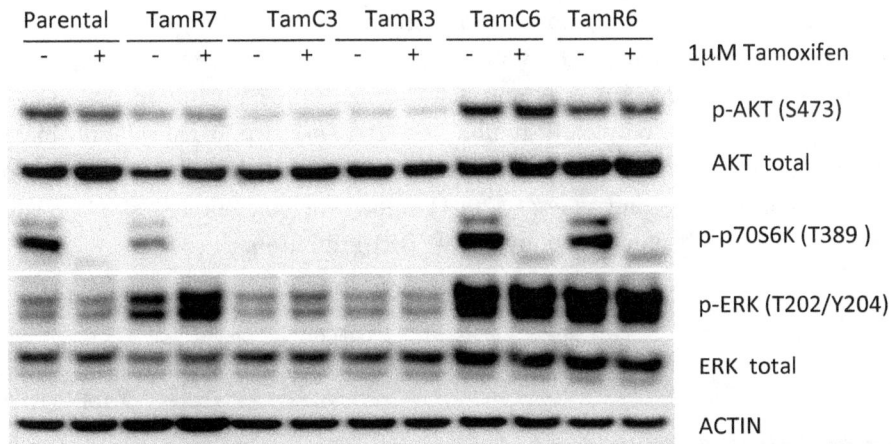

Figure 4: Phosphorylation of p70S6K and ERK by MCF-7 lines. Immunoblots for p-p70S6K (T389), p-Erk(T202/Y204), Erk total antibodies are indicated below the corresponding control. MCF-7 and its sub-lines were treated with and without 1 µM tamoxifen overnight. Actin is the loading control. Figure reproduced with permission from previously published data (Leung *et al.*, 2010).

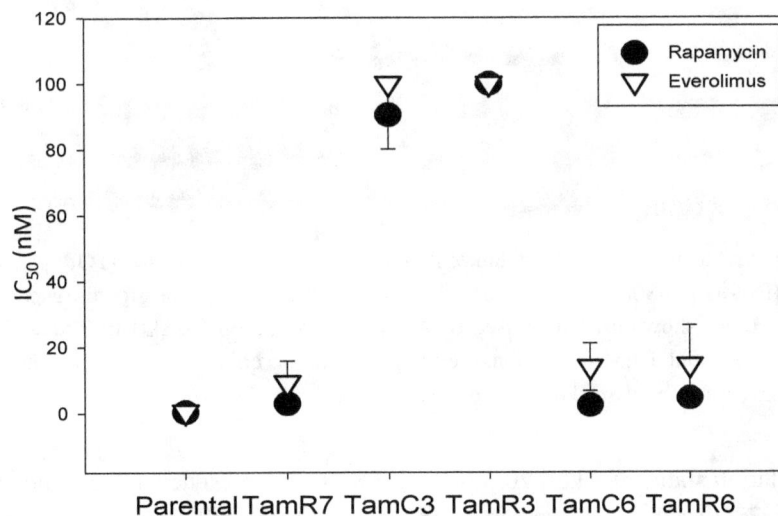

Figure 5: IC50 values for rapamycin and everolimus in MCF-7 and its sub-lines. Cells were treated with rapamycin or everolimus for 4 days with [3H]-thymidine added for the last 6 hours. Bars indicate SE (duplicate experiments). IC50 values of rapamycin for all the MCF-7 lines correlated significantly to those of everolimus (r =0.995; p<0.0001).

4.3   Effects of Allosteric mTOR Inhibitors on Akt, p70S6K, rpS6 and 4EBP1 Phosphorylation

Rapamycin alone or in combination with tamoxifen increased the level of phospho-Akt in parental MCF-7 cells and TamR7, TamC6 and TamR6 (Figure 6) (Leung *et al.*, 2010). Increases in phospho-Akt in some cells may be due to inhibitory feedback mechanisms between the mTOR effector p70S6K and the insulin receptor substrate-PI3K upstream of Akt (Shi *et al.*, 2005). Inhibition of mTOR signaling by rapamycin also increases Akt phosphorylation in MCF-7 cells (O'Reilly *et al.*, 2006; S. Y. Sun *et al.*, 2005; Wang *et al.*, 2008). Since rapamycin caused dephosphorylation of mTOR signaling proteins in all the cell lines tested regardless of tamoxifen or rapamycin sensitivity, the mTOR pathway is not a useful molecular predictor of the effects of rapamycin on tumor growth. Furthermore, rapamycin alone was unable to resensitize cell lines to tamoxifen (deGraffenried *et al.*, 2004). These results suggest that the downstream targets are not inhibited concordantly and that rapamycin response is mediated by other factors. Interestingly, rapamycin did not completely inhibit 4EPB1 (Thr70) phosphorylation in MCF-7 and its sub-lines (Figure 6) (Leung *et al.*, 2010). There was no differential difference in dephosphorylation of 4EBP1 (Thr70) phosphorylation (Gingras *et al.*, 2001) among the cell line tested, suggesting that the resistance in TamC3 and TamR3 is unlikely to involve 4EBP1 inhibition.

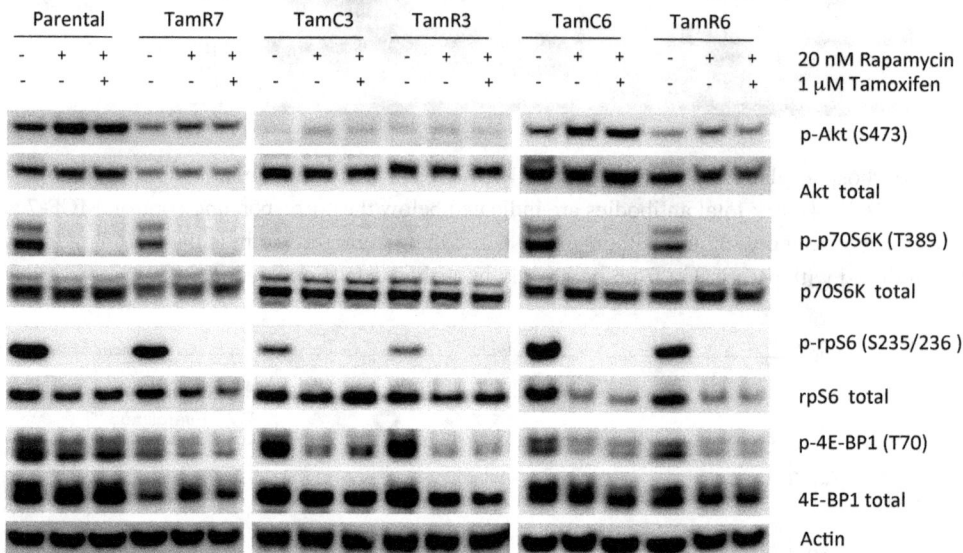

Figure 6: Rapamycin with or without tamoxifen inhibits signals through mTOR pathway and its downstream effectors p70S6k, rpS6 and 4EBP1 irrespective of the cellular growth response to the inhibitors. Immunoblot showing an increased of Akt phosphorylation (p-Akt) treated with 20 nM rapamycin with or without 1 μM tamoxifen. Actin is the loading control. Figure reproduced with permission from previously published data (Leung *et al.*, 2010).

The phosphorylation status of Akt, p70 S6K and rpS6 in the presence and absence of everolimus are compared in Figure 7. Everolimus increased the phospho-Akt in cell lines tested, suggesting a similar inhibitory mechanism to that of rapamycin. Differences in basal expression of phosphorylated proteins including Akt and p70 S6K (Figures 4, 6, and 7) within the same cell line could be due to different chemiluminescence detection sensitivities, different serum lots used and different cell passage numbers. However, the drug-induced changes in signaling activities are consistent.

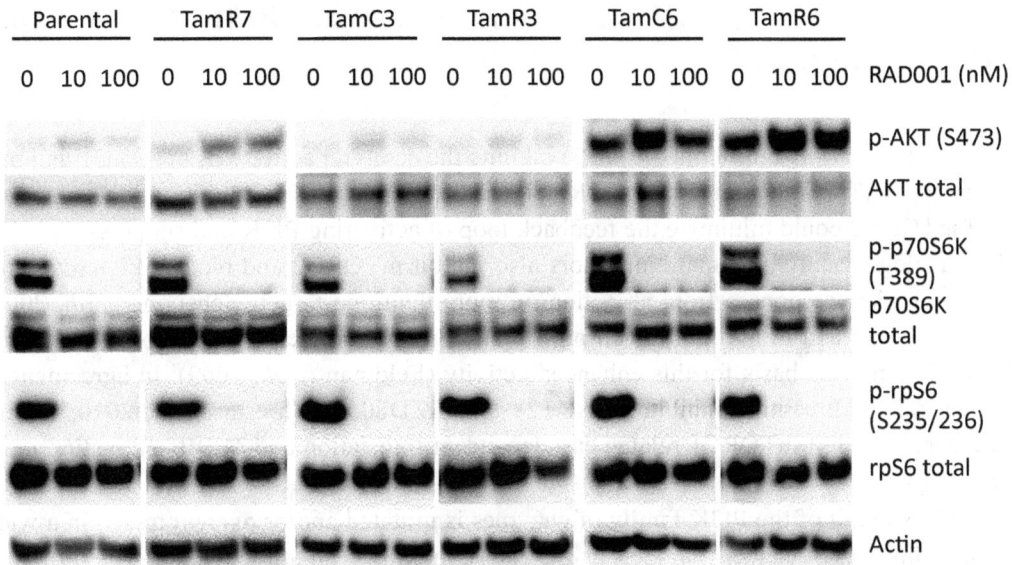

Figure 7: Everolimus inhibits signals through mTOR pathway and p70S6k and rpS6, irrespective of the cellular growth response. Immunoblot showing an increased of Akt phosphorylation (p-Akt) treated with 10 nM or 100 nM Everolimus, which also completely dephosphorylated p70S6K and rpS6. Actin is the loading control. Figure reproduced with permission from previously published data (Leung *et al.*, 2011).

4.4   Clinical Trials of mTOR Allosteric Inhibitors

The finding that the PI3K/Akt/mTOR pathway is often altered in breast cancer (Vivanco & Sawyers, 2002) led to growing interest in rapamycin and rapalogs as anti-cancer drugs (Carraway & Hidalgo, 2004). Rapamycin was initially used clinically as an immunosuppressant but inhibited growth of in estrogen receptor positive breast cancer cells (Chang *et al.*, 2007; Fasolo & Sessa, 2008). And everolimus was shown to be effective in renal cell carcinoma (http://www.pharma.us.novartis.com/product/pi/pdf/afinitor.pdf). However, rapamycin and rapalogs as single agents showed limited efficacy in clinical trials (Wang & Sun, 2009). Combination studies of rapamycin with other therapeutic agents are currently underway. One trial combines rapamycin with trastuzumab (an antibody to HER2) for human epidermal growth receptor 2 (HER2) positive metastatic breast cancers (NCT00411788). Another has combined everolimus with an aromatase inhibitor, with improved progression-free survival in postmenopausal patients in ER+ advanced breast cancer (Baselga *et al.*, 2012). Trials have also combined everolimus with trastuzumab for metastatic HER2 over-expressing breast cancer (NCT00317720), everolimus with carboplatin (cross-linking of DNA) for triple negative metastatic breast cancer (NCT01127763) and everolimus with bevacizumab (anti-VEGF) and lapatinib (anti-EGFR and anti-HER2) for primary breast cancer (NCT00567554) are also underway. Clinical studies using temsirolimus and neratinib for metastatic HER2-amplified or triple negative breast cancer (NCT01111825), ridaforolimus with trastuzumab for HER2 positive Trastuzumab-refractory metastatic breast cancer (NCT00736970) and ridaforolimus with dalotuzumab for ER+ breast cancer (NCT01234857) are also under investigation.

5   ATP-competitive mTOR Inhibitors and Dual PI3K/ATP-competitive mTOR Inhibitors

A new generation of mTOR inhibitors (Table 2) inhibits the catalytic activity of mTORC1 and mTORC2 by binding to the ATP-binding sites of mTOR (Figure 3). Some of these inhibitors also inhibit PI3K; inhibition of mTORC2 could minimize the feedback loop of activating PI3K and suppress the Akt activation. Unlike rapalogs, catalytic domain inhibitors also inhibit mTORC2 and block Akt activation, resulting in better biological responses from an action on more than one target (Schenone *et al.*, 2008). Two such inhibitors, PP242 and PP30, inhibit cell proliferation more completely than rapamycin, but surprisingly, mTORC2 is not the basis for this enhanced activity (Feldman *et al.*, 2009). In agreement with results for other ATP-competitive inhibitors INK128 and AZD8055 (Chresta *et al.*, 2010; Hsieh *et al.*, 2012), these agents inhibit mTORC1 related cap-dependent translation and 4EBP1 activation that are resistant to rapalogs.

The PI3Kα subunit of the PI3K family of enzymes is mutated and/or overexpressed in a wide range of cancers including breast cancer (Samuels *et al.*, 2004), making it an attractive target. Furthermore, the PI3K pathway is activated as a consequence of mTOR inhibition. Thus, dual PI3K/mTOR inhibitors abrogate the compensatory effect of mTOR inhibition responsible for their strong antiproliferative effect (Maira *et al.*, 2008). Since mTOR shares high sequence homology with PI3K, some compounds that were originally developed as PI3K inhibitors have also been found to target mTOR (Table 2). BEZ235 and GSK2126458 are highly selective and potent small molecule inhibitors that target both multiple class I PI3K isoforms and mTOR kinase activity (Knight *et al.*, 2010; Maira *et al.*, 2008). BEZ235 blocks PI3K/mTOR pathway and induces G1 cell cycle arrest (Leung *et al.*, 2011; Maira *et al.*, 2008).

5.1   Cell Lines for Studying Dual PI3K/ATP-competitive Catalytic mTOR Inhibitors

In contrast to their response to rapalogs, tamoxifen-resistant lines do not show significant increased sensitivity to PI3K/mTOR inhibitors BEZ235 and GSK2126458. While one sub-line, (TamR7) resembled the parental line in its sensitivity to the PI3K/mTOR inhibitors, four other sub-lines (TamC3, TamR3, TamC6 and TamR6) were significantly more resistant (Figure 8)(Leung *et al.*, 2011). Observation of PARP cleavage in MCF-7 parental and TamR7 correlated with their decrease in cell density in response to BEZ235 or GSK212.

5.2   Growth Inhibitory Action of BEZ235 and GSK2126458

Analysis of the cellular responses of MCF-7 and its sub-lines to BEZ235 and GSK2126458 shows that the predominant effect is the inhibition of the transition from G1-phase to S-phase rather than the induction of apoptosis (Leung *et al.*, 2011). Apoptosis, as measured by PARP induction, was observed only in the parental line and one sub-line following exposure to drugs at concentrations above those required to inhibit individual signaling pathways (Figure 8) (Leung *et al.*, 2011). Other studies have shown that individual breast cancer cell lines vary in sensitivity to BEZ235-induced apoptosis, with some cell lines more susceptible than others (Brachmann *et al.*, 2009; Serra *et al.*, 2008). A recent study reported a significant increase in apoptosis induced by BEZ235 in MCF-7 and MCF-7/LTED (long term estrogen deprived) cells but not HCC-1428 and HCC-1428/LTED cells. Studies of the effect of ZSTK474, another PI3K inhibitor, on PC3 prostate cancer cells indicated that cell cycle arrest was the dominant cellular response to this class of agents. The protein p27KIP1, an inhibitor of cyclin-dependent kinase-2, was induced by ZSTK474 and may be responsible to the arrest of cells in G1-phase (Dan *et al.*, 2009).

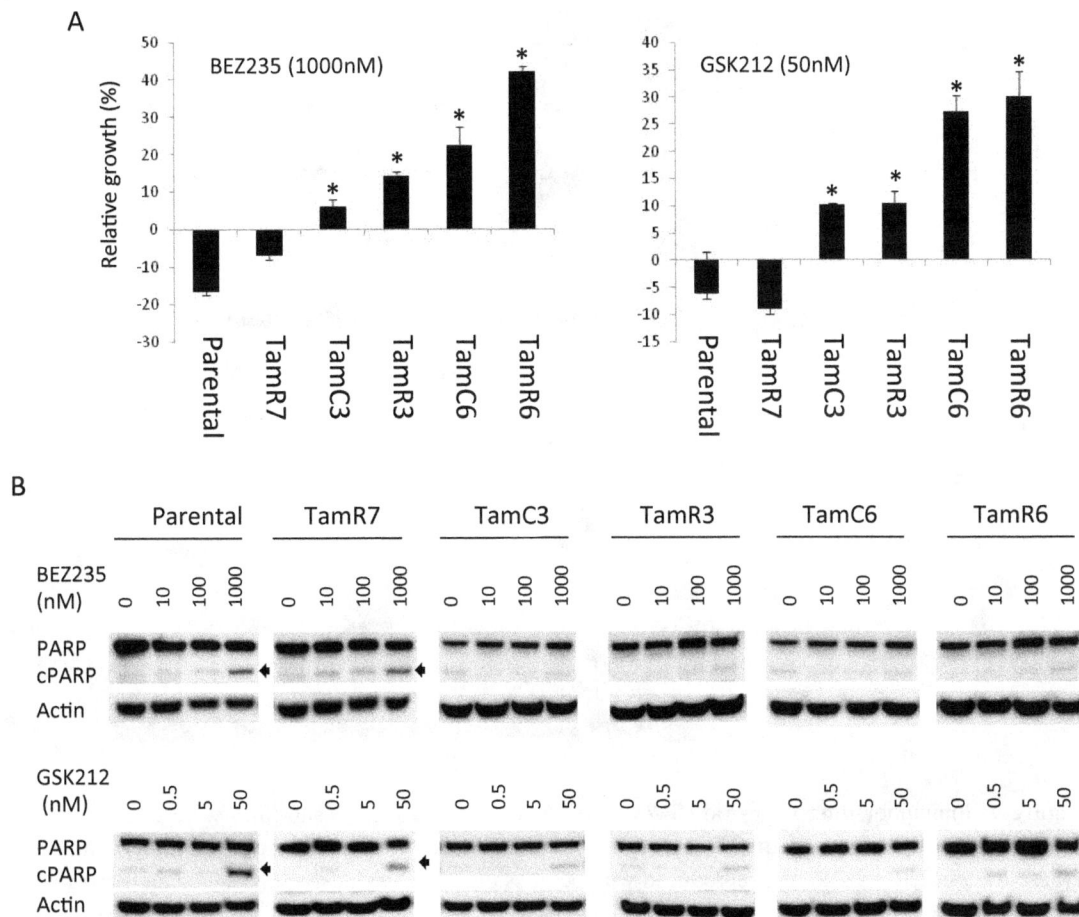

Figure 8: Effects of BEZ235 and GSK212 in MCF-7 parental and its derived sub-lines in proliferation and apoptosis. MCF-7 parental and its sub-lines were exposed to the indicated concentrations of BEZ235 and GSK212 (A) for 3 days, and cell proliferation was measured by the sulforhodamine B assay. Bars represent percentage changes in cell density after 72 h compared with initial amount present at the treatment start and expressed as the mean ± standard error from three experiments. Immunoblotting for cleaved PARP (cPARP) in MCF-7 cell lines treated with different concentration of (B) BEZ235 or GSK212 for 72 h. Actin is the loading control. Figure reproduced with permission from previously published data (Leung et al., 2011).

5.3   Effect of Inhibition of PI3K/mTOR Activation on Estrogen Receptor Expression

The MCF-7 line is ER-positive and it is of interest that all of the derived tamoxifen-resistant sub-lines expressed ER, generally at levels higher than that of the parent line, observation supporting the hypothesis that the tamoxifen resistance of the sub-lines is associated with increased ER expression and consequent maintenance of ER signaling pathways (Miller et al., 2010; Noguchi et al., 1993; Webb et al., 1995). ER expression was also modulated by exposure to PI3K/mTOR inhibitors (Figure 9) (Leung et al., 2011), emphasizing the high degree of cross-talk that exists in these cellular signaling pathways. However, ER expression levels did not correlate to PI3K pathway utilization in MCF-7 parental and the tamoxifen resistant sub-lines (Leung et al., 2011).

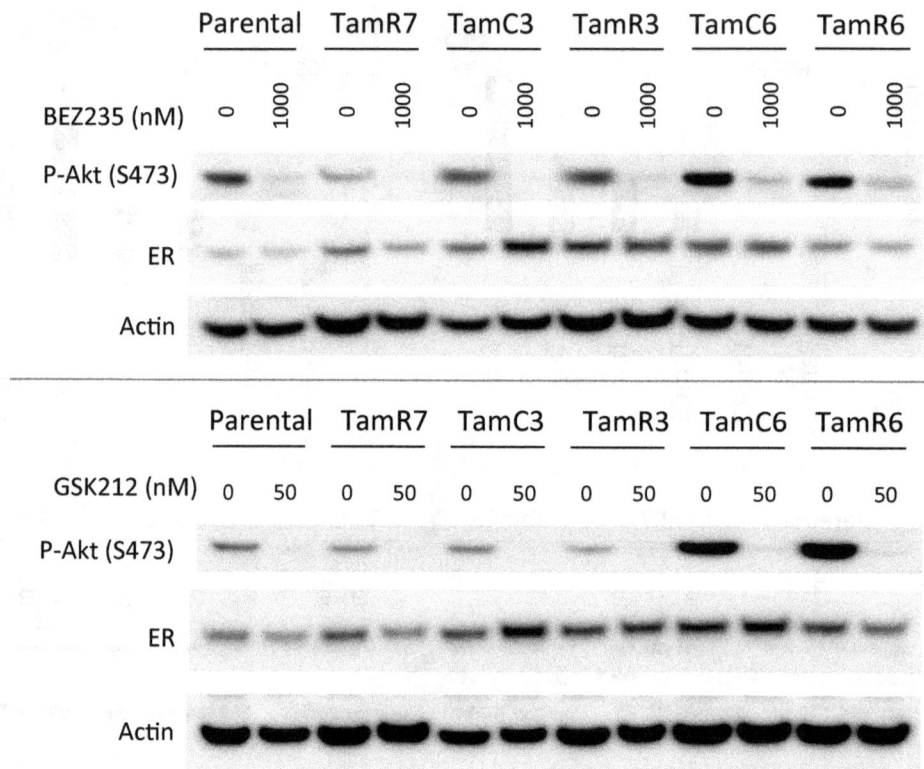

Figure 9: Immunoblotting for p-Akt (S473) and ER antibodies. MCF-7 sub-lines were treated with the indicated concentrations of BEZ235 or GSK2126458 overnight. Actin is the loading control. GSK212, GSK2126458. Figure reproduced with permission from previously published data (Leung *et al.*, 2011).

5.4   Effects of Inhibition on Akt, rpS6, p70S6K and ERK Phosphorylation

Downstream cellular responses to BEZ235 and GSK2126458 were assessed by measuring phosphorylation of Akt, p70S6K, rpS6 and ERK (Figure 10). BEZ235 significantly inhibited Akt phosphorylation in MCF-7 parental, TamR7, TamC3 and TamR3 cells but no significant change in phosphorylation of Akt was observed in TamC6 and TamR6 cells (Leung *et al.*, 2011). Although GSK2126458 significantly inhibited Akt phosphorylation in all six cell lines (Figure 10A), TamC6 and TamR6 showed lower responses to GSK2126458 as compared to MCF-7 parental cells. The downstream signals in phospho-p70S6K and phospho-rpS6 were significantly suppressed in all sub-lines tested, irrespective of their differential growth response to BEZ235 or GSK2126458 (Figures 10B and C). While p70S6K is a known modulator of a PI3K pathway feedback loop (O'Reilly *et al.*, 2006), no correlation was observed between p70S6K phosphorylation and active Akt levels. This might be expected since both BEZ235 and GSK2126458 are dual PI3K/mTOR inhibitors. Inhibition of mTOR signaling can lead to increased activation of ERK, presumably via a p70S6K/PI3K/RAS feedback loop (Wan & Helman, 2007). PI3K and MAPK signaling pathways have reciprocal pathway activation induced by inhibitor mediated release of negative feedback loops (Aksamitiene *et al.*, 2010; Sos *et al.*, 2009). Although all cell lines tested showed higher activated ERK levels (phospho-ERK) in response to inhibitors, no significant change in ERK activation was observed (Figure 10D).

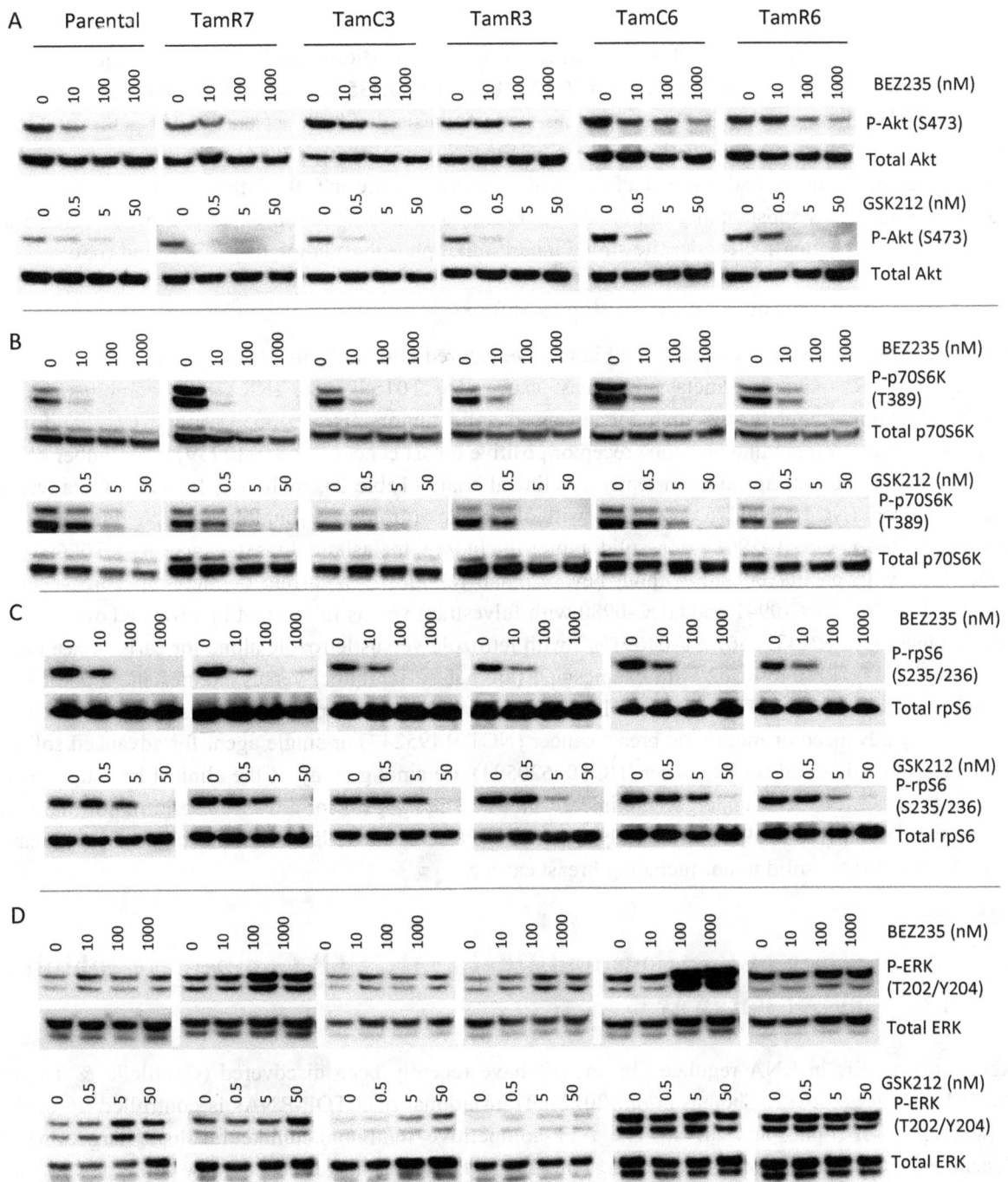

Figure 10: Immunoblots of PI3K pathway signaling proteins in MCF-7 cell lines treated with BEZ235 or GSK212 for 24 h. BEZ235 and GSK212 inhibit signaling through PI3K/mTOR, Akt (A), p70S6K (B), rpS6 (C). ERK activation was assessed (D). Immunoblotting for antibodies for p-Akt(S473), p-p70S6K(T389), p-rpS6 (S235/236), p-ERK(T202/Y204) and their respective proteins (which were used as loading controls). GSK212, GSK2126458. Figure reproduced with permission from previously published data (Leung *et al.*, 2011).

5.5   Growth Inhibitory Effect and Inhibition of the mTOR Signaling Pathway

The IC50 values for GSK2126458, as well as the drug concentrations required to inhibit the PI3K pathway, are lower than those for BEZ235, but IC50 values of BEZ235 and GSK2126458 are correlated ($r=0.93$, $p=0.008$) (Leung et al., 2011), supporting the hypothesis that both act on the Akt pathway. On the other hand, BEZ235 was more active than GSK2126458 in inhibiting p70S6K phosphorylation; inhibition of the Akt pathway had a larger effect than inhibition of the mTOR pathway on cell growth. The TamR7 sub-line was substantially inhibited by BEZ235 and GSK2126458 while growth of TamC6 and TamR6 was largely unaffected, despite strong inhibition of phosphorylation of p70S6K and rpS6.

5.6   Clinical Trials Using ATP-competitive Inhibitors

Selective ATP-competitive catalytic inhibitors have entered clinical trials (Table 2). AZD-2014 and fulvestrant for ER+ advanced metastatic breast cancer (NCT01597388), INK128 in combination with paclitaxel, with/without trastuzumab for advanced solid tumors (NCT01351350) and CC-223 for advanced solid tumor including hormone receptor positive breast cancer (NCT01177397). A number of dual PI3K/mTOR inhibitors are also currently in clinical trials (Table 2), including BGT266 for advanced breast cancer (NCT00600275), XL765 with letrozole (aromatase inhibitor) with breast cancer (NCT01082068), GSK1059615 for solid tumor including metastatic breast cancer (NCT00695448), GDC-0980 with paclitaxel with/without bevacizumab for locally recurrent or metastatic breast cancer (NCT01254526), GDC-0941 and GDC-0980 with fulvestrant versus fulvestrant in advanced or metastatic breast cancer (NCT01437566), PF-04691502 with letrozole versus letrozole alone for early breast cancer (NCT01430585), PF-04691502 with exemestane (aromatase inhibitor) versus exemestane alone for advanced breast cancer (NCT01658176). BEZ235 as combination therapy with paclitaxel for HER2 negative, locally advanced or metastatic breast cancer (NCT01495247) or single agent for advanced solid tumor including advanced breast cancer (NCT00620594) are among many of the clinical investigations of this drug. GSK2126458 is undergoing clinical trial as a single agent for advanced solid tumor malignancy, or lymphoma (NCT00972686). Lastly, PKI-587 (PF-05212384) is also under clinical investigation (NCT00940498) for solid tumor including breast cancer.

6   Combination of Rapalogs and Dual PI3K/ATP-Competitive Inhibitors of the mTOR Pathway

Regulatory motifs in RNA regulated by mTOR have recently been discovered (Gentilella & Thomas, 2012; Hsieh et al., 2012; Thomas et al., 2012). Translational of 5'TOP-RNAs is controlled by mTOR-dependent 4EBP1 phosphorylation. The ATP-competitive inhibitors, unlike rapalogs, target mTOR-dependent 4EBP1 phosphorylation (Hsieh et al., 2012). However, this effect could be cell type specific as 4EBP1 dephosphorylation by rapamycin was observed in our MCF-7 cell lines irrespective of the differential growth effect (Figure 6).

Several studies suggested that the variable anti-proliferative effects of rapalogs in cancer cells might be due to the incomplete mTORC1 inhibition in some tumor types (Feldman et al., 2009; Hsieh et al., 2012). Everolimus has been found to have good efficacy of growth inhibition in basal-like triple negative breast cancer cell lines (Yunokawa et al., 2012), while BEZ235 has been identified as an effective agent for growth inhibition in mesenchymal stem-like triple negative breast cancer cell lines (Lehmann et al.,

2011). Targeting both mTOR and PI3K/Akt signaling using rapamycin and LY294002 prevents mTOR inhibition initiated Akt activation and enhances anticancer activity in cell cultures and in xenograft models (Wang *et al.*, 2008). Akt activation that was induced by mTOR inhibition has been reported to be independent of mTORC2 activity (Wang *et al.*, 2008). Moreover, LY294002 is a dual PI3K/mTOR inhibitor that inactivates mTOR kinase as well as PI3K at similar concentrations (Ballou *et al.*, 2007). Recently, combination of everolimus with BEZ235 showed synergistic inhibition in the proliferation of a number cancer cell lines (Shoji *et al.*, 2012; Thomas *et al.*, 2012; Xu *et al.*, 2011). Although the exact mechanism has yet to be understood, it has been suggested that the synergy involved the down-regulation in genes involved in autophagy (Thomas *et al.*, 2012).

6.1   Cell Line Models for Studying Combinations of Everolimus and BEZ235

We have examined the combination of everolimus and BEZ235 on cell growth of MCF-7 TamC3 and TamR3 by (Figure 11). We also tested the growth response using the drug combination on the triple negative MDA-MB-231 breast cancer cell line since it has low PI3K/mTOR pathway utilization and showed IC50 value for everolimus exceeding 100 nM (Yunokawa *et al.*, 2012). The everolimus and BEZ235 combination exhibited growth inhibitory effects that are greater than that caused by each single agent of sub-optimal concentration in a 4 day culture assay. Proliferation was reduced to 41%, 34% and 33% at the suboptimal dose of 10 nM everolimus and 10 nM of BEZ235 in TamC3, TamR3 and MDA-MB-231, respectively. Further study is required to investigate the combination effects on PI3K/mTOR signaling pathway in order to determine the synergy in growth inhibition followed Akt, rpS6 or 4EPB1 dephosphorylation, and whether autophagy is involved.

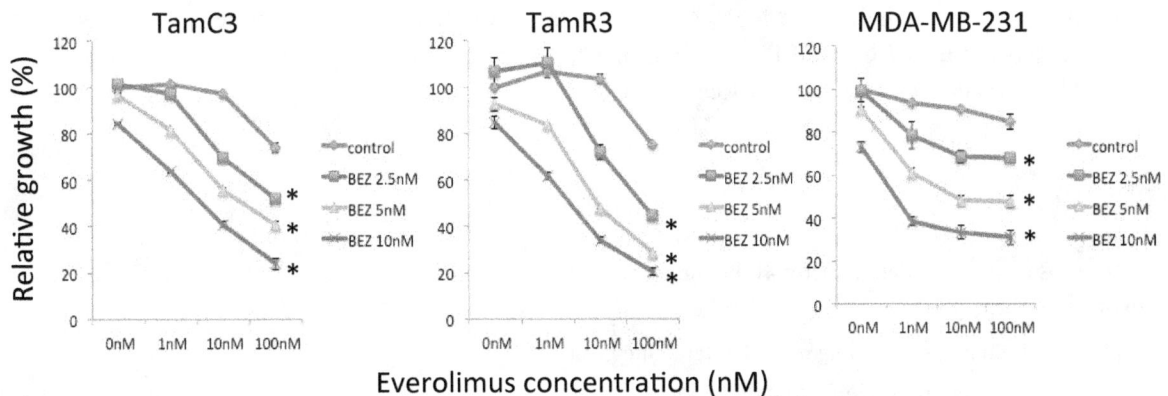

Figure 11: Everolimus and BEZ235 synergistically decrease proliferation in MCF-7 TamC3 and TamR3 sub-lines, the MDA-MB-231 cell line. Cells were treated with the indicated concentrations of everolimus and/or BEZ235 for 96 hours. Cells were treated with rapamycin or everolimus for 4 days with [3H]-thymidine added for the last 6 hours. Mean ± standard error (two experiments). *Significant difference from treatment control ($p < 0.01$). The methodology has been previously published (Leung *et al.*, 2010).

6.2   Clinical Trials Using Combinations of Everolimus and ATP-competitive Inhibitors

Considerable efforts have been dedicated to targeting the PI3K/Akt/mTOR pathway for cancer treatment. There is emerging evidence that multiple inhibition of pathway may provide better responses without inducing unacceptable toxicity. BEZ235 in combination with everolimus in advanced solid tumors including breast cancer (NCT01482156 and NCT01508104) is currently under investigation.

7   Conclusion

Breast cancer is increasingly being recognized as a disease characterized by a high degree of heterogeneity. Molecular subtype profiling of breast cancer provides prognostication and prediction, complementary to clinicopathological parameters, for selection of targeted therapies in breast cancer (Weigelt *et al.*, 2010). However, identification of tumor subtype from biopsy samples may underestimate the intratumor heterogeneity. Breast cancer sub-lines developed from small subpopulations may therefore provide useful tools to investigate such heterogeneity, particularly as a basis for the development of drug resistance. Such an approach may be particularly useful in developing combinations of drugs that target the mTOR pathway and drugs that target other pathways such as the PI3K/AKT pathway. An important challenge for the future is to identify and validate biomarkers to detect the emergence of resistant sub-populations, with the ultimate goal of tailoring chemotherapy sequences to individual cancer patients.

Acknowledgements

The authors thank Paul Oei (IGENZ, New Zealand) assistance on fluorescence in situ hybridization and cytogenetic analysis, and Gordon W. Rewcastle for discussions on PI3K/mTOR inhibitors. Funding for this work was obtained from Cancer Society of New Zealand and its Auckland Division, the New Zealand Breast Cancer Foundation, the New Zealand Lottery Commission, the Maurice and Phyllis Paykel trust, Auckland Medical Research Foundation, and the Genesis Oncology Trust, and this work is also supported by Auckland Cancer Society Research Centre.

Abbreviations

4E-BP1	Eukaryotic initiation factor 4E binding protein 1
BEZ235	NVP-BEZ235
DEPTOR	dEP domain-containing mTOR-interacting protein
eIF4E	Eukaryotic translation initiation factor 4E
eIF4F	Eukaryotic translation initiation factor 4F
ER	Estrogen receptor
ERK	Extracellular signal-regulated kinases
FAT	FRAP, ATM and TTRAP
FATC	C-terminal FAT domain
FKBP12	FK506 Binding Protein 12
FRB	FKBP12/rapamycin-binding
GSK212	GSK2126458
HEAT	Huntington, elongation factor 3, protein phosphatase 2A, TOR1

HER2	Human Epidermal Growth Factor Receptor 2
IGF-1	Insulin-like growth factor 1
MAPK	Mitogen-activated protein kinases
mLST8	Mammalian lethal with SEC13 protein 8
mSIN1	Mammalian stress-activated map kinase-interacting protein 1
mTOR	Mammalian target of rapamycin
mTORC1	mTOR complex 1
mTORC2	mTOR complex 2
PARP	Poly ADP-ribose polymerase
PI3K	Phosphatidylinositide 3-kinases
PKC	Protein kinase C
PRAS40	40 kDa Pro-rich Akt substrate
rapalogs	Rapamycin and its analogues
RAPTOR	mTOR regulatory-associated protein of mTOR
RICTOR	Rapamycin-insensitive companion of mTOR
S6K1	S6 kinase 1
SGK1	Serine/threonine-protein kinase 1
TSC1	Tuberous sclerosis protein 1
TSC2	Tuberous sclerosis protein 2
VEGF	Vascular endothelial growth factor

References

Aksamitiene, E., Kholodenko, B. N., Kolch, W., Hoek, J. B., & Kiyatkin, A. (2010). PI3K/Akt-sensitive MEK-independent compensatory circuit of ERK activation in ER-positive PI3K-mutant T47D breast cancer cells. Cell Signal, 22(9), 1369-1378.

Astle, M. V., Hannan, K. M., Ng, P. Y., Lee, R. S., George, A. J., Hsu, A. K., Haupt, Y., Hannan, R. D., & Pearson, R. B. (2012). AKT induces senescence in human cells via mTORC1 and p53 in the absence of DNA damage: implications for targeting mTOR during malignancy. Oncogene, 31(15), 1949-1962.

Baguley, B. C., & Leung, E. (2012). Heterogeneity of phenotype in breast cancer cell lines (Vol. Book 1): Intech Publishers

Ballou, L. M., & Lin, R. Z. (2008). Rapamycin and mTOR kinase inhibitors. J Chem Biol, 1(1-4), 27-36.

Ballou, L. M., Selinger, E. S., Choi, J. Y., Drueckhammer, D. G., & Lin, R. Z. (2007). Inhibition of mammalian target of rapamycin signaling by 2-(morpholin-1-yl)pyrimido[2,1-alpha]isoquinolin-4-one. J Biol Chem, 282(33), 24463-24470.

Baselga, J., Campone, M., Piccart, M., Burris, H. A., 3rd, Rugo, H. S., Sahmoud, T., Noguchi, S., Gnant, M., Pritchard, K. I., Lebrun, F., Beck, J. T., Ito, Y., Yardley, D., Deleu, I., Perez, A., Bachelot, T., Vittori, L., Xu, Z., Mukhopadhyay, P., Lebwohl, D., & Hortobagyi, G. N. (2012). Everolimus in postmenopausal hormone-receptor-positive advanced breast cancer. N Engl J Med, 366(6), 520-529.

Benjamin, D., Colombi, M., Moroni, C., & Hall, M. N. (2011). Rapamycin passes the torch: a new generation of mTOR inhibitors. Nat Rev Drug Discov, 10(11), 868-880.

Brachmann, S. M., Hofmann, I., Schnell, C., Fritsch, C., Wee, S., Lane, H., Wang, S., Garcia-Echeverria, C., & Maira, S. M. (2009). Specific apoptosis induction by the dual PI3K/mTor inhibitor NVP-BEZ235 in HER2 amplified and PIK3CA mutant breast cancer cells. Proc Natl Acad Sci U S A, 106(52), 22299-22304.

Cai, Q., Lin, T., Kamarajugadda, S., & Lu, J. (2012). Regulation of glycolysis and the Warburg effect by estrogen-related receptors. Oncogene.

Carraway, H., & Hidalgo, M. (2004). New targets for therapy in breast cancer: mammalian target of rapamycin (mTOR) antagonists. Breast Cancer Res, 6(5), 219-224.

Chang, S. B., Miron, P., Miron, A., & Iglehart, J. D. (2007). Rapamycin inhibits proliferation of estrogen-receptor-positive breast cancer cells. J Surg Res, 138(1), 37-44.

Chresta, C. M., Davies, B. R., Hickson, I., Harding, T., Cosulich, S., Critchlow, S. E., Vincent, J. P., Ellston, R., Jones, D., Sini, P., James, D., Howard, Z., Dudley, P., Hughes, G., Smith, L., Maguire, S., Hummersone, M., Malagu, K., Menear, K., Jenkins, R., Jacobsen, M., Smith, G. C., Guichard, S., & Pass, M. (2010). AZD8055 is a potent, selective, and orally bioavailable ATP-competitive mammalian target of rapamycin kinase inhibitor with in vitro and in vivo antitumor activity. Cancer Res, 70(1), 288-298.

Coser, K. R., Wittner, B. S., Rosenthal, N. F., Collins, S. C., Melas, A., Smith, S. L., Mahoney, C. J., Shioda, K., Isselbacher, K. J., Ramaswamy, S., & Shioda, T. (2009). Antiestrogen-resistant subclones of MCF-7 human breast cancer cells are derived from a common monoclonal drug-resistant progenitor. Proc Natl Acad Sci U S A, 106(34), 14536-14541.

Dan, S., Yoshimi, H., Okamura, M., Mukai, Y., & Yamori, T. (2009). Inhibition of PI3K by ZSTK474 suppressed tumor growth not via apoptosis but G0/G1 arrest. Biochem Biophys Res Commun, 379(1), 104-109.

deGraffenried, L. A., Friedrichs, W. E., Russell, D. H., Donzis, E. J., Middleton, A. K., Silva, J. M., Roth, R. A., & Hidalgo, M. (2004). Inhibition of mTOR activity restores tamoxifen response in breast cancer cells with aberrant Akt Activity. Clin Cancer Res, 10(23), 8059-8067.

Dowling, R. J., Topisirovic, I., Alain, T., Bidinosti, M., Fonseca, B. D., Petroulakis, E., Wang, X., Larsson, O., Selvaraj, A., Liu, Y., Kozma, S. C., Thomas, G., & Sonenberg, N. (2010). mTORC1-mediated cell proliferation, but not cell growth, controlled by the 4E-BPs. Science, 328(5982), 1172-1176.

Encarnacion, C. A., Ciocca, D. R., McGuire, W. L., Clark, G. M., Fuqua, S. A., & Osborne, C. K. (1993). Measurement of steroid hormone receptors in breast cancer patients on tamoxifen. Breast Cancer Res Treat, 26(3), 237-246.

Fasolo, A., & Sessa, C. (2008). mTOR inhibitors in the treatment of cancer. Expert Opin Investig Drugs, 17(11), 1717-1734.

Feldman, M. E., Apsel, B., Uotila, A., Loewith, R., Knight, Z. A., Ruggero, D., & Shokat, K. M. (2009). Active-site inhibitors of mTOR target rapamycin-resistant outputs of mTORC1 and mTORC2. PLoS Biol, 7(2), e38.

Fingar, D. C., Richardson, C. J., Tee, A. R., Cheatham, L., Tsou, C., & Blenis, J. (2004). mTOR controls cell cycle progression through its cell growth effectors S6K1 and 4E-BP1/eukaryotic translation initiation factor 4E. Mol Cell Biol, 24(1), 200-216.

Fox, E. M., Miller, T. W., Balko, J. M., Kuba, M. G., Sanchez, V., Smith, R. A., Liu, S., Gonzalez-Angulo, A. M., Mills, G. B., Ye, F., Shyr, Y., Manning, H. C., Buck, E., & Arteaga, C. L. (2011). A kinome-wide screen identifies the insulin/IGF-I receptor pathway as a mechanism of escape from hormone dependence in breast cancer. Cancer Res, 71(21), 6773-6784.

Gentilella, A., & Thomas, G. (2012). Cancer biology: The director's cut. Nature, 485(7396), 50-51.

Gerlinger, M., Rowan, A. J., Horswell, S., Larkin, J., Endesfelder, D., Gronroos, E., Martinez, P., Matthews, N., Stewart, A., Tarpey, P., Varela, I., Phillimore, B., Begum, S., McDonald, N. Q., Butler, A., Jones, D., Raine, K., Latimer, C., Santos, C. R., Nohadani, M., Eklund, A. C., Spencer-Dene, B., Clark, G., Pickering, L., Stamp, G., Gore, M., Szallasi, Z., Downward, J., Futreal, P. A., & Swanton, C. (2012). Intratumor heterogeneity and branched evolution revealed by multiregion sequencing. N Engl J Med, 366(10), 883-892.

Gingras, A. C., Raught, B., Gygi, S. P., Niedzwiecka, A., Miron, M., Burley, S. K., Polakiewicz, R. D., Wyslouch-Cieszynska, A., Aebersold, R., & Sonenberg, N. (2001). Hierarchical phosphorylation of the translation inhibitor 4E-BP1. Genes Dev, 15(21), 2852-2864.

Hietakangas, V., & Cohen, S. M. (2008). TOR complex 2 is needed for cell cycle progression and anchorage-independent growth of MCF7 and PC3 tumor cells. BMC Cancer, 8, 282.

Hsieh, A. C., Liu, Y., Edlind, M. P., Ingolia, N. T., Janes, M. R., Sher, A., Shi, E. Y., Stumpf, C. R., Christensen, C., Bonham, M. J., Wang, S., Ren, P., Martin, M., Jessen, K., Feldman, M. E., Weissman, J. S., Shokat, K. M., Rommel, C., & Ruggero, D. (2012). The translational landscape of mTOR signalling steers cancer initiation and metastasis. Nature, 485(7396), 55-61.

Hsu, P. P., Kang, S. A., Rameseder, J., Zhang, Y., Ottina, K. A., Lim, D., Peterson, T. R., Choi, Y., Gray, N. S., Yaffe, M. B., Marto, J. A., & Sabatini, D. M. (2011). The mTOR-regulated phosphoproteome reveals a mechanism of mTORC1-mediated inhibition of growth factor signaling. Science, 332(6035), 1317-1322.

Johnston, S. R. (2006). Clinical efforts to combine endocrine agents with targeted therapies against epidermal growth factor receptor/human epidermal growth factor receptor 2 and mammalian target of rapamycin in breast cancer. Clin Cancer Res, 12(3 Pt 2), 1061s-1068s.

Johnston, S. R. (2010). New strategies in estrogen receptor-positive breast cancer. Clin Cancer Res, 16(7), 1979-1987.

Jordan, V. C. (2008). Tamoxifen: catalyst for the change to targeted therapy. Eur J Cancer, 44(1), 30-38.

Knight, Steven D., Adams, Nicholas D., Burgess, Joelle L., Chaudhari, Amita M., Darcy, Michael G., Donatelli, Carla A., Luengo, Juan I., Newlander, Ken A., Parrish, Cynthia A., Ridgers, Lance H., Sarpong, Martha A., Schmidt, Stanley J., Van Aller, Glenn S., Carson, Jeffrey D., Diamond, Melody A., Elkins, Patricia A., Gardiner, Christine M., Garver, Eric, Gilbert, Seth A., Gontarek, Richard R., Jackson, Jeffrey R., Kershner, Kevin L., Luo, Lusong, Raha, Kaushik, Sherk, Christian S., Sung, Chiu-Mei, Sutton, David, Tummino, Peter J., Wegrzyn, Ronald J., Auger, Kurt R., & Dhanak, Dashyant. (2010). Discovery of GSK2126458, a Highly Potent Inhibitor of PI3K and the Mammalian Target of Rapamycin. ACS Medicinal Chemistry Letters, 1(1), 39-43.

Laplante, M., & Sabatini, D. M. (2012). mTOR signaling in growth control and disease. Cell, 149(2), 274-293.

Leary, A. F., Drury, S., Detre, S., Pancholi, S., Lykkesfeldt, A. E., Martin, L. A., Dowsett, M., & Johnston, S. R. (2010). Lapatinib restores hormone sensitivity with differential effects on estrogen receptor signaling in cell models of human epidermal growth factor receptor 2-negative breast cancer with acquired endocrine resistance. Clin Cancer Res, 16(5), 1486-1497.

Lehmann, B. D., Bauer, J. A., Chen, X., Sanders, M. E., Chakravarthy, A. B., Shyr, Y., & Pietenpol, J. A. (2011). Identification of human triple-negative breast cancer subtypes and preclinical models for selection of targeted therapies. J Clin Invest, 121(7), 2750-2767.

Leung, E., Kannan, N., Krissansen, G. W., Findlay, M. P., & Baguley, B. C. (2010). MCF-7 breast cancer cells selected for tamoxifen resistance acquire new phenotypes differing in DNA content, phospho-HER2 and PAX2 expression, and rapamycin sensitivity. Cancer Biol Ther, 9(9), 717-724.

Leung, E., Kim, J. E., Rewcastle, G. W., Finlay, G. J., & Baguley, B. C. (2011). Comparison of the effects of the PI3K/mTOR inhibitors NVP-BEZ235 and GSK2126458 on tamoxifen-resistant breast cancer cells. Cancer Biol Ther, 11(11), 938 - 946.

Ma, X. M., & Blenis, J. (2009). Molecular mechanisms of mTOR-mediated translational control. Nat Rev Mol Cell Biol, 10(5), 307-318.

Maira, S. M., Stauffer, F., Brueggen, J., Furet, P., Schnell, C., Fritsch, C., Brachmann, S., Chene, P., De Pover, A., Schoemaker, K., Fabbro, D., Gabriel, D., Simonen, M., Murphy, L., Finan, P., Sellers, W., & Garcia-Echeverria, C. (2008). Identification and characterization of NVP-BEZ235, a new orally available dual phosphatidylinositol 3-kinase/mammalian target of rapamycin inhibitor with potent in vivo antitumor activity. Mol Cancer Ther, 7(7), 1851-1863.

212   Chapter 10 – mTOR Signaling in Endocrine Resistance Growth Control

Miller, T. W., Hennessy, B. T., Gonzalez-Angulo, A. M., Fox, E. M., Mills, G. B., Chen, H., Higham, C., Garcia-Echeverria, C., Shyr, Y., & Arteaga, C. L. (2010). Hyperactivation of phosphatidylinositol-3 kinase promotes escape from hormone dependence in estrogen receptor-positive human breast cancer. J Clin Invest, 120(7), 2406-2413.

Noguchi, S., Motomura, K., Inaji, H., Imaoka, S., & Koyama, H. (1993). Up-regulation of estrogen receptor by tamoxifen in human breast cancer. Cancer, 71(4), 1266-1272.

O'Reilly, K. E., Rojo, F., She, Q. B., Solit, D., Mills, G. B., Smith, D., Lane, H., Hofmann, F., Hicklin, D. J., Ludwig, D. L., Baselga, J., & Rosen, N. (2006). mTOR inhibition induces upstream receptor tyrosine kinase signaling and activates Akt. Cancer Res, 66(3), 1500-1508.

Perez-Tenorio, G., & Stal, O. (2002). Activation of AKT/PKB in breast cancer predicts a worse outcome among endocrine treated patients. Br J Cancer, 86(4), 540-545.

Peterson, T. R., Laplante, M., Thoreen, C. C., Sancak, Y., Kang, S. A., Kuehl, W. M., Gray, N. S., & Sabatini, D. M. (2009). DEPTOR is an mTOR inhibitor frequently overexpressed in multiple myeloma cells and required for their survival. Cell, 137(5), 873-886.

Samuels, Y., Wang, Z., Bardelli, A., Silliman, N., Ptak, J., Szabo, S., Yan, H., Gazdar, A., Powell, S. M., Riggins, G. J., Willson, J. K., Markowitz, S., Kinzler, K. W., Vogelstein, B., & Velculescu, V. E. (2004). High frequency of mutations of the PIK3CA gene in human cancers. Science, 304(5670), 554.

Schenone, S., Brullo, C., & Botta, M. (2008). Small molecules ATP-competitive inhibitors of FLT3: a chemical overview. Curr Med Chem, 15(29), 3113-3132.

Schenone, S., Brullo, C., Musumeci, F., Radi, M., & Botta, M. (2011). ATP-competitive inhibitors of mTOR: an update. Curr Med Chem, 18(20), 2995-3014.

Serra, V., Markman, B., Scaltriti, M., Eichhorn, P. J., Valero, V., Guzman, M., Botero, M. L., Llonch, E., Atzori, F., Di Cosimo, S., Maira, M., Garcia-Echeverria, C., Parra, J. L., Arribas, J., & Baselga, J. (2008). NVP-BEZ235, a dual PI3K/mTOR inhibitor, prevents PI3K signaling and inhibits the growth of cancer cells with activating PI3K mutations. Cancer Res, 68(19), 8022-8030.

Shi, Y., Yan, H., Frost, P., Gera, J., & Lichtenstein, A. (2005). Mammalian target of rapamycin inhibitors activate the AKT kinase in multiple myeloma cells by up-regulating the insulin-like growth factor receptor/insulin receptor substrate-1/phosphatidylinositol 3-kinase cascade. Mol Cancer Ther, 4(10), 1533-1540.

Shoji, K., Oda, K., Kashiyama, T., Ikeda, Y., Nakagawa, S., Sone, K., Miyamoto, Y., Hiraike, H., Tanikawa, M., Miyasaka, A., Koso, T., Matsumoto, Y., Wada-Hiraike, O., Kawana, K., Kuramoto, H., McCormick, F., Aburatani, H., Yano, T., Kozuma, S., & Taketani, Y. (2012). Genotype-dependent efficacy of a dual PI3K/mTOR inhibitor, NVP-BEZ235, and an mTOR inhibitor, RAD001, in endometrial carcinomas. PLoS One, 7(5), e37431.

Sos, M. L., Fischer, S., Ullrich, R., Peifer, M., Heuckmann, J. M., Koker, M., Heynck, S., Stuckrath, I., Weiss, J., Fischer, F., Michel, K., Goel, A., Regales, L., Politi, K. A., Perera, S., Getlik, M., Heukamp, L. C., Ansen, S., Zander, T., Beroukhim, R., Kashkar, H., Shokat, K. M., Sellers, W. R., Rauh, D., Orr, C., Hoeflich, K. P., Friedman, L., Wong, K. K., Pao, W., & Thomas, R. K. (2009). Identifying genotype-dependent efficacy of single and combined PI3K- and MAPK-pathway inhibition in cancer. Proc Natl Acad Sci U S A, 106(43), 18351-18356.

Sun, Q., Chen, X., Ma, J., Peng, H., Wang, F., Zha, X., Wang, Y., Jing, Y., Yang, H., Chen, R., Chang, L., Zhang, Y., Goto, J., Onda, H., Chen, T., Wang, M. R., Lu, Y., You, H., Kwiatkowski, D., & Zhang, H. (2011). Mammalian target of rapamycin up-regulation of pyruvate kinase isoenzyme type M2 is critical for aerobic glycolysis and tumor growth. Proc Natl Acad Sci U S A, 108(10), 4129-4134.

Sun, S. Y., Rosenberg, L. M., Wang, X., Zhou, Z., Yue, P., Fu, H., & Khuri, F. R. (2005). Activation of Akt and eIF4E survival pathways by rapamycin-mediated mammalian target of rapamycin inhibition. Cancer Res, 65(16), 7052-7058.

Thomas, H. E., Mercer, C. A., Carnevalli, L. S., Park, J., Andersen, J. B., Conner, E. A., Tanaka, K., Matsutani, T., Iwanami, A., Aronow, B. J., Manway, L., Maira, S. M., Thorgeirsson, S. S., Mischel, P. S., Thomas, G., & Kozma, S. C. (2012). mTOR Inhibitors Synergize on Regression, Reversal of Gene Expression, and Autophagy in Hepatocellular Carcinoma. Sci Transl Med, 4(139), 139ra184.

Thoreen, C. C., Chantranupong, L., Keys, H. R., Wang, T., Gray, N. S., & Sabatini, D. M. (2012). A unifying model for mTORC1-mediated regulation of mRNA translation. Nature, 485(7396), 109-113.

Visvader, J. E. (2009). Keeping abreast of the mammary epithelial hierarchy and breast tumorigenesis. Genes Dev, 23(22), 2563-2577.

Vivanco, I., & Sawyers, C. L. (2002). The phosphatidylinositol 3-kinase AKT pathway in human cancer. Nat Rev Cancer, 2, 489 - 501.

Wan, X., Harkavy, B., Shen, N., Grohar, P., & Helman, L. J. (2007). Rapamycin induces feedback activation of Akt signaling through an IGF-1R-dependent mechanism. Oncogene, 26(13), 1932-1940.

Wan, X., & Helman, L. J. (2007). The biology behind mTOR inhibition in sarcoma. Oncologist, 12(8), 1007-1018.

Wang, X., & Sun, S. Y. (2009). Enhancing mTOR-targeted cancer therapy. Expert Opin Ther Targets, 13(10), 1193-1203.

Wang, X., Yue, P., Kim, Y. A., Fu, H., Khuri, F. R., & Sun, S. Y. (2008). Enhancing mammalian target of rapamycin (mTOR)-targeted cancer therapy by preventing mTOR/raptor inhibition-initiated, mTOR/rictor-independent Akt activation. Cancer Res, 68(18), 7409-7418.

Webb, P., Lopez, G. N., Uht, R. M., & Kushner, P. J. (1995). Tamoxifen activation of the estrogen receptor/AP-1 pathway: potential origin for the cell-specific estrogen-like effects of antiestrogens. Mol Endocrinol, 9(4), 443-456.

Xu, C. X., Li, Y., Yue, P., Owonikoko, T. K., Ramalingam, S. S., Khuri, F. R., & Sun, S. Y. (2011). The combination of RAD001 and NVP-BEZ235 exerts synergistic anticancer activity against non-small cell lung cancer in vitro and in vivo. PLoS One, 6(6), e20899.

Yamnik, R. L., & Holz, M. K. (2010). mTOR/S6K1 and MAPK/RSK signaling pathways coordinately regulate estrogen receptor alpha serine 167 phosphorylation. FEBS Lett, 584(1), 124-128.

Yunokawa, M., Koizumi, F., Kitamura, Y., Katanasaka, Y., Okamoto, N., Kodaira, M., Yonemori, K., Shimizu, C., Ando, M., Masutomi, K., Yoshida, T., Fujiwara, Y., & Tamura, K. (2012). Efficacy of everolimus, a novel mTOR inhibitor, against basal-like triple-negative breast cancer cells. Cancer Sci.

Zinzalla, V., Stracka, D., Oppliger, W., & Hall, M. N. (2011). Activation of mTORC2 by association with the ribosome. Cell, 144(5), 757-768.

Zoncu, R., Efeyan, A., & Sabatini, D. M. (2011). mTOR: from growth signal integration to cancer, diabetes and ageing. Nat Rev Mol Cell Biol, 12(1), 21-35.

Reduced Growth of Human Breast and Prostate Cancer Cells *in vitro* by Extracts from Different Tomato Varieties and from Broccoli

Jiri A. Mejsnar
GENNET Ltd., Kostelni 9, Prague 7, Czech Republic

Kamila Balusikova
*Department of Cell and Molecular Biology & Center for Research of
Diabetes Metabolism and Nutrition, Third Faculty of Medicine
Charles University in Prague, Czech Republic*

Pavlina Cejkova
*Department of General Biology and Genetics, Third Faculty of Medicine
Charles University in Prague, Czech Republic*

Vlasta Fiedlerova
Food Research Institute Prague, Czech Republic

Marie Holasova
Food Research Institute Prague, Czech Republic

1   Introduction

Breast cancer is recognized as having a multifactorial and polygenic (Brunner & Dano, 1993; Lo *et al.*, 2007) mode of inheritance, both in familial and sporadic cases. Similarly, prostate carcinoma has a polygenic inheritance (at least two genes identified on chromosomes 1 and 8) and the incidence of it in a population is affected by dietary intake and the style of life. Such complicated systems for breast and prostate tumor progression justify studies of the epidemiological evidence (Block *et al.*, 1992) that dietary intake of some fruits and vegetables may reduce the risk of certain human malignancies, including breast cancer (Terry *et al.*, 2001). Health benefits of tomatoes are believed to be derived, from its prominent carotenoid, lycopene, and for broccoli, from its isothiocyanate metabolite, sulforaphane. However, as a therapy consideration, considerable experimental data present/s at least three groups of problems.

First, there are contradictory facts about these compounds, especially lycopene. On one side, the accumulated data from in vitro and physiological models show that lycopene reduces the growth rate of cancer cells. Lycopene increases apoptotic rates in some types of malignant cells (Salman *et al.*, 2007), inhibits cell cycle progression at the G_1 phase in breast and endometrial cancers (Nahum *et al.*, 2001), inhibits breast tumor cell growth by modulation of gap junctions in cell lines (Fornelli *et al.*, 2007; Livny *et al.*, 2002), inhibits endometrial, breast, and lung cancer cell proliferation (Salman *et al.*, 2007; Fornelli *et al.*, 2007), decreases plasma concentration of risky insulin-like growth factors in colon cancer patients (Walfisch *et al.*, 2007), changes intercellular communication by up-regulated expression of a connexin gene in breast cancer cells (Chalabi *et al.*, 2007), and inhibits signaling of platelet-derived growth factor by trapping (Wu *et al.*, 2007). On the other side, older data that lycopene has no in vivo protection as an antioxidant (Dugas *et al.*, 1999; Sutherland *et al.*, 1999), especially in relation to prostate cancer, have been deemed insufficient of evidence for health claim approval by the US Food and Drug Administration (Schneeman, 2005). Adding to the lycopene controversy, some studies (Diplock, 1991; Giovannucci, 1999) have shown that lycopene is the only carotenoid associated with a preventive role relative to cancer. However, this appears unlikely when over 600 compounds constitute the carotenoid family isolated from natural sources (During & Harrison, 2006), among which seven, beside lycopene, are abundant in tomato products (Roldan-Gutierrez & Luque de Castro, 2007), followed by a large number of other active phytochemicals.

Second, tomato juice contains largely unidentified growth factor(s) that act as mitogens for some bacteria (Peeler *et al.*, 1949; Garvie & Mabbitt, 1967). This old information, widely accepted in microbiology, has been extended by a finding that green tomato extract stimulates angiogenesis, *i.e.*, endothelial cell proliferation and blood vessel growth (Heeschen *et al.*, 2001). This finding indicates a possibility for a more generalized effect of tomato growth factors on eukaryotic cells. If this is the case, then the question remains, how would these contradictory roles interact *i.e.*, the antiproliferative agents coupled with growth factors such as mitogens, together within a single phytochemotherapeutical extract.

Third, contextually with the above mentioned importance of natural phytochemicals, various methods have been investigated to extract the active agents, principally carotenoids, from plant tissues, using conventional extraction methods with organic solvents, saponification, absorption, and supercritical carbon dioxide flow rates (Roldan-Gutierrez & Luque de Castro, 2007; Wei *et al.*, 2005). The methods have different advantages and disadvantages with regard to solubilization and stabilization of the extracted carotenoids in general, and lycopene in particular:

This study comprises four objectives: 1) to develop a standard extraction method, yielding tomato products which are suitable for cell cultures, and enable product comparison of different tomato varieties;

2) to compare antiproliferative potencies of products prepared in a standardized manner from five tomato varieties and broccoli; 3) to determine whether, relative to breast and prostate cancer cells, tomato and broccoli products *substitute* each other due to their common effector when administered simultaneously, or whether there is an additive relationship existing between them, which results in a (*summation*) *summation* of effects. The summation relationship might be expected, since mechanisms of sulforaphane antiproliferative action via induction of phase II detoxication enzymes (Zhang *et al.*, 1992; Zhang & Talalay, 1998), or by affecting spindle microtubule function (Azarenko *et al.*, 2008) are likely different from the above mentioned actions associated with tomato extract; 4) to test the opposing antiproliferative and mitogenic effects of standardized tomato extract on breast cancer cells and on nontransformed cells which retain some growth potential in culture, *i.e.*, on human fetal cells.

2   Materials and Methods

The effects of tomato purée extracts plus juice from five tomato varieties (Proton, Sejk, 441, 444, 447) and broccoli were examined on proliferation of the human *breast cancer* cell line SK-BR-3, on the human *prostate cancer* cell line DU-145, and on human *fetal cells*. SK-BR-3 as well as DU-145 was obtained from the ATCC (American Type Culture Collection, Manassas, VA, USA). For cultivations, cells were maintained in FBS medium (Musilkova & Kovar, 2001), based on RPMI 1640 medium and supplemented with 10% (v/v) fetal bovine serum, at 37°C in humidified air with 5% CO_2. During actual experiments, FBS medium containing broccoli juice (22.5 μl/ml), tomato supernatant (40 μl/ml) and tomato products (40 μl/ml of tomato supernatant with 4 μl/ml of tomato extract) in dimethylformamide (DMF) or combinations of these vegetable products were used. FBS medium without additives was used when measuring control growth rates. For testing with vegetable products, cells were harvested and then seeded in 1 ml into 12-well plates. The culture medium was replaced with experimental or control medium, after 24 hr, necessary for cell adhesion. Cell growth and survival were evaluated after 48 hours. The number of living cells was determined by hemocytometer counting after trypan blue staining.

Human fetal cells, provided by Cytolab Ltd., were obtained prenatally from amniotic fluid sampling (amniocentesis). After clinical cytogenetic analysis, further culturing was performed based on approval from the donor mother, for anonymous use in medical research. For examination, harvested fetal cells were cultured in incubation flasks containing 5 ml of AMNIOMAX (Gibco) medium, supplemented with 14% (v/v) fetal bovine serum, for a (average) period of 89 hr, with respect to the slightly different growth rates of harvested cells for an each couple of the control and the experimental cultivation.

Preparation of tomato products for cell cultures started with a purée, obtained by homogenization, autoclaved at 121°C for 20 min and subsequently frozen at −18°C. Broccoli was pressed, the juice filtered (0.20 μm Filtropur S, Sarstedt) and frozen. In experiments, 10 g of the tomato purée was centrifuged, the supernatant decanted, the sediment was milled into fine powder in liquid nitrogen and extracted with a solution (6 ml) containing hexane-ethanol (1:1, v/v) for 40 min at room temperature. After centrifugation, the hexane-ethanol suspension was dried under nitrogen gas and in the last step resuspended in 800 μl of DMF. Prior to treatment, all tomato products were sterilized via filtration.

Growth of fetal cells is unaffected up to 70 μl of DMF in 5 ml of incubation medium, at which point some cells start to be deliberated into the medium, but cell shape was fine and practically all of them grew at the bottom of the cultivation flask. The breast cancer cells were more sensitive, a maximum volume of 4 μl of DMF within 1 ml of the incubation medium, when cells are still morphologically "nice" and after trypsinization there were no dead cells in the suspension. The prostate cancer cells manifested a similar sensitivity when tested by six points' DRC (dose-response curve), and thus revealed applicability of the same 4µl DMF/ml volume ratio.

Lycopene was assayed, after nitrogen drying of the particular tomato extract, when subsequently dissolved in DMF solution, by high–performance liquid chromatography (HP 1 100, Hewlett Packard); just, according to our definition, as a quantitative indicator of extraction efficiency during nine subsequently tested procedures progressing toward a final standardized method, and in experiments – together with assayed supernatant – for preparation of 1 µM concentrations of lycopene in cellular cultures (Hwang & Bowen, 2005).

Data are presented as mean ± standard error of the mean (S.E.M.) of experimental values obtained in triplicates of two and more independent experiments. Statistical significance of differences was determined using paired T-test for cancer cells and non-parametric Wilcoxon signed-rank test for fetal cells. The significance level was set at 0.05.

3   Results

The individual effects of two tomato varieties and broccoli upon the growth rates and thus proliferation of breast cancer cells are shown in Figure 1. In experimental cultivations (48 hr) with Proton's or Sejk's tomato products or with broccoli juice (see Materials and Methods), cell numbers per ml reached $5.61 \times 10^5 \pm 1.56 \times 10^4$ S.E.M., $6.01 \times 10^5 \pm 7.98 \times 10^4$ S.E.M., and $4.44 \times 10^5 \pm 0$ S.E.M., respectively. Control cell numbers reached $8.07 \times 10^5 \pm 2.21 \times 10^4$ S.E.M. cells/ml.

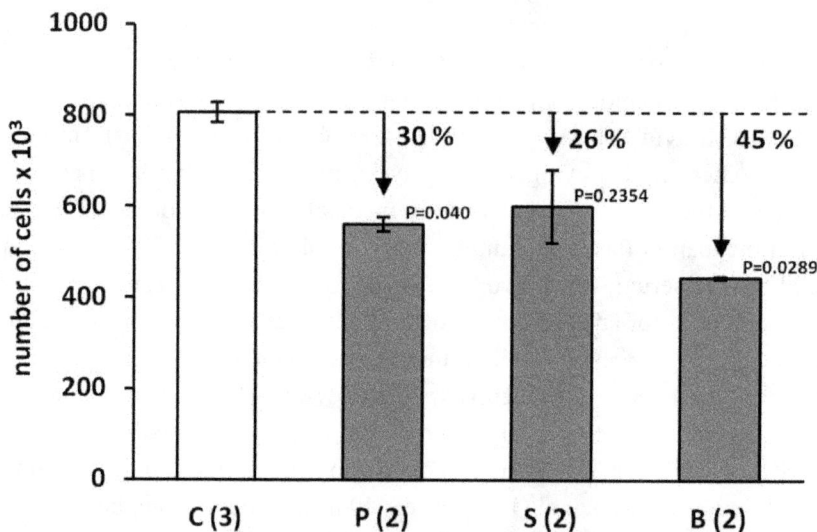

Figure 1: Breast cancer cell number ± S.E.M. after 48 hr cultivation of controls (C) and influenced by products from tomato Proton (P) and Sejk (S) varieties and from broccoli (B). The culture medium contained 44 µl/ml of individual tomato product or 22.5 µl/ml of broccoli juice (see Materials and Methods). Respective inhibition extents by the products are evaluated as percentage decrease of the control cells number considered as 100%. Paired T-test was used to compare experimental values. Number of cultivations in brackets

As for the determination whether effects of tomato and broccoli products substitute each other, or whether their additive relationship results in a summation of effects, data indicating a cumulative effect of products from tomato varieties and broccoli are presented in Figure 2. In comparison with the braking power rates evaluated in Figure 1, the results in Figure 2 overshadow the summation of effects due to the active products in tomatoes and broccoli, where the cumulative effect of Sejk and broccoli products reached 66% difference between control ($8.88 \times 10^5 \pm 3.87 \times 10^4$ S.E.M. cells/ml) and experimental ($3.02 \times 10^5 \pm 1.71 \times 10^4$ S.E.M. cells/ml) growth rates of breast cancer cells.

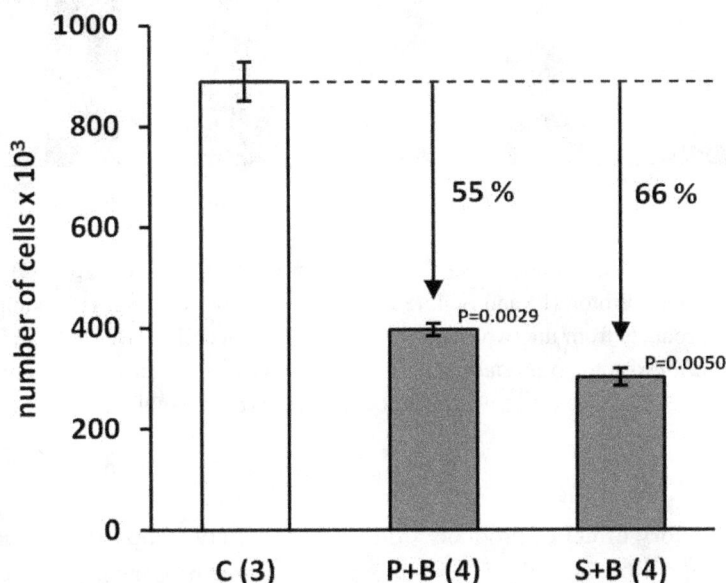

Figure 2: The braking power on breast cancer cell growth due to a cumulative effect of products from tomato varieties Proton (P) or Sejk (S) and broccoli (B). The combinations of 44 μl/ml of tomato product and 22.5 μl/ml of broccoli juice were used (see Materials and Methods). Respective changes are evaluated as percentage decrease of the control cells number. Paired T-test was used to compare experimental values. Number of cultivations in brackets

Macroscopic comparison of the two tomato varieties, at first glance, suggests structural differences. The Sejk variety has a more delicate tissue structure yielding more lycopene in the eluate (0.1832 μg/4 μl DMF) and less lycopene in juice (0.3898 μg/40 μl DMF). Sejk products used together in 1 ml of incubation medium (see Materials and Methods) provide a lycopene concentration of 1.07 μM. The Proton variety, with its tougher tissue, yielded less lycopene in the eluate (0.1054 μg/4 μl DMF) and more lycopene in juice (0.4364 μg/40 μl DMF). In combination in 1 ml of incubation medium, Proton products reached practically the same final concentration of lycopene (1.009 μM) as Sejk variety.

The individual effects of the same two tomato varieties and broccoli upon the growth rates of prostate cancer cells and the cumulative effect of simultaneously acting tomatoes and broccoli products are evaluated in Figure 3. In comparison with results presented in Figure 1 and 2, the inhibitory effect of both tomato varieties on breast and prostate cell proliferation is approximately same. For the breast carcinoma, the inhibitory effect of Proton and Sejk variant reached 30% and 26%, respectively. For the prostate carcinoma, the inhibitory effect of Proton and Sejk variant reached 27% and 21%, respectively. There is a

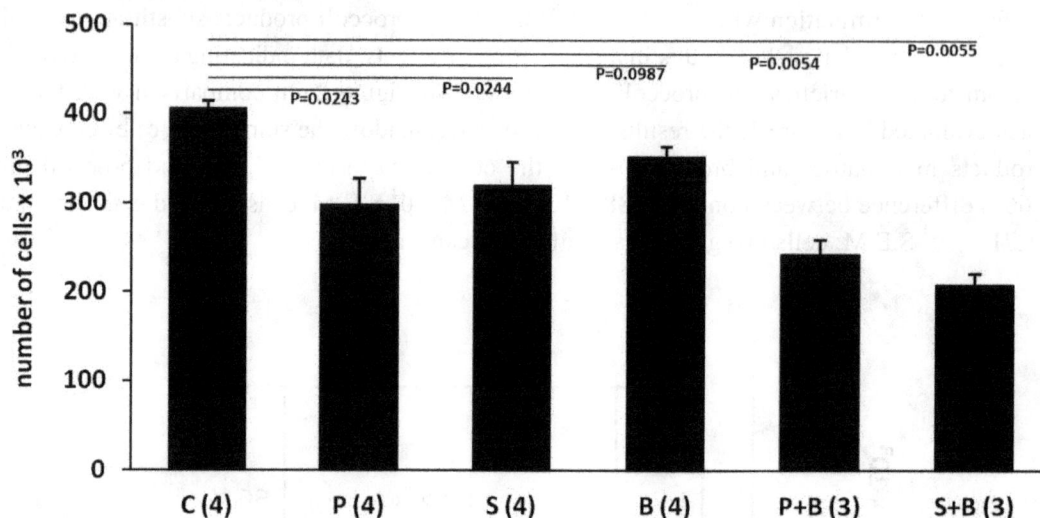

Figure 3: Prostate cancer cell number ± S.E.M. after 48 hr cultivation of controls (C) and influenced by products from tomato Proton (P) and Sejk (S) varieties and from broccoli (B), completed by a cumulative effect of products from the two tomato varieties and broccoli (P+B, S+B). The culture medium contained 44 µl/ml of tomato product, 22.5 µl/ml of broccoli juice or combinations of both (see Materials and Methods). Paired T-test was used to compare experimental values. Number of cultivations in brackets

marked cumulative inhibitory effect of products from tomato varieties and broccoli on both types of cancer cells, reaching 66% and 49% for Sejk variety in breast and prostate cancer cells, respectively.

Individual inhibitory effects of five tomato varieties upon the growth rates of prostate cancer cells (growth rate of controls = 100%) ranged from 18% to 36% (see Figure 4). The magnitude of individual inhibitory effect is not proportional to concentrations of lycopene, achieved by the respective varieties in cellular cultures. The varieties' lycopene content (in mg/100g of a sample) equaled: Proton = 10.10 mg, Sejk = 8.87 mg, 447 = 10.94 mg, 444 = 8.66 mg and 441 = 10.22 mg. These comparative data show that lycopene is not the only carotenoid associated with the inhibitory role relative to prostate cancer.

In six control cultivations (average time 89 hr) of slightly different numbers of seeded *fetal cells,* the average cell number reached $3.71 \times 10^5 \pm 1.95 \times 10^4$ S.E.M. per cultivation flask, which represents (calculated as the average of the percentage increases in each cultivation) a nearly 35% increase. In parallel six experimental cultivations (89 hr) with 200 µl of Proton extract, cell numbers reached $7.41 \times 10^5 \pm 2.59 \times 10^4$ S.E.M., which represents more than a 115% increase. Thus, the percentage difference of the two growth rates at the end of cultivation equaled 80%, which evaluates as the *stimulatory* effect of the Proton supernatant.

The effect of the Proton extract on *breast cancer cells* was tested and evaluated in an analogous manner. In three control cultivations, 2×10^5 breast cells were plated per well. After 48 hr, average cell numbers reached $8.067 \times 10^5 \pm 2.21 \times 10^4$ S.E.M. cells/well which represents a 403% increase. In three parallel experimental cultivations (48 hr) with 40 µl/well of Proton extract, cell numbers reached $5.69 \times 10^5 \pm 2.31 \times 10^4$ S.E.M. cells/well which represents a 285% decrease. Thus, the percentage difference of the two growth rates equals 118% as a measure of Proton extract *inhibitory* effects. Both effects of Proton extract on breast cancer and fetal cells are illustrated in Figure 5.

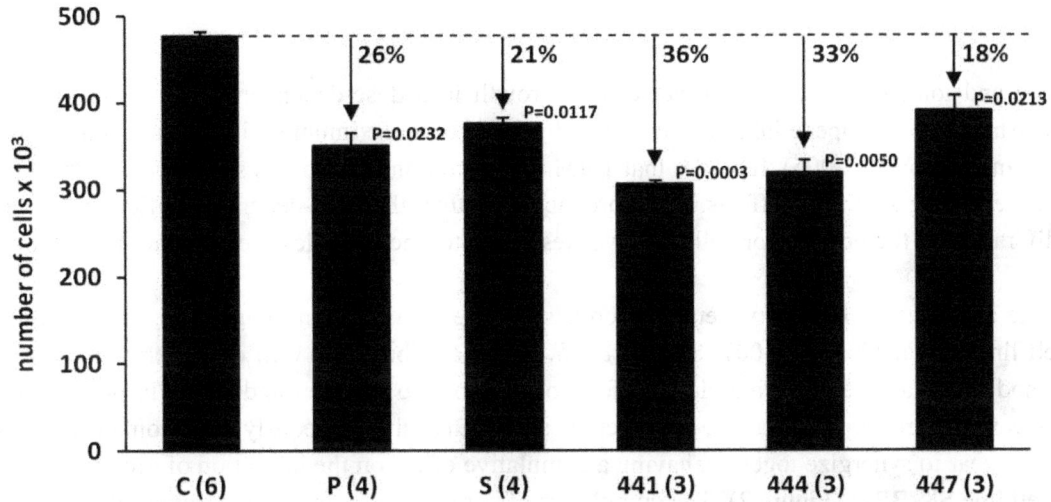

Figure 4: Prostate cancer cell number ± S.E.M. after 48 hr cultivation of controls (C) and influenced by products from Proton (P), Sejk (S), 441, 444 and 447 tomato varieties. The culture medium contained 44 µl/ml of tomato product (see Materials and Methods). Paired T-test was used to compare experimental values. Number of cultivations in brackets

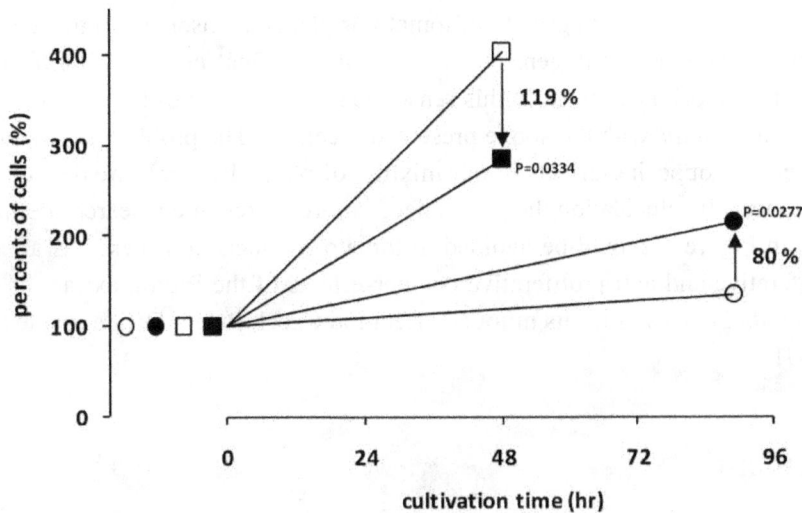

Figure 5: Opposing-effects of the tomato Proton variety supernatant on growth rates of breast cancer and fetal cultured cells. The culture medium contained 40 µl/ml of tomato supernatant during three and six independent experiments with breast cancer and fetal cells, respectively. Breast cancer cells – control growth (□) (100% = 2 x 105 cells per well). Breast cancer cells – growth with the supernatant (■) (100% = 2 × 105 cells per well). Fetal cells – control growth (○) (100% = 2.65 × 105 cells per cultivation flask). Fetal cells – growth with the supernatant (●) (100% = 4.67 × 105 cells per cultivation flask). The supernatant stimulates proliferation of fetal cells by 80% and inhibits proliferation of breast cancer cells by 119%. Paired T-test and non-parametric Wilcoxon signed-rank test was used to compare experimental values of breast cancer and fetal cells, respectively.

4   Discussion

Lycopene and tomato extract inhibit cancer cell growth in a dose-dependent (0.1 – 50 µM lycopene) manner, when 1 µM lycopene inhibits the growth by 69% (of a maximum inhibition at a concentration 50 µM) (Hwang & Bowen, 2005). It means that 1 µM concentration used in this study represents an onset of a plateau regarding saturation effects. In accordance with that, the dose-dependent influence of lycopene on proliferation of the both tumor cell lines was tested up to one order less concentration (Fornelli *et al.,* 2007).

The anti-cancer effect of vegetable products will be of a different magnitude on different malignant cell lines (Chalabi *et al.,* 2007; Salman *et al.,* 2007) and based as well on differences in vegetable species and even varieties. The individual effects of two tomato varieties and broccoli, presented in Figure 1, are very similar. Importantly, however, it seems that simultaneously used tomato and broccoli products appear to synergize together, having a cumulative effect on the inhibition of growth of the breast tumor cell line SK-BR-3 (Figure 2). The cumulative effect of 66% is definitely stronger than the separate effects of each product. This conclusion emphasizes the benefits of a combination of various micronutrients in various proportions are not only the basis of the disease-prevention activity of a diet rich in vegetables (Levy & Sharoni, 2004), but could be also the basis for a mixture of phytochemotherapeutical extracts.

During the time of this study, databases retrieved four thousand records for the keywords *tomato growth factor*. Surprisingly all of them were either connected with growth factors of different tomato anti-proliferative mechanisms, or with growth of tomato or plants themselves. In this context, our finding that tomato supernatant acts as a mitogen, means it stimulates fetal cells division (Figure 5), and can therefore be considered an original result. In this sense the result substitutes the keywords *tomato mitogen factor* for *tomato growth factor* with the above presented meaning. The problem arises, how the proliferative and anti-proliferative opposing-effects of our mixture of phytochemicals are dependent on cell transformation toward cancer. Its elucidation, however, needs more systematic research. Perhaps, the proliferative effect shown in Figure 5 should be avoided in tomato products considered as an anti-proliferative mixture. The proliferative and anti-proliferative counter-effects of the Proton extract has been published recently (Mejsnar *et al.,* 2010) and for its mitogen effect the Czech Patent Office granted an Utility Model No.: CZ 20005 U1.

Acknowledgement

The authors acknowledge the fetal cell cultivations performed by Mrs. Jarmila Sulcova. This study was supported in part by the Ministry of Agriculture, Czech Republic grant No. QH 72 149 and by Cytolab Ltd.

References

Azarenko, O., Okouneva, T., Singletary, K. W., Jordan, M. A., &Wilson, L. (2008). *Suppression of microtubule dynamic instability and turnover in MCF7 breast cancer cells by sulforaphane. Carcinogenesis, 29, 2360-2368.*

Block, G., Patterson, B., &Subar, A. (1992). Fruit, vegetables and cancer prevention: a review of the epidemiological evidence. Nutrition and Cancer, 18, 1-29.

Brunner, N., &Dano, K. (1993).Invasion and metastasis factors in breast cancer.Breast Cancer Research and Treatment, 24, 173-174.

Chalabi, N., Delort, L., Satih, S., Dechelotte, P., Bignon, Y. J., &Bernard-Gallon, D. J. (2007). Immunohistochemical expression of RARalpha, RARbeta, and Cx43 in breast tumor cell lines after treatment with lycopene and correlation with RT-QPCR.Journal of Histochemistry and Cytochemistry, 55, 877-883.

Diplock, A. T. (1991). Antioxidant nutrients and disease prevention: an overview. American Journal of Clinical Nutrition, 53(Suppl 1), 189-193.

Dugas, T. R., Morel, D. W., &Harrison, E. H. (1999).Dietary supplementation with beta-carotene, but not with lycopene, inhibits endothelial cell-mediated oxidation of low-density lipoprotein. Free Radical Biology and Medicine, 26, 1238-1244.

During, A., &Harrison, E. H. (2006).Digestion and intestinal absorption of dietary carotenoids and vitamin A. In: Physiology of the gastrointestinal tract, 4th edition(pp. 1735-1752), Academic Press New York.

Fornelli, F., Leone, A., Verdesca, I., Minervini, F., &Zacheo, G. (2007).The influence of lycopene on the proliferation of human breast cell line (MCF-7).ToxicoogyIn Vitro, 21, 217-223.

Garvie, E. I.,&Mabbitt, L. A. (1967).Stimulation of the growth of Leuconostocoenos by tomato juice.ArchivfürMikrobiologie, 55, 398-407.

Giovannucci, E. (2006). Tomatoes, tomato-based products, lycopene, and cancer: review of the epidemiologic literature. Journal of National Cancer Institute, 91, 317-331.

Heeschen, C., Jang, J. J., Weis, M., Pathak, A., Kaji, S., Hu, R. S., Tsao, P. S., Johnson, F. L., &Cooke, J. P. (2001).Nicotine stimulates angiogenesis and promotes tumor growth and atherosclerosis. Nature Medicine, 7, 833-839.

Hwang, E. S., &Bowen, P. E. (2005).Effects of lycopene and tomato paste extracts on DNA and lipid oxidation in LNCaP human prostate cancer cells. Biofactors, 23, 97-105.

Levy, J., &Sharoni, Y. (2004).The functions of tomato lycopene and its role in human health.HerbalGram, 62, 49-56.

Livny, O., Kaplan, I., Reifen, R., Polak-Charcon, S., Madar, Z., &Schwartz, B. (2002).Lycopene inhibits proliferation and enhances gap-junction communication of KB-1 human oral tumor cells. Journal of Nutrition, 132, 3754-3759.

Lo, Y. L., Yu, J. C., Chen, S. T., Hsu, G. C., Mau, Y. C., Yang, S. L., Wu, P. E., &Shen, C. Y. (2007). Breast Cancer Risk Associated with Genotypic Polymorphism of the Mitotic Checkpoint Genes: a Multigenic Study on Cancer Susceptibility. Carcinogenesis, 28, 1079-1086.

Mejsnar, J.A., Balusikova, K., Cejkova, P., Fiedlerova, V., &Holasova, M. (2010). Tomato supernatant in a microenviroment has the proliferative and antiproliferative opposing effects on breast cancer and fetal cultured cells. BioMedCentral Proceedings, 4(Suppl 2), P18.

Musilkova, J.,&Kovar, J. (2001).Additive stimulatory effect of extracellular calcium and potassium on non-transferrin ferric iron uptake by HeLa and K562 cells.BiochimicaetBiophysicaActa, 1514, 117-126.

Nahum, A., Hirsch, K., Danilenko, M., Watts, C. K. W., Prall, O. W. J., Levy, J., &Sharoni, Y. (2001). Lycopene inhibition of cell cycle progression in breast and endometrial cancer cells is associated with reduction in cyclin D levels and retention of p27 (Kip1). in the cyclin E-cdk2 complexes. Oncogene, 20, 3428-3436.

Peeler, H. T., Yacowitz, H., &Norris, L. C. (1949).A microbiological assay for vitamin B12 using Lactobacillus leichmannii.Proceedings of the Society for Experimental Biology and Medicine, 72, 515-521.

Roldan-Gutierrez, J. M., &Luque de Castro, M. D. (2007).Lycopene: The need for better methods for characterization and determination. Trends on Analytical Chemistry, 26, 163-170.

Salman, H., Bergman, M., Djaldetti, M., &Bessler, H. (2007).Lycopene affects proliferation and apoptosis of four malignant cell lines. Biomedicine and Pharmacotherapy, 61, 366-369.

Schneeman, B. O. (2005). Qualified Health Claims: Letter Regarding Tomatoes and Prostate Cancer (Lycopene Health Claim Coalition), Docket No. 2004Q-0201 Center for Food Safety and Applied Nutrition. Food and Drug Administration.Silver Spring USA.

Sutherland, W. H., Walker, R. J., De Jong, S. A., &Upritchard, J. E. (1999).Supplementation with tomato juice increases plasma lycopene but does not alter susceptibility to oxidation of low-density lipoproteins from renal transplant recipients. Clinical Nephrology, 52, 30-36.

Terry, P., Wolk, A., Persson, I., &Magnusson, C. (2001).Brassica Vegetables and Breast Cancer Risk.Journal of the American Medical Association, 285, 2975-2977.

Walfisch, S., Walfisch, Y., Kirilov, E., Linde, N., Mnitentag, H., Agbaria, R., Sharoni, Y., &Levy, J. (2007).Tomato lycopene extract supplementation decreases insulin-like growth factor-I levels in colon cancer patients. European Journal of Cancer Prevention, 16, 298-303.

Wei, P. C., May, C. Y., Ngan, M. A., &Hock, C. C. (2005). Supercritical fluid extraction of palm carotenoids.American Journal of Environmental Sciences, 1, 264-269.

Wu, W. B., Chiang, H. S., Fang, J. Y., &Hung, C. F. (2007).Inhibitory effect of lycopene on PDGF-BB-induced signalling and migration in human dermal fibroblasts: a possible target for cancer. Biochemical Society Transactions, 35, 1377-1378.

Zhang, Y., &Talalay, P. (1998).Mechanism of differential potencies of isothiocyanates as inducers of anticarcinogenic Phase 2 enzymes.Cancer Research, 58, 4632-4639.

Zhang, Y., Talalay, P., Cho, C. G., &Posner, G. H. (1992).A major inducer of anticarcinogenic protective enzymes from broccoli: isolation and elucidation of structure. Proceedings of the National Academy of Sciences USA, 89, 2399-2403.

NMR-based Metabolomics: Global Analysis of Metabolites to Address Problems in Prostate Cancer

Matthew J. Roberts
Centre for Clinical Research / Centre for Advanced Imaging
The University of Queensland, Australia

Horst Joachim Schirra
Centre for Advanced Imaging
The University of Queensland, Australia

Martin F. Lavin
Centre for Clinical Research
The University of Queensland, Australia
Radiation Biology and Oncology
Queensland Institute of Medical Research, Australia

Robert A. Gardiner
Centre for Clinical Research
The University of Queensland, Australia
Department of Urology
Royal Brisbane and Women's Hospital, Queensland, Australia

1   Introduction

Cancer significantly contributes to the worldwide burden of disease and premature death across many countries. Consequently, current oncology research focuses on discovering and validating new biomarkers to improve early detection. These efforts are of worldwide importance in detecting significant cancer while it is still localised and in lessening associated morbidities and death.

Biomarkers have mostly been sourced from non- or minimally invasive biofluids, such as blood, urine, and biopsy tissue. Traditionally, biomarkers were limited to circulating end-products of altered cellular function in cancer. However, technology advances and emergence of the –omics sciences have improved analysis of genes, gene expression, proteins and metabolites alike – on both an individual and system-wide scale. This field of research, termed "systems biology", has allowed for molecules at all levels of the cellular hierarchy to be considered as biomarkers. Continuous improvements in sensitivity, resolution and precision of these analytical techniques produces large datasets, allowing for simultaneous characterisation of, ideally all, compounds in a single sample. Subsequent statistical analysis of these datasets and their interpretation with respect to cellular function is the basis of the different -omics technologies, such as genomics, transcriptomics, proteomics and metabolomics.

In this chapter, we will describe principles and processes that are involved in investigating biological or clinical problems with nuclear magnetic resonance (NMR)-based metabolomics - an approach that involves the global analysis of metabolites. In writing for the scope of this book, we have broken this chapter into three sections: (1) First we will describe and illustrate the methods commonly used in NMR-based metabolomics, including spectral processing, data treatment and subsequent statistical analysis. (2) Secondly, we will use prostate cancer (PCa) as a case study to illustrate how NMR-based metabolomics can be applied to a clinical problem. PCa is the second most common type of cancer and the sixth leading cause of cancer-related death worldwide (Center *et al.*, 2012; Ferlay *et al.*, 2010; Siegel *et al.*, 2012). The diagnosis of prostate cancer is currently problematic for a number of reasons that include lack of sensitive and specific tumour markers as well as limitations due to morbidity inherent with the biopsy diagnosis process. Furthermore, many patients harbour early prostate cancer with insignificant tumours that may not progress to produce clinical problems. (3) Lastly, we will briefly outline the future directions for the role of NMR-based metabolomics, including personalized medicine and integration with other –omics datasets, in order to create a holistic, systems biology approach to solving clinical problems.

Outlining the processes, applications and potential of metabolomics will be of assistance to biostatisticians and bioinformaticians who may be interested in expanding into this area of research. Similarly, we aim to inspire scientists and clinicians who are interested in applying this approach to a scientific or clinical problem.

2   Metabolomics: History and Methods

2.1   What is Metabolomics?

Metabolomics has been highlighted as a technique that is unique and exciting in biomarker discovery (Abate-Shen & Shen, 2009; Bino *et al.*, 2004; Nicholson & Lindon, 2008). It is the quantification of all small molecular weight metabolites to accurately define the metabolite composition of a biological sample (Fiehn, 2002).   The term "metabolomics" is often used interchangeably with "metabonomics", which is defined as 'the quantitative measurement of the dynamic multiparametric metabolic response of living systems to pathophysiological stimuli' (Nicholson *et al.,* 1999). The technical approach to both metabonomics and metabolomics is similar, involving measurement and analysis of metabolite data for a given sample. Conceptually, however, the objective and application of these techniques is slightly different: Metabolomics seeks to describe the composition of complex biological samples, while metabonomics aims to map and understand the change of a biological system in response to external or artificial stimuli. In the current chapter, we will use the term "metabolomics", while both metabolomics and metabonomics will be discussed. The advent and development of metabolomics/metabonomics has largely been possible due to advances in analytical techniques, such as nuclear magnetic resonance (NMR) spectroscopy and mass spectrometry (MS), as well as chromatographic separation techniques. As the authors have expertise in NMR spectroscopy, the focus of this chapter will be on NMR-based techniques within the field of metabolomics. We refer the reader to several excellent reviews that detail the application of MS in metabolomics and systems biology (Lu *et al.*, 2008; Pasikanti *et al.*, 2008; Theodoridis *et al.*, 2008)

2.2   Historical Perspective

While "metabolomics" is a recently coined term, the analysis of metabolic end products is a long-practiced ancient scientific process. About 2000-1500 BCE, analysis of urine by human taste or animal behaviour (due to the high urinary glucose concentration) helped diagnose patients with diabetes mellitus (van der Greef & Smilde, 2005). In 1506, a "urine wheel" by Ulrich Pinder linked crude changes detected by human senses (colour, smell, taste) with various medical conditions (Pinder, 1506; Weiss & Kim, 2012). Although qualitative measures of metabolism have been performed for centuries, the origins of quantitative studies stem from the measurement of insensible perspiration and other hydration losses in medieval Italy (Eknoyan, 1999). Technological limitations in analytical chemistry hindered further advances until the early 20th century. At this time, the development of sensitive analytical methods allowed quantification of key compounds/metabolites in urine and other sample types (Simoni *et al.*, 2002). This quantitative approach continued to develop with the introduction of various analytical techniques, such as mass spectrometry (Griffiths, 2008; Thomson, 1912) and NMR (Bloch *et al.*, 1946; Freeman, 1995; Purcell *et al.*, 1946), and with the application of these techniques to metabolic research (Gates & Sweeley, 1978; Hoult *et al.*, 1974). The integration of medical science and analytical chemistry at this time led to a greater understanding of metabolic perturbations in medical conditions, e.g. kidney stones among many others (Reginato & Kurnik, 1989). Further improvements in metabolite profiling in the latter half of the 20th century were aided by advances in chemometrics, the foundation behind data analysis in analytical chemistry (Geladi & Esbensen, 1990). Appropriate data processing and interpretation was achieved by multivariate statistical methods, which will be outlined in more detail below.

2.3   Modern Metabolomics and its Varieties/Applications

Metabolomics continues to evolve as a field and is increasingly used in a variety of applications. Initially, biofluids were analyzed specifically to quantify metabolic perturbations due to drug toxicity, disease, and other internal and external influences. For example, perturbations in steroid metabolism were used for anti-doping testing during the Los Angeles Summer Olympics in 1984 (Fitch, 2008). In the following section, the diverse applications of metabolomics are briefly described; more comprehensive accounts are available in other sources (Duarte & Gil, 2012; Ma *et al.,* 2012b; Ng *et al.,* 2011; Rhee & Gerszten, 2012; Spratlin *et al.*, 2009).

2.3.1   Biofluid and Excretion Analysis

Metabolomics has been used to quantify endogenous metabolites in many human biofluids, with those most commonly analyzed being urine and blood (serum, plasma). Analysis of urine metabolites has shown early promise in diagnosing kidney (Ganti & Weiss, 2011) and bladder tumors (Hyndman *et al.*, 2011), as well as more systemic conditions such as type 2 diabetes mellitus (Salek *et al.*, 2007). Indeed, distinct serum metabolite patterns have been characterized for abnormal clinical states including breast cancer (Oakman *et al.*, 2011), leukemia (MacIntyre *et al.*, 2010), sepsis and acute lung injury (Serkova *et al.*, 2011), coronary artery disease (Brindle *et al.*, 2002) and obesity (Oberbach *et al.*, 2011; Xie *et al.*, 2012). Furthermore, cardiovascular health has been assessed by metabolomic analysis of feces, linking perturbations in the metabolite profiles of gut flora to the metabolic syndrome and dyslipidemia (Wang *et al.*, 2011). Seminal fluid and expressed prostatic secretions (EPS), have been used to characterize disturbed metabolism in prostate cancer (Averna *et al.*, 2005; Kline *et al.*, 2006; Lynch *et al.*, 1994, 1997; Serkova *et al.*, 2008) and infertility (Deepinder *et al.*, 2007; Hamamah *et al.*, 1993, 1998). Studies on cerebrospinal fluid have associated metabolite changes with brain tumors and neurodegenerative disorders, such as multiple sclerosis and Alzheimer's disease (Han *et al.*, 2011). Salivary metabolomics has been used to investigate oral cancer and pre-malignant changes, such as leukoplakia (Wei *et al.*, 2011). Thus, this minimally invasive approach has enormous potential in providing valuable scientific and clinical information for medical professionals and researchers.

2.3.2   NMR Spectroscopy of Tissues and *in vivo* Imaging Techniques

High-resolution magic-angle spinning (HR-MAS) NMR spectroscopy can be used to perform nondestructive metabolite profiling of tissue or other solid samples (Keifer, 2007). That means that after HR-MAS NMR spectroscopy, further testing of tissue samples can be performed such as histopathological evaluation, the current gold standard in disease diagnosis, or genome and protein sequencing. As a result, HR-MAS NMR has been used to investigate a number of disease states (Brown *et al.*, 2012; Dittrich *et al.*, 2012; Kurhanewicz *et al.*, 2002; Martínez-Bisbal *et al.*, 2004; Maxeiner *et al.*, 2010; Millis *et al.*, 1997; Sitter *et al.*, 2002).

Metabolomic analysis can also be performed directly *in vivo*, largely owing to advances in magnetic resonance spectroscopic imaging and positron emission tomography (PET). A standard clinical magnetic resonance imaging (MRI) scan uses similar physical concepts to NMR, but takes many scans across a section of living tissue. This data is processed to produce an anatomically correct image based on physical properties of the tissue. A magnetic resonance spectroscopy imaging sequence is able to produce NMR-like spectra for a targeted volume segment in the body, allowing for visualization of metabolite content in that anatomical location. Metabolic alterations measured *in vivo* have been shown to correlate with histopathology (Delongchamps *et al.*, 2011; Kwock *et al.*, 2006). Furthermore, *in vivo* metabolomics is being used to monitor the response to various therapies, such as radiotherapy and chemotherapy (Coy *et al.*, 2011; Lodi & Ronen, 2011).

Different MRI techniques allow the investigation of different phenomena. Dynamic contrast-enhanced MRI uses the uptake and elimination of contrast agents, such as gadolinium, to distinguish between different tissues. The use of dynamic contrast-enhanced MRI in oncology is based on the premise that cancer cells have a higher metabolism, and thus a higher uptake and elimination of gadolinium contrast (Vargas *et al.*, 2012). Diffusion weighted imaging, initially used to investigate connectivity between different brain regions (Behrens *et al.*, 2003), uses slower water diffusion in cancerous tissues compared with surrounding healthy cells due to a higher nuclear content and cellular density coupled with extracellular changes (Lim & Tan, 2012). Recently, these MRI techniques have been combined into multiparametric MRI, which has been shown to increase accuracy in cancer detection (Hoeks *et al.*, 2011). The value of these *in vivo* applications and their role in oncology is commonly described and reviewed in radiology literature (Hoeks *et al.*, 2011; Hoh *et al.*, 1997; Koh & Collins, 2007; Padhani, 2002).

Further understanding of altered metabolism in cancer and identification of abnormal pathways facilitates imaging using PET in combination with computed tomography (CT) via PET/CT (Basu *et al.*, 2011; Jones & Price, 2012). After identifying metabolites, that are either preferentially used or upregulated within particular pathways, nuclear isotopes can be chemically attached either to these metabolites or to metabolite analogues. The emission of positrons from these isotopes can then be measured as gamma rays and superimposed on a CT scan during PET/CT scanning. For example, most cancer cells display heightened glycolysis. Thus, fluoro-deoxy-glucose, containing a radiolabeled positron emitter such as ^{18}F, can be administered and taken up by cancer cells, which are highlighted (Costello & Franklin, 2005). In addition, PET is able to distinguish specific cancers, e.g. ^{11}C-choline PET is used to detect prostate cancer (Evangelista *et al.*, 2012; Reske *et al.*, 2006).The application of PET in other clinical scenarios is diverse, but widespread use is limited by logistical and financial constraints (Fletcher *et al.*, 2008; Kelloff *et al.*, 2005; Rohren *et al.*, 2004).

Recently, a novel method has been proposed to perform *in vivo* metabolomics during surgery by using real-time MS analysis of the smoke produced from electric cautery to biochemically recognize malignant/diseased tissue in which macroscopic changes are not present (Balog *et al.*, 2010; Kinross *et al.*, 2011). Although major development is required before clinical use, the initial concept is intriguing in its potential to improve surgical accuracy and treatment outcomes following cancer surgery.

2.4 Integration with other -Omics Sciences

Metabolites are part of the complex and interconnected cellular hierarchy involving DNA, RNA, proteins and metabolites, as outlined in Figure 1. Consequently, providing an understanding of the mutual relationships between genomic, transcriptomic, proteomic and metabolomic data is a major aim of systems biology.

Integration of multi-omics data sets is already providing insight into biological processes. This integration is enabled by the availability of new statistical methods to correlate information contained in multiple large datasets (Rantalainen *et al.*, 2006). Furthermore, ever increasing genome-wide association studies (GWAS) are identifying multiple risk loci associated with various disease states. However, the penetrance of these loci, and therefore their relevance, remains unclear. By integrating metabolomics and other –omics sciences with GWAS, it is anticipated that identification of loci with a high penetrance/phenotypic manifestations will be unveiled (Suhre *et al.*, 2011; Weckwerth, 2011). Integration of –omics data sets has major potential in oncology (Casado-Vela *et al.*, 2011) and some studies have used a targeted approach in relating datasets obtained by different analytical methods (Rantalainen *et al.*, 2006). A recently published study related metabolomic changes to genomic disturbances in PCa tissue to demonstrate alterations in m-aconitase and acetyl citrate lyase. Phospholipase A2 group VII and choline kinase α were responsible for altered citrate and choline levels, respectively (Bertilsson *et al.*, 2012). Other integrative works investigated colorectal cancer (Ma *et al.*, 2012a), heart failure (Lin *et al.*, 2011) and other diseases (Adamski, 2012; Chen *et al.*, 2012). These studies show impressive proof of concept of this new approach. As a result, multivariate statistical analysis and integration of large and multi-omics data sets are a valuable strategy for further investigation.

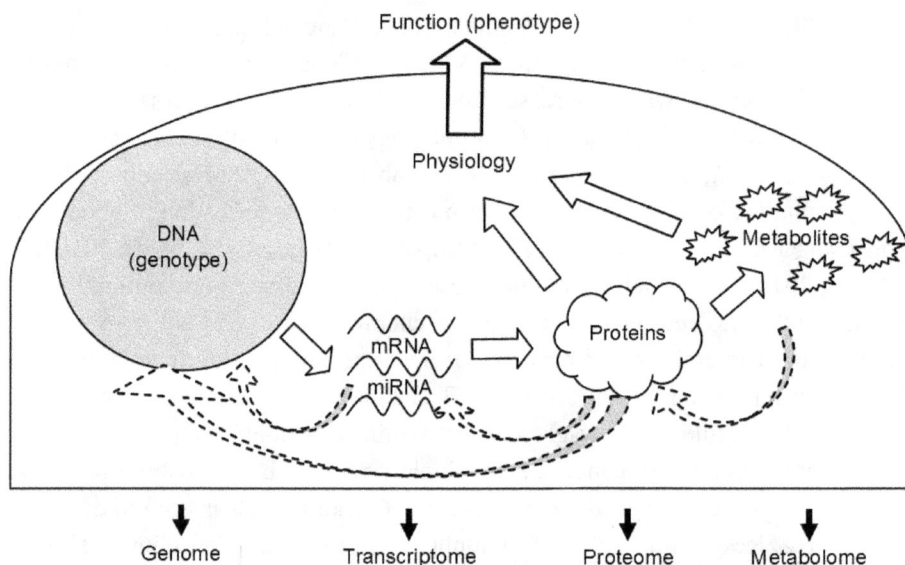

Figure 1: Major targets for exploratory analysis in systems biology. The flow of information and bio-chemical processes between various levels in cellular organisation illustrates the progression from genotype to phenotype (solid arrows). The individual levels of cellular organisation are also regulated by complex intrinsic feedback mechanisms (dashed arrows). Adapted from (Roberts *et al.*, 2011)

Another key frontier in systems biology is the creation of genome-wide *in silico* models of cellular metabolism that are able to incorporate and integrate multi-omic data (Bordbar & Palsson, 2012). Such reconstructed metabolic networks have already suggested improvements for targeted treatment strategies of cholesterol homeostasis in human cellular models (Mo *et al.*, 2007).

The first genome-scale model of human metabolism published in 2007 was a promising milestone (Duarte *et al.*, 2007). The next step in metabolic modeling in oncology will be to construct cancer-specific metabolic models that will incorporate –omics data. This daunting task requires improved cura-tion and annotation of genome databases, as well as integration of high quality –omics datasets from stud-ies of specific cancer types, or of other disease states to create disease-specific reconstructions. Public accessibility and maintenance of data from publicly funded research is critical to these efforts (Field *et al.*, 2009), as is data management (Sansone *et al.*, 2012) and interpretation (Leader *et al.*, 2011).

2.5 Analytical Techniques

Of the many analytical techniques that are used in metabolomics to investigate physiological and pathological states, NMR spectroscopy and gas chromatography (GC) or liquid chromatography (LC) combined with MS are the two most commonly used methods. Both have low running costs, are diverse in sample type and allow for accurate metabolite identification. Other techniques in use are ultra-performance LC-MS, inductively coupled plasma MS, Fourier-transform MS, Fourier-transform infrared spectrometry and thin layer chromatography (Zhang *et al.*, 2012). We will briefly describe the processes involved in MS-based metabolomics, with more extensive reviews available elsewhere (Dunn *et al.*, 2005; Dunn & Ellis, 2005; Lu *et al.*, 2008; Mishur & Rea, 2012; Pasikanti *et al.*, 2008; Theodoridis *et al.*, 2008). Subsequently, we will focus on NMR-based metabolomics, describing the basic principles and statistical approaches that are currently in use.

2.5.1   GC-/LC-MS

Mass spectrometry detects ionized compounds in biological samples according to their mass/charge (m/z) ratio following chromatographic (e.g. GC or LC) separation, and metabolites can be identified in the resulting mass spectrum with reference to internal standards (Wilson *et al.*, 2005). LC- and GC-MS are well used techniques in metabolite analysis and have similar sensitivity, with the major difference being that GC requires more sample preparation (derivatization) and higher analysis temperatures, thus LC may be preferred for this reason (Issaq *et al.*, 2009; Mishur & Rea, 2012). We will briefly outline the basic processes in MS-based metabolomics, which are sample preparation, separation (via liquid-/gas-chromatography), ionization, mass analysis and detection, and finally, data processing.

Sample preparation for MS is dependent on the type of sample. Simple biofluid preparation often involves removing macromolecules through protein precipitation and centrifugation or filtration. Similarly, sampling of the exometabolome (metabolites secreted by cells or organisms into the growth medium) is straightforward. In contrast, to obtain intracellular metabolites, tissues or cells need to be extracted in an appropriate solvent system (Mishur & Rea, 2012). As different solvent systems are biased towards particular classes of metabolites (e.g. polar extraction systems yielding predominantly polar metabolites), the exact choice of solvent depends upon the metabolites of interest. To achieve consistency between samples, internal standards are typically added during/after extraction (Mishur & Rea, 2012).

In GC-MS, derivatization is a further necessary preparation step, which is applied to non-volatile metabolite classes, such as amino and organic acids, sugars, amines and lipids, to render them volatile and thermally stable for GC (Dunn *et al.*, 2005; Dunn & Ellis, 2005; Mishur & Rea, 2012). Derivatization can introduce bias towards individual metabolites if the derivatizing agents are not provided in excess, as the derivatizing reactions have different efficiencies with different metabolites (Mishur & Rea 2012). In addition, metabolites with multiple exchangeable protons will create multiple derivatization products that will show up as separate peaks, thus complicating the final mass spectrum. For GC-MS, electron impact ionization is almost exclusively used (Dunn *et al.*, 2005).

LC-MS is rapidly replacing GC-MS as method of choice in metabolomics, as both methods are similarly sensitive, but sample preparation for LC-MS is simpler, because derivatization is not required (Griffin & Shockcor, 2004). LC typically runs as reverse-phase high-performance LC (HPLC), or recently even as ultra-performance LC (UPLC), and electrospray ionization is typically used in LC-MS systems (Mishur & Rea, 2012). Electrospray ionization MS can run in positive or negative ionization mode, and because individual metabolites are generally only detected in one of those two modes, both ionization modes need to be run to improve coverage of the metabolome (Dunn & Ellis, 2005).

In the resulting mass spectrum, metabolites are quantified by external calibration or by comparison with internal standards (Dunn & Ellis, 2005). GC-MS experiments may also require the use of deconvolution software to adequately analyse overlapping chromatographic peaks (Dunn & Ellis, 2005). To allow comparable results between experiments, data may also undergo further pre-treatment steps, including spectral alignment and automated picking of metabolite peaks (Dettmer *et al.*, 2007). The subsequent multivariate analysis of processed MS data is similar to data obtained by NMR-spectroscopy.

2.5.2   NMR Spectroscopy

NMR spectroscopy is a quantitative technique used to accurately determine metabolite concentrations in samples. Chemical compounds in biological samples are identified by their characteristic peak patterns and signal positions in the NMR spectrum with the aid of online databases (Wishart *et al.*, 2009) (http://www.metabolomicssociety.org/database). More comprehensive accounts of NMR theory and application in metabolomics are available in dedicated texts (Ross *et al.*, 2007). A comparison of the strengths and limitations of NMR and MS is provided in Table 1.

Technique	Advantages	Limitations
NMR	- high reproducibility - high resolution - non-destructive - quantitative - low running costs - minimal sample preparation/no derivatization - unbiased metabolite profile - analysis of tissue (HR-MAS) - translation to *in vivo* (MRI) - rapid analysis - ability for automation - structural identification (2D, 3D)	- low sensitivity - peak overlap - libraries of limited use due to complex matrix - long acquisition times for heteronuclear techniques, e.g. ^{13}C - high initial capital cost - reduced availability
GC-MS	- high sensitivity - large linear range - robust - identification of wide range of metabolites (wider range with LC-MS) - analysis of complex biofluids - non-targeted - established databases - widely available and comparably low capital cost - preferred for targeted analysis	- slow - sample unable to be re-used - requires chemical derivatization - potentially multiple derivatization products for metabolites - many analytes thermally unstable - metabolite weight limitation (<1400 Da)
LC-MS	- high sensitivity - high reproducibility - large linear range - no chemical derivatization needed	- slow - limited commercial libraries - sample unable to be re-used - generation of adducts - higher capital cost (HPLC-MS)

Table 1: Comparison of the advantages and disadvantages of NMR, GC-MS, and LC-MS (Issaq *et al.*, 2009; Shepherd *et al.*, 2011; Shulaev, 2006; Zhang *et al.*, 2012).

2.6   Processing of NMR Data

Processing of NMR data comprises four steps: Fourier transformation, phase correction, baseline correction and calibration. Fourier transformation transforms the raw real-time data into the frequency domain, and phase correction corrects the phase of the resulting NMR spectrum. Baseline correction ensures a constant zero baseline across an NMR spectrum, and calibration is needed to ensure a consistent chemical shift scale/axis across all spectra. Inadequate processing introduces artifacts that confound statistical analysis and jeopardize data integrity (see Figure 2). Minimum standards for reporting and processing have been outlined (Goodacre *et al.*, 2007), and continue to be a good guide for authors publishing metabolomics research.

Usually, NMR spectra require a phase correction following Fourier transformation in order to achieve pure absorptive line shapes for all peaks in a NMR spectrum. Where possible, phasing should be performed automatically or by the same operator across all samples to ensure consistency. Incorrect phasing can distort peak integrals and thus, the subsequent multivariate statistical analysis (MVSA; see Figure 2A/2B).

Baseline correction is the third critical processing step in producing consistent, comparable and reliable data in NMR spectroscopy. At a minimum, the y-offset of the entire spectrum is corrected to be zero. However, baseline corrections are often more complex, using spline, polynomial or other mathematical functions to accomplish a zero baseline over the whole spectrum. As signal intensities are calculated with reference to zero, inadequate baseline correction will distort spectral peak intensities (Figure 2B/2C), and compromise the subsequent MVSA.

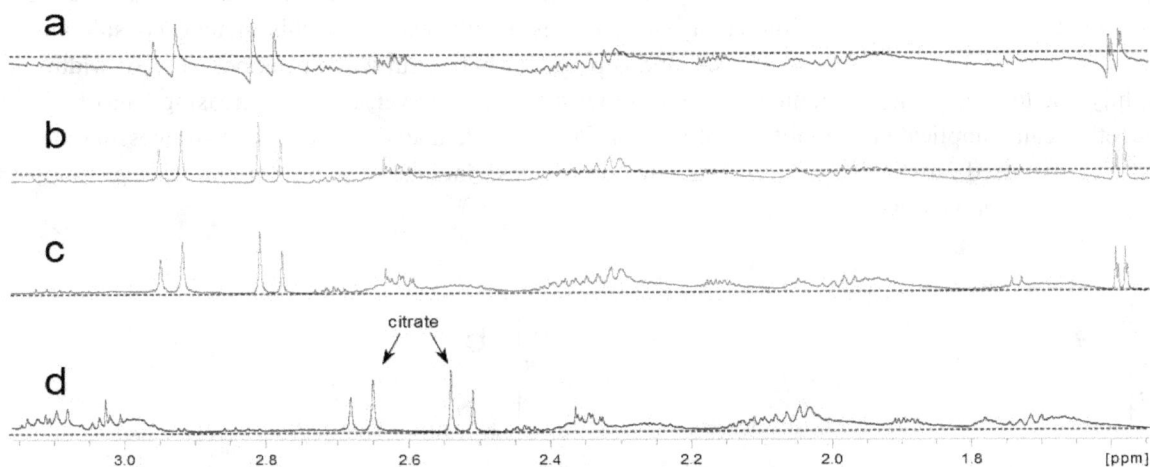

Figure 2: Sequential steps of processing NMR spectra. Shown is a spectrum of human ejaculate in the region of citrate (2.45 – 2.65 ppm) as example. Correct baseline position is illustrated with dotted lines. a - Spectrum after Fourier transformation. The phases of the NMR signals are partly dispersive and in need of phase correction. b - Spectrum after phase correction. Globally reduced metabolite peak intensities and negative values for the baseline occur across the entire spectrum. c - Spectrum after baseline correction, but requiring calibration to a chemical shift standard. Chemical shift values are incorrect across the entire spectrum, resulting in incorrect metabolite identification. d - Correctly processed spectrum suitable for data reduction.

Importantly, the chemical shift axis of each NMR spectrum must be adequately calibrated using a chemical shift standard, such as (deuterated) 4,4-dimethyl-4-silapentane-1-sulfonic acid-d_6 (DSS). In samples containing a high protein content (such as plasma), DSS cannot be used as internal standard. Thus, other endogenous metabolites that are present across all samples, such as lactate, glucose or formate, are used as internal reference. The alternative is to use DSS as an *external* standard by either inserting a capillary with DSS in deuterium oxide (D_2O) into the NMR tube, or inserting the sample in a capillary into a tube containing DSS in D_2O. The use of 4,4-dimethyl-4-silapentane-1-ammonium trifluoroacetate (DSA) has also been suggested as chemical shift standard that is not affected by protein binding (Alum *et al.*, 2008). Chemical shift calibration ensures consistent global alignment of spectra in a metabolomics data set which is critical for statistical analysis. In addition, correct spectral alignment is required for reliable metabolite identification. However, even in correctly calibrated spectra, individual peaks can still exhibit differences in chemical shift between individual spectra due to differences in sample pH and ionic strength. These can be corrected post-processing by various automatic peak alignment procedures (Anderson *et al.*, 2011; Giskeødegård *et al.*, 2010; MacKinnon *et al.*, 2012; Savorani *et al.*, 2010; Staab *et al.*, 2010; Wright *et al.*, 2012).

2.7   Statistical Pre-processing

2.7.1   Data Reduction

After processing of raw NMR data, further processing steps are needed to prepare data for MVSA, which are usually termed "statistical pre-processing". Reducing the full resolution data into small segments of equal width, called bins, or "buckets" (Figure 3), is the most widespread method of data reduction in chemometrics (Wishart, 2008). Compared with analysis at full resolution, this method considerably reduces the size of the data matrix in MVSA, and is particularly helpful when peak positions or widths vary slightly due to changes in pH, ionic strength or other factors. However, due to decreasing data resolution, bucketing can complicate metabolite identification following data analysis. Other pre-processing methods that can be used, particularly in targeted metabolomics, include deconvolution, peak-picking, and weighting factors (Goodacre *et al.*, 2007).

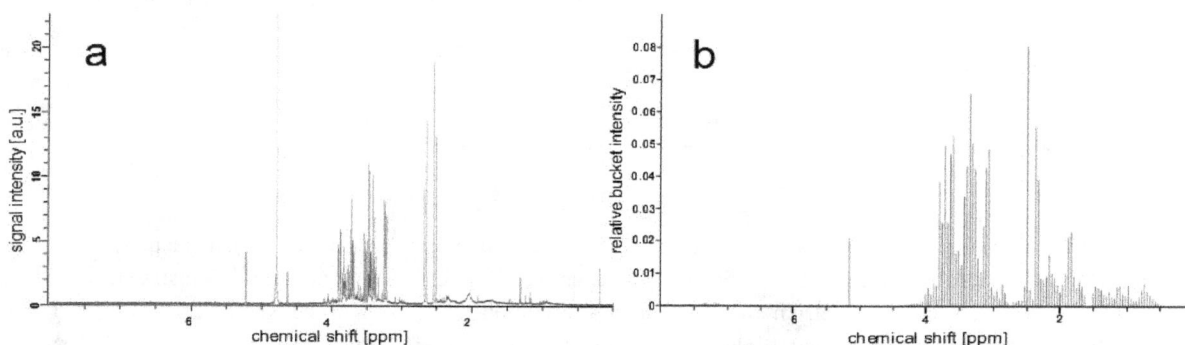

Figure 3: Illustration of data reduction by "bucketing". a - NMR spectrum of human ejaculate with suitable pre-processing (segment shown). b – Same spectrum segmented/data reduced into buckets of 0.04 ppm width across the region 8 – 0 ppm. The region around the water signal from 5.08 – 4.52 ppm was excluded due to artifacts from imperfect water suppression. Note that the area in each individual bucket is integrated across the spectral width of 0.04 ppm and then normalized, yielding intensities similar to a histogram.

2.7.2   Normalization

After data reduction, data need to be normalized to produce data that are comparable between samples (Craig *et al.*, 2006). Normalization is a row operation in the data matrix, and different normalization methods are used to obtain the best representation of the data. In total integral normalization, or normalizing to total intensity, the spectral intensity in each bucket is divided by the total intensity of each spectrum. This procedure normalizes differences between spectra due to sample concentration/dilution, e.g. due to different water content between samples. However, total integral normalization is vulnerable to distortions when one or a few intense signals change considerably between spectra.

Another method involves normalization to an internal reference compound. For metabolomics analysis of urine, normalization to creatinine has been widely used (Akira *et al.*, 2008; Jentzmik *et al.*, 2010). For physiological reasons, urine creatinine is believed to be a suitable indicator of urine concentration as creatinine excretion is constant. However, creatinine normalization has limitations because it will be confounded by any background pathophysiology that alters serum creatinine levels or creatinine excretion, such as in kidney disease. In these cases, creatinine normalization is not suitable. Furthermore, variations in chemical properties within the sample can distort creatinine alignment, so that other metabolites, especially creatine, will overlap with the creatinine signal and thus impede the proper measurement of creatinine concentration (Ross *et al.*, 2007).

Probabilistic quotient normalization (PQN) is a method that reduces variation caused by large changes in the intensity of one or a few signals across samples, as shown in Figure 4. Thus, PQN can overcome the main weakness of total integral normalization. In PQN, which is usually performed after total integral normalization, each variable (bucket) in a spectrum is first divided by the intensity of the same variable in a reference spectrum. Afterwards the full spectrum is divided by the median of these quotients. This procedure is repeated for all spectra in a data set, using the same reference spectrum (Dieterle *et al.*, 2006).

Recently, Kohl *et al.* compared many normalization methods, with some derived from genomic data analysis, and recommended more advanced methods, such as quantile normalization for datasets of $n \geq$ 50, as well as Cubic Spline Normalization and Variance Stabilisation Normalization (Kohl *et al.*, 2012).

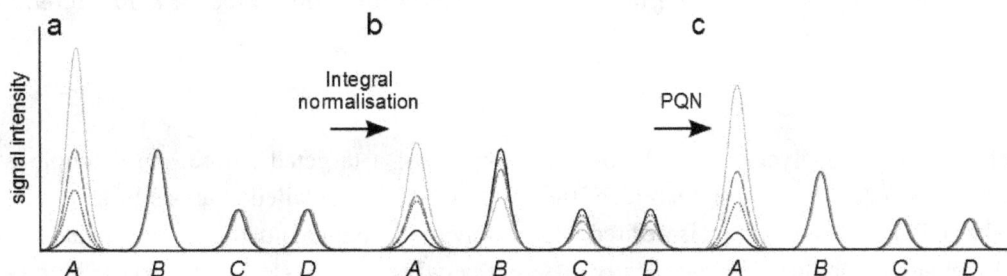

Figure 4: Schematic depiction of spectra containing four NMR signals *A-D*, following two different normalization methods. a – raw spectra with marked intensity variation present in the first peak *A* and identical intensities of remaining peaks between all spectra. b - Integral normalization (normalization to total intensity) reduces variation, and therefore influence of the dominant signal *A*, but also alters relative intensities of the smaller, previously identical signals. c - Probabilistic quotient normalization (PQN) partially reduces variation and influence of the larger signal *A*, while maintaining the original relationships between smaller peaks to allow optimal comparison during MVSA.

2.7.3   Scaling Effects

Following normalization, metabolomic data must be appropriately scaled, or transformed in a column operation in a way that changes how much signals of large and small intensity, respectively, influence the data analysis (Craig *et al.*, 2006; Goodacre *et al.*, 2007). The objective is to reduce noise and maximize information content in the data. Inappropriate scaling may lead to results that highlight parts of the data unrelated to a biological factor, thus compromising the analysis and biological interpretation of the data. In metabolomics statistical analysis, three scaling methods are largely used.

Centre scaling, or mean centering, subtracts the mean value of each variable/bucket from the original data of that bucket (Craig *et al.*, 2006). This method is the least manipulative, and is also best at minimizing background noise, but large relative variations in small signals may not be detected. Mean centering is usually performed mandatorily. Thus, this method is also sometimes referred to as "no scaling", as no further scaling is performed after mean centering.

Univariate, or unit variance, scaling divides the raw data obtained after mean centering by the standard deviation of each variable. Univariate scaling gives each variable equal weighting, such that variables with small absolute but large relative variation are highlighted, but this also means that background noise and other unrelated data variation may be overemphasized and thus confound the analysis (Craig *et al.*, 2006).

Pareto scaling is performed by dividing each variable by the square root of its standard deviation (Erikson *et al.*, 1999). This is the recommended scaling method for NMR-based metabolomic data, as it is able to increase the weighting on metabolites with smaller amplitudes, but does not overemphasize the influence of background noise.

2.8   Statistical Analysis

Statistical analysis of metabolomic data depends on the biological question studied and the design of the particular project, thus, the choice of data analysis methods varies between different projects. In addition, the methods for data analysis are continually evolving. Nevertheless, there is a core set of methods of univariate and multivariate statistical analysis that is in use for metabolomics, and minimum reporting standards for data analysis have been established (Goodacre *et al.*, 2007; Liberati *et al.*, 2009; Schulz *et al.*, 2010).

2.8.1   Univariate Statistical Analysis

The role of univariate analysis in metabolomics is largely of a targeted nature. An example would be where metabolites of interest have been identified by MVSA, and detailed analysis of statistical significance of the individual metabolites is desired. Basic univariate methods can be used to analyze whether or not individual metabolites are significantly different between two classes. However, as with any statistical analysis, the distribution of the data determines the type of analysis used. If the data are normally distributed, t-tests, z-tests, and analysis of variance (ANOVA) may be used. In cases where the distribution is not normal, non-parametric methods such as the Kruskal-Wallis test are used (Goodacre *et al.*, 2007). However, given the high number of variables within a metabolomics dataset, use of multiple hypothesis testing corrections, such as Bonferroni correction or false discovery rate/Benjamini-Hochberg are absolutely imperative (Noble, 2009). This means that, to be significant, p-values need to be much smaller (e.g. $p \leq 5 \times 10^{-5}$) after correcting for multiple hypothesis testing compared to standard univariate statistical analysis (Broadhurst & Kell, 2006).

2.8.2   Multivariate Statistical Analysis (MVSA)

Modern day metabolomics is largely based on data sets incorporating many variables, between several hundred in the case of bucketed data and up to 65,536 if 1D-NMR spectra are used at full resolution.

Thus, MVSA methods which simultaneously analyze all these variables are preferred (Broadhurst & Kell, 2006). MVSA determines whether there are inherent patterns or groupings within the data that correspond to biological states and also which variables are important in discriminating between the different groupings. Thus, this approach is well suited to analyzing metabolomics datasets, where the aim is to correlate multiple metabolite changes with alterations in biology.

There are two general classes of MVSA methods: unsupervised methods, which analyze patterns within a data matrix X, and supervised methods in which the patterns in X are correlated with other external data (e.g. clinical data) contained in a Y matrix or Y table. The advantages and disadvantages of the most common MVSA methods are summarized in Table 2, and will be discussed in the following sections. Some examples of software programs, both commercial and free/open-source, that are available to perform MVSA are given in Table 3.

Approach	Method	Advantages	Disadvantages
Unsupervised	Principal components analysis (PCA)	• Simplifies data • Describes variation in original data without bias • Groups samples with similar metabolite profiles	• Variation might be unrelated to biological question • Influenced by *any* confounders
Supervised	Partial least squares (PLS)	• Simplifies data • Groups samples with similar metabolite profiles • Extracts variation that is correlated with external data/identifiers • more directed to the biological question	• Possibility of introducing bias • Require rigorous validation
	Orthogonal projections to latent structures (OPLS)	• As PLS • Removes orthogonal (unrelated) variation • Improved knowledge extraction	
	2-way OPLS (O2PLS)	• As OPLS • Two-way data correlation between X and Y • Potential for unsupervised analysis (when analyzing two large datasets without external Y table)	
	Kernel OPLS	• As OPLS • Improved model prediction	
	O*n*PLS	• As O2PLS • Simultaneous data correlation from multiple (n) matrices	• Possibility of introducing bias • Require rigorous validation • Not widely available (commercial/open source)
	Bi-modal O*n*PLS	• As O*n*PLS • Data correlation between variables (columns) and samples (rows)	
	O*n*PLS path modelling	• As O*n*PLS • Linkage of matrices along statistically related paths	

Table 2: Summary of multivariate statistical analysis methods used in metabolomics for information recovery. The advantages and disadvantages of unsupervised and supervised methods are outlined.

Software Package	Use in NMR/MS	Reference/Source
Commercial		
SIMCA	Both	http://www.umetrics.com
MATLAB	Both	http://www.mathworks.com
MarkerLynx/MassLynx	MS	http://www.waters.com
STATISTICA Data Miner	Both	http://www.statsoft.com
AMIX	Both	http://www.bruker.com
Agilent Mass Profiler Professional	MS	http://metabolomics.chem.agilent.com
Progenesis CoMet	MS	http://www.nonlinear.com
Free/Open Source		
R	Both	http://www.r-project.org
Metaboanalyst	Both	http://www.metaboanalyst.ca (Xia *et al.*, 2012)
MAVEN	MS	http://maven.princeton.edu (Melamud *et al.*, 2010)
MZmine	MS	http:// mzmine.sourceforge.net (Pluskal *et al.*, 2010)
MeltDB	MS	https://meltdb.cebitec.uni-bielefeld.de/ (Neuweger *et al.*, 2008)
MetabolomeExpress	MS	https://www.metabolome-express.org (Carroll *et al.*, 2010)

Table 3: Examples of software packages used to perform multivariate statistical analysis in metabolomics.

2.8.3   Unsupervised Methods in Multivariate Statistical Analysis

Often, unsupervised analysis methods are initially used in MVSA as they are excellent data exploration tools that can be either used to simplify the data (dimensionality reduction – principal- or independent-components analysis) or to group samples with similar metabolite patterns (clustering – hierarchal, partitional). Although many different methods exist, principal components analysis (PCA) is the most commonly used method of unsupervised analysis in metabolomics.

PCA simplifies the original multivariate data which form a swarm of data points in a high-dimensional statistical space, by projecting them down into a new space with comparatively few dimensions called principal components (PCs). These PCs are latent variables that describe the variation in the original data. The first PC indicates the direction in which most variation occurs in the data. Subsequent PCs are all orthogonal to each other and sorted in order of descending amount of variation. This arrangement describes the majority of variation in the data within the first few PCs. PCA is visualized by two types of plots, the scores and loadings plots (Figure 5).

The scores plot illustrates the relationship and similarity of samples to each other, and allows for inspection of groupings and outliers. Outliers can be visually identified on the scores plot, or statistically defined as being outside the Hotelling's 95% confidence range across all components. Further statistical validation can be obtained using the residual variance of the model, known as distance to model plot (Erikson *et al.*, 1999; Trygg *et al.*, 2007). The variables (buckets, ultimately metabolites) attributable to each component in the model are illustrated in the loadings plot (see Figure 5; Denkert *et al.*, 2006; Pan *et al.*, 2007).

The inherent advantage of unsupervised methods is that they are unbiased, i.e. they detect *any* statistical variation in the data, whether or not it is related to the underlying biological effect (e.g. differences between cancer and non-cancer samples). This property is also their most noticeable limitation, because when confounding effects are larger than the biological effect, unsupervised analyses will pre

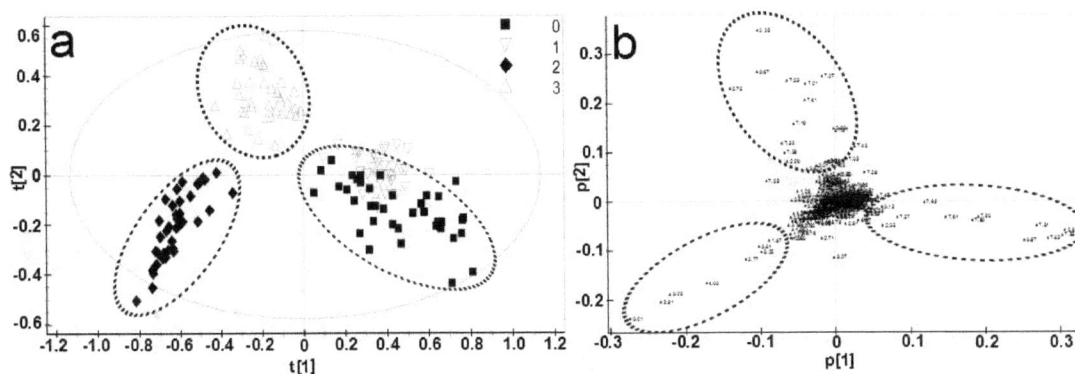

Figure 5: Visualization of a typical multivariate analysis (e.g. PCA, PLS etc.). Sheep urine samples before and after road transport of 12 and 48 hours are shown as an example (Li *et al.*, 2010). a – Scores plot – shows any relationships between samples, such as the presence of separate groups or outliers. This scores plot shows similarity of the pre-transport groups for both transport durations (open inverted triangle = 12 h, black squares = 48 h), and differences between both post-transport groups (48 hours = black diamonds, 12 hours = open triangles). b – Loadings plot – displays the relationship of influential variables that are responsible for the position of outliers or groups seen in the scores plot. Note that the positions/directions of groupings/outliers in the scores plot and responsible variables in the loadings plot correspond to each other (Trygg *et al.*, 2007).

dominantly show the effects of these confounding factors. Distorting variation may also come from un-correlated background variation, or from noise. For this reason, robust experimental design that limits confounding factors and appropriate pre-processing prior to data analysis are vitally important to ensure meaningful results.

2.8.4   Supervised Methods in Multivariate Statistical Analysis (MVSA)

MVSA can be improved by including external data, such as clinical data, in a *Y* table or *Y* matrix. This data inclusion then makes it possible to use a different class of MVSA methods, which are called supervised analysis methods. The biggest advantage of supervised methods is that they can identify the variation (and associated variables) in the biological data that is *correlated* (or co-varies) with the external data, i.e. they improve information recovery and thus interpretation of the biological data. The main supervised methods used in metabolomics-based biomedical research are partial least squares (PLS) and orthogonal projections to latent structures (OPLS) (Gu *et al.*, 2011; Pan *et al.*, 2007; Trygg & Lundstedt, 2007).

PLS is a method that seeks to identify correlation between the dataset matrix (*X*) and one or multiple variables (contained in *Y*). *Y* data may be categorical (class identities, e.g. healthy vs. disease) or continuous (blood pressure, height etc.). If the external variable(s) are qualitative, then the method will discriminate between the corresponding classes and is known as PLS discriminant analysis (PLS-DA) (Trygg *et al.*, 2007). Figure 6 illustrates this distinction. Supervised analyses in metabolomics can be affected by systematic variation that is unrelated to the class, as this affects any correlation found by the analysis method.

0.5	0.46	0.42	0.38	0.34	0.3	0.26	STATUS	SerumPSA
-0.00026	-0.00029	-0.00022	-0.00024	-0.0002	-0.00015	-0.00023	A	6.7
-0.00079	-0.00081	-0.00078	-0.00081	-0.00087	-0.0008	-0.00081	A	5.1
-0.00034	-0.00033	-0.00045	-0.00041	-0.00045	-0.00045	-0.00049	A	8.2
6.37E-07	3.44E-05	1.58E-05	-2.4E-05	-2.1E-05	1.13E-06	-3.8E-05	A	3.4
1.67E-05	-1.7E-05	-4.2E-05	-6.9E-05	-9E-05	-8.1E-05	-9.6E-05	A	5.4
-0.00025	-0.00031	-0.00031	-0.00031	-0.00031	-0.0003	-0.00034	A	11
-0.00048	-0.00053	-0.00052	-0.00054	-0.00058	-0.00059	-0.00062	A	8.2
3.64E-05	5.5E-05	2.67E-05	-3.4E-06	-2E-05	2.86E-05	-3.7E-05	A	6
0.00017	0.000109	0.000103	6.84E-05	3.05E-05	4.6E-05	3.34E-05	A	2.5
-0.00037	-0.00037	-0.00036	-0.00041	-0.00041	-0.00041	-0.00044	A	8.3
1.51E-05	-3.6E-05	-6.5E-05	-9.2E-05	-0.00013	-0.00015	-0.00016	A	4.7
7.17E-05	4.02E-05	1.94E-05	5.16E-06	-9.5E-06	-4E-05	-6.1E-05	A	2.2
-0.00056	-0.00053	-0.0005	-0.00047	-0.00049	-0.00047	-0.00045	A	6.4
3.4E-05	-1.2E-05	5.92E-06	-6.8E-05	-6.5E-05	-8.5E-05	-0.00011	A	0.78
-0.00013	-0.00018	-0.00014	-0.00019	-0.00016	-0.00013	-0.0002	B	4.1
0.000497	0.000455	0.000421	0.000418	0.000276	0.000294	0.000266	B	7.9
0.000208	0.000193	0.000153	0.000141	0.000113	0.00011	5.38E-05	B	5.6
-0.00016	-0.00019	-0.00014	-0.0002	-0.00023	-0.00024	-0.0002	B	6.7
-0.00023	-0.0002	-0.0002	-0.00022	-0.00024	-0.00021	-0.00022	B	2.7
-0.00067	-0.00069	-0.00067	-0.00066	-0.00081	-0.00074	-0.00071	B	5.2
-0.00013	-0.0001	-0.00016	-0.00016	-0.00014	-0.00014	-0.00013	B	10.5
-0.00039	-0.00039	-0.00041	-0.00043	-0.00038	-0.0004	-0.00039	B	5.4
0.000446	0.000427	0.000348	0.00034	0.000294	0.000285	0.000267	B	5.6
1.33E-05	-3.8E-06	-2E-05	-2.1E-05	-4.1E-05	-3.7E-05	-4.4E-05	C	8.6
0.000109	7.26E-05	8.2E-05	8.7E-05	6.78E-05	1.65E-05	-9.6E-06	C	5.6
-8.5E-05	-0.0001	-0.00011	-0.00017	-0.00018	-0.00016	-0.00016	C	3.6
5.66E-05	7.49E-05	2.74E-05	-2.4E-05	-2.1E-06	-9.9E-06	-9.9E-06	C	2.8
0.000171	0.000123	0.000103	8.17E-05	6.53E-05	6.1E-05	3.62E-05	C	7.3
-0.00023	-0.00034	-0.00026	-0.00013	-0.0003	-0.00032	-0.00027	C	8.9
-0.00013	-7.7E-05	-0.00015	-0.00015	-0.00015	-0.00013	-0.00017	C	11.9

$\longmapsto$ —— X —————— $\longmapsto$ Y Y
PLS-DA   PLS

Figure 6: Data included in a PLS analysis. The X table/matrix comprises the metabolomic data following pre-processing. Depending on the objective of the analysis, the Y table/matrix can include continuous (PLS) or categorical (PLS-DA) data to which the X data are correlated.

OPLS is an improvement on PLS that separates variation in the data into two parts: one that is correlated with the biological factor(s) and one that is unrelated/orthogonal, i.e. OPLS separates X into variation that is predictive of Y and variation that is orthogonal to Y (Brindle et al., 2002; Trygg et al., 2002, 2003, 2007; Wagner et al., 2005). A further development of OPLS is 2-way OPLS (O2PLS). While OPLS only correlates data in X with Y, O2PLS is able to correlate X and Y with each other in both directions (Trygg & Wold, 2003). In addition, individual variables from an O2PLS analysis can be visualized as a bivariate 1D loadings plot facilitating identification of potential metabolites (Cloarec et al., 2005). Both, OPLS and O2PLS have recently been preferred to PLS, as separation and correlation of predictive variation to the Y table has been shown to optimize discriminant analysis, improving overall knowledge extraction (Bylesjö et al., 2006; Pinto et al., 2012; Wiklund et al., 2008). This is because both predictive and orthogonal variation can be examined, which may provide more detailed insight into the factors influencing the biological system (Kirwan et al., 2012). Furthermore, O2PLS can be used to correlate two different data sets with each other, e.g. metabolomic and proteomic datasets in an animal model of prostate cancer (Rantalainen et al., 2006). If applied in this way, O2PLS is essentially an unsupervised analysis that is able to correlate variables of different datasets, providing further insight into related structures and pathways in altered metabolic states (Bylesjö et al., 2007).

Different extensions of OPLS or O2PLS have been published, including kernel-OPLS, which improves model prediction (Rantalainen et al., 2007). OnPLS is an extension of O2PLS which determines correlation not only between two, but multiple (n) matrices, allowing for integration of any number of datasets for a given study (Löfstedt & Trygg, 2011). Bi-modal O*n*PLS is an extension to O*n*PLS that is not only able to analyze orthogonal variation in variables (columns), but also in samples (rows) (Löfstedt *et al.*, 2012a). This bi-modal approach should provide more informed data analysis, of both, the variables associated to the biological question, and of confounding factors associated to particular samples. Finally, O*n*PLS path modeling is a method of linking multiple matrices along a set of paths that flow between data blocks. These paths are assumed to be due to a specific causative mechanism, e.g. changes over time, and are able to extract the minimum number of predictive components that have maximum covariance and correlation (Löfstedt, *et al.*, 2012b). Use of these recent extensions of O2PLS is not yet widespread, but highly promising in improving metabolomic data analysis.

One inherent problem of any supervised MVSA method is that, because they attempt to correlate the experimental data (X) with external data (Y), they are prone to introducing bias in the analysis. This can happen due to overemphasis of spurious correlations in the data that are only coincidental and not caused by biology. As a result, MVSA models have to be rigorously validated when compared to unsupervised analysis methods. The value of a validated supervised model may be higher than that of a model originating from unsupervised methods because supervised methods are more directed toward the biological question. There are several methods of validation. The gold standard is the use of an independent set of data to test the predictive power of the original (training) set of data, combined with external cross-validation of the training data set. An established alternative is permutation analysis in which the data in the Y table are repeatedly permuted at random and the model recalculated with the permuted Y data (Westerhuis *et al.*, 2008). If the model is stable and correlations to Y are only of biological origin, randomization and permutation of Y data will reduce the fit and predictability of the model (see Figure 7A). Weak models in which correlations to Y are due to chance, rather than biology, will produce permuted models that may provide similar or superior prediction than the original model and are thus invalid (see Figure 7B).

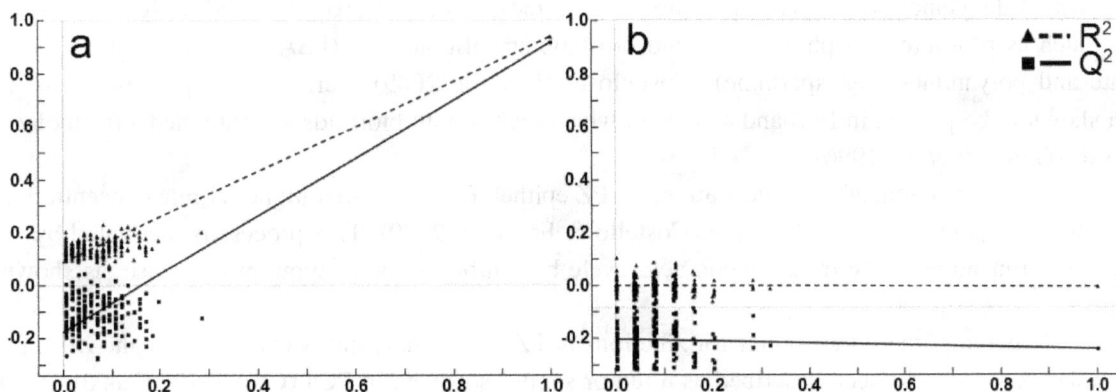

Figure 7: Validation by permutation analysis. a – Example of a valid model (original R^2 and Q^2 plotted on right side of panel), with permutations resulting in models that are less predictive (plotted on left side of panel). The *x*-axis indicates the distance of the permuted model to the original model, and the *y*-axis indicates R^2 and Q^2. b – Example of an invalid model, with permutations resulting in models with similar or improved predictability.

Measures of validity in this context are the R^2 value, which measures goodness of fit, and Q^2, which measures model prediction ability. However – similar to cross-validation – permutation analysis becomes less trustworthy the lower the ratio between number of samples (n) and variables (k) is. The turning point may be near a ratio of n/k of $< 0.02 - 0.04$, although this is not applicable for all data sets, and each study has to be evaluated on its own merits (Rubingh $et\ al.$, 2006). In situations where validation via permutation analysis is not easily accessible, cross-validated ANOVA can be used which uses cross-validated $predictive$ residuals using two degrees of freedom for each component, and is more reliable than ANOVA which uses $fitted$ residuals (Eriksson $et\ al.$, 2008).

3   Current Evidence: Metabolomics in Prostate Cancer

3.1   Prostate Cancer Pathophysiology

Prostate cancer (PCa) is the most common internal cancer in men worldwide and is more prevalent and lethal in Western countries (Siegel $et\ al.$, 2012). Continually evolving methods for early PCa detection have improved outcomes due to earlier treatment and a better prognosis for patients. Current methods of detection (serum prostate-specific antigen (PSA) and/or digital rectal examination) leading to diagnosis (via trans-rectal ultrasound (TRUS) guided biopsy) require improvement due to limited diagnostic sensitivity and specificity. Improved methods will help to avoid morbidity in men for whom a diagnosis of PCa remains elusive due to limitations and problems associated with TRUS-guided biopsy, as is the current situation. Thus, PCa pathogenesis has been extensively studied to facilitate the discovery of new methods for determining the presence of PCa.

The prostate gland sits in the pelvis below the bladder and in front of the rectum. It is a secretory gland that contributes to the seminal fluid component of ejaculate/semen to facilitate sperm motility and egg fertilization $in\ utero$. The secretory portion of the gland is called the peripheral zone (PZ), and constitutes 70% of the gland volume. The epithelium within the PZ secretes prostatic fluid, which contains proteins, such as prostatic acid phosphatase and prostatic specific antigen (PSA), and metabolites, such as citrate and polyamines (e.g. spermine) (Costello & Franklin, 2009). Furthermore, prostatic cells have been shown to be present in EPS and ejaculate, which makes both biofluids suitable media for molecular analysis (Gardiner $et\ al.$, 1996).

Citrate production, after sequestration, by PZ epithelium results in a higher citrate concentration in EPS when compared with blood plasma (Costello & Franklin, 2009). This process is facilitated by zinc-dependent truncation of the tricarboxylic acid cycle by inhibiting the enzyme m-aconitase, as shown in Figure 8.

ZIP1 is the primary transporter for zinc ions in PZ epithelium, and is expressed by the $ZIP1$ gene, which has consequently been described as a tumor suppressor gene in PCa (Costello & Franklin, 2006). The expression of ZIP1 and other zinc transporters recently has been described as being regulated by the micro-RNA cluster miR-183-96-182 (Mihelich $et\ al.$, 2011). Zinc ions inhibit m-aconitase, which converts citrate to isocitrate, the first step of the citric acid cycle. As a result, the preferential sequestration of zinc ions in the PZ epithelium causes citric acid cycle truncation, producing an increased glucose requirement within the PZ epithelium.

The resulting high citrate and Zn^{2+} concentrations in PZ epithelium are reflected in EPS. Citrate is important in seminal ion homeostasis, and is the predominant regulator of calcium ions, which are important in the motility, metabolism and fertilization functions of sperm (Owen & Katz, 2005). Levels of zinc ions are correlated with those of other cations, such as calcium and magnesium, but are considerably higher in concentration. In semen, these cations are largely redistributed in binding to negatively charged seminal vesicle proteins, such as seminogelins, which are vital in regulating sperm function (de Lamirande, 2007). In seminal fluid, zinc ions are bound mostly to metallothionein, with changes in levels

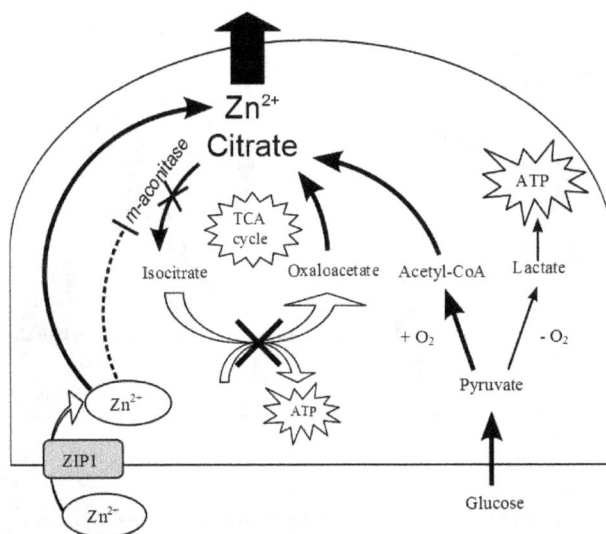

Figure 8: Pertinent physiology of the healthy PZ epithelium. Biochemical reactions are shown by solid/open arrows and regulatory interactions by dashed arrows. When healthy, ZIP1 mediated uptake of zinc inhibits isomerization of citrate to isocitrate by m-aconitase. The result is high intracellular concentrations of zinc ions and citrate, which are secreted to aid in fertilization. Adapted from (Costello & Franklin, 2009; Roberts *et al.*, 2011).

of zinc being paralleled by those of this protein which is mostly derived from the prostate itself (Suzuki *et al.*, 1994).

3.1.2   The Malignant Prostate

Malignant transformation of cells is the result of irreversible genetic alterations, most commonly due to mutations. Specific to PCa, malignant transformation impairs Zn^{2+} accumulation, removing zinc-mediated inhibition of m-aconitase. The result is completion of the citric acid cycle and increased ATP production via oxidative phosphorylation. This is reflected by low zinc and citrate concentrations present in PZ epithelium and prostatic fluid, which have been investigated as potential biomarkers (Costello & Franklin, 2009). Further alterations in gene expression impair normal mitochondrial functioning. Coupled with the relatively rapid division and increased basal metabolic rate in cancer cells, increased glycolysis and lactate fermentation in the presence of oxygen occurring in the malignant state increases glucose uptake, as well as proteolysis and subsequent alanine production. Pyruvate is produced in excess of what can be processed by the tricarboxylic acid cycle, and is converted to lactate. This is known as the Warburg effect, and is seen as a marker of advanced disease in prostate and other cancers (Bayley & Devilee, 2012; Warburg, 1956). This process is outlined in Figure 9. Furthermore, increased membraneogenesis accompanying increased cellular proliferation adds to the changes in the metabolite profile with malignant transformation, and requires synthesis of choline and creatine, which have been shown to be elevated in malignant prostate tissues (Noworolski *et al*., 2008).

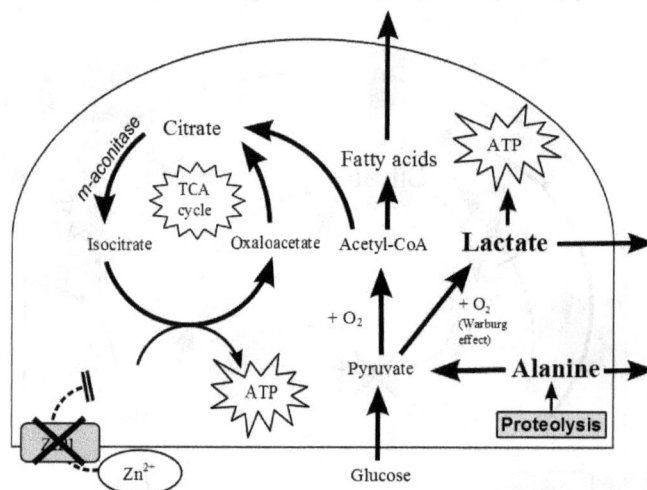

Figure 9: Pathophysiology of the PZ epithelium after malignant transformation. Impaired zinc uptake reduces inhibition of *m-aconitase*, resulting in citrate isomerization and completion of the TCA cycle. Alanine is produced secondary to proteolysis and lactate as a consequence of the Warburg effect. Adapted from (Costello & Franklin, 2009; Israël & Schwartz, 2011; Roberts *et al*., 2011).

3.2   Individual Biomarkers

A single biomarker that is able to confirm the presence of an altered biological process or indicates progression of a disease is a valuable asset in prompting appropriate management for any medical condition to improve the outcome for a particular patient. For instance, extremely high serum levels of the human hormone β-chorionic gonadotropin (β-hCG, a marker normally used in pregnancy) in a male patient with a small testicular mass strongly indicate the presence of choriocarcinoma. While this is an example of an ideal biomarker, such biomarkers do not currently exist for most scenarios in oncology, particularly in PCa (Cole, 2009).

3.2.1   Serum

The most widely used biomarker for PCa is serum human kallikrein 3, also known as prostatic-specific antigen (PSA). PSA is a serine protease that is normally secreted in seminal fluid to catalyze proteolysis of seminal proteins, such as seminogelin (Lilja, 1985). PSA is elevated in blood in the presence of PCa as well as with other prostatic conditions, such as bacterial prostatitis and benign prostatic hyperplasia (BPH). Despite not being specific for cancer, PSA is clinically valued and widely used (Clarke *et al*., 2010).

The normal range of serum PSA, based on population studies, is defined as <1.0 ng/ml. Serum PSA is not only frequently elevated in other disease states, but can also change in the absence of pathology due to other confounders, such as racial and environmental variables (Henderson *et al*., 1997; Marks *et al*., 2006; Vollmer, 2004). In biomarker research, often a cut-off point is derived from studies to determine the optimal sensitivity (i.e. the ability of the test to accurately predict true negative patients) and specificity (i.e. the ability of the test to predict accurate true positive patients). A vast body of evidence has shown that a safe cut-off value for PSA does not exist (Schröder *et al.*, 2000; Thompson *et al.*, 2004). Safety in this context refers to a level that is low enough to detect the majority of men with cancer, but not so low as to cause extensive and unnecessary investigation of men without cancer. This finding of the absence of a safe cut-off value for PSA has been used as one of the major arguments against population screening for PCa using PSA (Catalona *et al.*, 2012; Moyer, 2012).

Serum PSA is a clinically valued test when used with discrimination, and various adaptations have been discovered and trialed with varying success, though none has been considered superior to total serum PSA itself (Auprich *et al.*, 2012; Roobol *et al.*, 2009). Examples include free to total PSA levels, PSA velocity and doubling time (time course of an increase by a factor of two), PSA density (serum PSA in relation to the prostate volume determined by TRUS) and, most recently, the prostate health index which incorporates serum PSA, pro-PSA and percentage free PSA (Catalona *et al.*, 2011; Hori *et al.*, 2012; Lughezzani *et al.*, 2012).

Other serum biomarkers in PCa diagnosis vary in type and size, from circulating tumor cells (Danila *et al.*, 2011; Doyen *et al.*, 2012), to microRNAs (Catto *et al.*, 2011; Sevli *et al.*, 2010), with small molecules and ions, such as sarcosine and zinc, having yielded inconsistent results as markers (Daragó *et al.*, 2011; Li *et al.*, 2005; Lucarelli *et al.*, 2012; Struys *et al.*, 2010).

3.2.2   Urine

Ideally, the perfect marker of PCa is sourced from a non-invasive sample/procedure and indicates both the presence and nature of the disease. Currently, the best urinary marker for PCa is PCA3, formerly known as differential display clone 3 (DD3) (Salagierski & Schalken, 2012). The PCA3 test relies on a patient having had a firm digital rectal examination or prostatic massage just before micturition with the flow of urine flushing dislodged prostatic cells in the prostatic urethra to beyond the external meatus with the void for collection, so there is some licence involved in calling this a urine test. PCA3 is a non-coding RNA which has been shown to be highly expressed in and specific for prostatic tissue (Bussemakers *et al.*, 1999; de Kok *et al.*, 2002; Landers *et al.*, 2005). PCA3 in urine is expressed as a ratio to PSA RNA, and improves detection compared with serum PSA. Use of recently described PCA3 isoforms may further improve results (Clarke *et al.* 2009; Haese *et al.*, 2008; Hessels *et al.*, 2003). PCA3 also contributes to and has been recommended for clinical decision making for men with previous negative biopsies but in whom clinical suspicion is high (Tombal *et al.*, 2012), however its role in PCa detection has yet to be established clinically. Inclusion of the TMPRSS2: ERG fusion gene also has been reported to improve detection of PCa with reference to biopsy (Tomlins *et al.*, 2011).

3.2.3   Seminal Fluid

The main concern with tests using EPS is that both firm DRE / prostatic massage and TRUS biopsy target the posterior part of the prostate, and neglect anterior and anterolateral aspects of the gland in which up to 30% of PCa's are sited (Quann *et al.*, 2010; Samaratunga *et al.*, 2007). In contrast, seminal fluid contains a prostatic component, which is the result of global smooth muscle contraction, and thus theoretically reflects the pathological status of the whole gland. Furthermore, the ability to produce seminal fluid via ejaculation is an indicator of cardiovascular status, as erectile dysfunction is a known event in deteriorating cardiovascular status (Chew *et al.*, 2011; Schouten *et al.*, 2008). Thus, men who produce seminal fluid are expected to have a more favorable mortality outcome following intervention with curative intent for PCa than men who are impotent since cardiovascular disease is the commonest cause of patient demise in this population. Prostatic tissue and prostatic fluid show similar levels of citrate and Zn^{2+}, further suggesting that prostatic fluid reflects intraprostatic pathophysiological status (Zaichick et al., 1996).

3.2.4   Metabolite Changes in Seminal Fluid

Historically, changes in citrate and Zn^{2+} in PCa have been the most pronounced and easily detectable in prostatic and seminal fluid (Cooper & Imfeld, 1959). Metabolite profiling and recent metabolomic analysis of seminal fluid and EPS have discovered alterations in other metabolites, summarized in Table 3. Disturbed zinc homeostasis removes the inhibition of m-aconitase, resulting in citrate oxidation in the citric acid cycle. This causes luminal Zn^{2+} and citrate depletion. Zinc depletion only occurs in PCa, and has been shown to be a stable indicator of PCa status and progression (Zaichick et al., 1996).

PCa-induced change	Metabolite	Role (normal)	Alteration hypothesis	Reference
Increase	Choline	Membrane phospholipid precursor	Increased membraneogenesis	(DeFeo & Cheng, 2010; Swanson et al., 2003, 2006, 2008)
	Lactate	End product of anaerobic glycolysis	Warburg effect	(DeFeo & Cheng, 2010; Swanson et al., 2006; Tessem et al., 2008)
	Alanine	End product of anaerobic glycolysis	Warburg effect	(DeFeo & Cheng, 2010; Swanson et al., 2006; Tessem et al., 2008)
	Omega-6 fatty acids	Cell membrane biosynthesis, fatty acid oxidation	Altered gene Expression	(Stenman et al., 2009)
	Cholesterol	Membrane biosynthesis, androgen regulated	Increased cell Turnover	(Thysell et al., 2010)
	Sarcosine	Glycine metabolism, purine synthesis	Cell invasion	(Sreekumar et al., 2009)
	(Choline + creatine) / citrate	Metabolite ratio	Increased ratio	(Kurhanewicz et al., 1995; van Asten et al., 2008)
	Choline / citrate	Metabolite ratio	Increased ratio	(van Asten et al., 2008)
	Choline / creatine	Metabolite ratio	Increased ratio	(van Asten et al., 2008)
Decrease	Citrate	Ion homeostasis, pH buffer	m-aconitase activation	(Serkova et al., 2008)
	Spermine	Polyamine synthesis	Oxidative stress, enzyme alteration	(Serkova et al., 2008; van der Graaf et al., 2000)
	Myo-inositol	Membrane biosynthesis		(Serkova et al., 2008)
	Citrate / spermine	Metabolite ratio	Decreased ratio	(Lynch & Nicholson, 1997)
	Citrate / creatine	Metabolite ratio	Decreased ratio	(van Asten et al., 2008)

Table 3: Summary of metabolite changes in prostate cancer. Changes generic to cancer, such as lactate and alanine, are listed together with changes specific to prostate physiology, such as citrate, sarcosine and spermine. Adapted from (Roberts et al., 2011).

Although citrate levels are altered in other pathophysiological states, such as BPH and prostatitis (Cooper & Farid, 1964), reduced citrate concentrations in histologically benign prostatic tissue is considered to precede microscopic evidence of PCa (Dittrich *et al.*, 2012). In poorly differentiated tumors, these normally abundant metabolites are present in very low concentrations (Kurhanewicz *et al.*, 1993). This metabolite relationship in PCa has also been correlated with the Gleason histological scoring system and is more accurate than serum PSA (Kline *et al.*, 2006). Such biochemical changes reflect early neoplastic processes that may not be histologically identifiable, a concept familiar in oncology as the "field effect" (Costello & Franklin, 2009). This further supports the role of metabolomics in identifying significant metabolic alterations in pre-malignant tissue.

Other metabolite changes seen in oncology that are not prostate-specific are also present in seminal fluid. Disturbed synthesis and intracellular depletion of polyamines, such as spermine, are reflected in prostatic fluid (Cheng *et al.*, 2001; Kline *et al.*, 2006; Serkova *et al.*, 2008; van der Graaf *et al.*, 2000). The prostate contains the highest levels of spermine in the body, and disturbances in ornithine-decarboxylase in polyamine metabolism have been a hypothesized mechanism for spermine depletion (Mohan *et al.*, 1999; Simoneau *et al.*, 2008; van der Graaf *et al.*, 2000). A role of increased reactive oxygen species production by increased expression of spermine oxidase in PCa has linked inflammation with PCa carcinogenesis (Goodwin *et al.*, 2008). Levels of myo-inositol, a molecule involved in membrane biosynthesis, have also been shown to be reduced in prostatic fluid (Lynch & Nicholson, 1997; Serkova *et al.*, 2008).

Some changes in metabolite levels in prostatic tissue are not reflected in prostatic fluid. Choline is upregulated in PCa tissue, both *in vitro* and *in vivo*, being hypothesized as another metabolite involved in membrane biosynthesis. The use of choline as a marker in prostatic fluid is compromised by the endogenous conversion of phosphocholine (from the seminal vesicles) to choline catalyzed by prostatic acid phosphatase (from the prostate) shortly following ejaculation. This produces a biological artefact in choline concentration. Lactate and alanine are also increased in PCa tissue as part of the Warburg effect. However, spermatozoa utilize fructose from the seminal vesicles and glucose via glycolysis to produce ATP to fuel flagellal movement *in utero* to aid fertilization, resulting in varying levels of lactate and alanine as metabolic by-products. This illustrates a confounding factor between external cellular components and intraprostatic metabolites.

3.3   Metabolomics in Prostate Cancer Diagnosis: Finding the Best Combination

Metabolite concentrations and ratios have aided in distinguishing PCa from benign prostates (Swanson *et al.*, 2003, 2008; Tessem *et al.*, 2008; van Asten *et al.*, 2008). Yet, despite promising preliminary results, there is currently no test available that is accepted as an accurate, stand-alone diagnostic or screening test. With improved data acquisition and processing technology, the concept of using entire metabolic profiles as a large-scale combination of biomarkers has become feasible. Furthermore, metabolite profiles have been shown to be more sensitive as predictors of PCa, and in predicting metastatic potential (Hricak *et al.*, 2007) (Cheng *et al.*, 2005; Mazaheri *et al.*, 2008; Wu *et al.*, 2010). This concept has been demonstrated by metabolomic imaging, in which multivoxel MR spectra of intact prostates were analysed with MVSA. This was able to detect highly significant changes between the global metabolite profiles of benign and malignant prostate tissue without the need to identify specific metabolites (Wu *et al.*, 2010). Similar relationships were demonstrated using freshly frozen PCa tissue when microarray gene expression data and metabolomic data were combined using PLS, providing further insight into mechanisms of metabolite alterations in PCa (Bertilsson *et al.*, 2012). In another study, metabolomic profiling provided an accurate prediction of biochemical recurrence of PCa, that is a rise in serum PSA, following intervention (Maxeiner *et al.*, 2010). This illustrates the potential of metabolomics as a suitable method for monitoring PCa behavior following clinical interventions (Roberts *et al.*, 2011).

The concept of multiple markers in cancer diagnosis has been examined for some time. Specific to PCa, panels of molecular and protein-based markers have been used to improve serum PSA-based PCa detection (Cao *et al.*, 2011; Cuperlovic-Culf *et al.*, 2010; Talesa *et al.*, 2009). The most widely publicized and promising appear to be the combination of PCA3 and TMPRSS2-ERG fusion transcripts in post-massage urine as previously described. Multiple studies have shown improved sensitivity when combining PCA3 and TMPRSS2-ERG compared with PCA3 or serum PSA alone (Hessels *et al.*, 2003; Tomlins *et al.*, 2011). Multiple mRNA markers (GalNAc-T3, PSMA, Hepsin and PCA3) in malignant prostate tissue have been able to provide optimal detection rates (Clarke *et al.*, 2010; Landers *et al.*, 2005, 2008). Other researchers have attempted to combine single markers of different origins to improve PCa diagnosis. For example, a multiplex model utilizing gene-, protein- and metabolite-based targets for PCa outperformed any single biomarker (Cao *et al.*, 2011). However, although these studies are promising in improving PCa diagnosis, many are impractical for use in a clinical setting, mostly due to financial and logistical constraints. Thus, in addition to improved accuracy, a further potential benefit of using metabolomics in PCa diagnosis is a reduction in cost and logistical requirements for each sample, although a high initial capital equipment financial outlay is required. Further limitations of this approach are outlined below.

3.4   Limiting/Confounding Factors

As previously discussed, detecting PCa is difficult. This is due to many confounding factors relating to the pathophysiology of PCa, but also due to concomitant prostatic disease mimicking PCa. In the majority of studies to date, the greatest interference arises from concomitant pathophysiology of the prostate, such as BPH and prostatitis. Serum PSA is known to be elevated in BPH: androgens contributing to BPH development drive PSA synthesis which is mirrored in serum levels. Prostatitis associated with inflammation and prostatic cell lysis, results in increased release of intracellular PSA into the bloodstream, elevating serum PSA. It is for these reasons that serum PSA lacks sensitivity (detecting many false positives) and that there is sustained criticism directed toward serum PSA testing.

Tissue and prostatic fluid levels of citrate were reported to be initially promising in PCa diagnosis compared with serum PSA, but were observed in the past to be depleted in prostatitis (Averna *et al.*, 2005; Kavanagh *et al.*, 1982; Kline *et al.*, 2006). Notwithstanding similar potential dilemmas as those experienced with serum PSA, diminished levels of both zinc and citrate in these samples may provide improved sensitivity in PCa detection, although conclusive evidence in conjunction with PSA elevations is lacking to date (Daragó *et al.*, 2011; Kavanagh *et al.*, 1982; Zaichick *et al.*, 1996). The relationship of citrate depletion in tissues following radiotherapy or hormonal therapy also relates to biochemical recurrence, defined as a rising serum PSA following intervention with curative intent (Menard *et al.*, 2001; Mueller-Lisse *et al.*, 2001). Furthermore, reduced specificity of serum PSA when compared with metabolite diagnosis may be due to pre-malignant disturbances in metabolic homeostasis that are not histologically visible (Costello & Franklin, 2009). The underlying issue of biochemical characterisation preceding histopathology creates ongoing uncertainty, as tissue histopathology is the current gold standard for PCa diagnosis.

Intra- and extracellular citrate levels are also known to increase in BPH, thus citrate estimation in biopsy tissue may be unreliable. In these circumstances, prostatic fluid may be a more appropriate sample to use since prostatic fluid is produced mostly in the peripheral zone, which is also where most PCa is located (Costello & Franklin, 2009), whereas BPH develops in the transition (central) zone of the prostate. A small proportion of transition zone tumors may be missed, but in the large majority of cases these are less aggressive and therefore of less significance (Grignon & Sakr, 1994).

4   Future Directions

4.1   Pharmacometabolomics and Theranosis: Towards Personalized Medicine

Pharmacometabolomics seeks to predict the metabolic response to exogenous therapeutic agents prior to or during drug administration, and theranosis is the identification and monitoring of optimal treatments for patients as guided by diagnostic tests (Clayton *et al.*, 2006; DeNardo & DeNardo, 2012; Nicholson *et al.*, 2012). Both are important aspects, given the recently emerging evidence of inter-individual differences in drug pharmacokinetics, being the ability of an individual to absorb, distribute, metabolize and excrete an administered drug (Suhre *et al.*, 2011). The result is reduced therapeutic efficacy, but may also be responsible for toxicity and adverse drug effects. The etiology of these differences in drug metabolism is diverse and is well understood in only a limited number of circumstances (e. g. Cytochrome p450 enzyme family (De Gregori *et al.*, 2010)). Gender, age, race and concomitant diseases have been suggested as inherent factors, but have yet to be substantiated (Nebert *et al.*, 2003). External factors such as dietary and lifestyle habits, as well as toxin exposure, may also have a large influence on therapeutic efficacy. Furthermore, less obvious but important factors may contribute, such as altered gut flora in various circumstances (Dumas *et al.*, 2006; Ley *et al.*, 2006; Wang *et al.*, 2011). As such, metabolic phenotypes are diverse and complex due to these many influencing factors (Holmes *et al.*, 2008). Although genetic profiling across different disorders is important, metabolite profiling promises to better reflect the phenotype of disease states, and advanced analysis between both methods may help to identify genes with significant penetrance.

As has been illustrated, the carcinogenic changes in various cancers will cause common changes to individual metabolic profiles that can be investigated with metabolomics. In contrast, each individual patient will exhibit inherently different metabolic profiles, while also responding differently to therapeutic interventions (Wilson, 2009). Thus, the concept of personalized medicine, where treatments are tailored to an individual's personal metabolic or genetic phenotype, is one that is exciting, and important in advancing medical treatments (Loscalzo *et al.*, 2007). Using metabolite profiles as a representation of metabolic phenotype promises to enable theranosis by providing the most useful information for predicting inter-individual variation that will guide and assess efficacy of treatment outcomes.

Early research focused on genetic predisposition to cancer or alterations in drug-metabolizing enzymes (Yong *et al.*, 2006). Recent research has focused on identifying varying metabolic profiles that indicate significantly affected drug metabolism, with links to altered gut flora homeostasis (Clayton *et al.*, 2006, 2009). This research related individual background urinary metabolic phenotype to biological and therapeutic outcomes of drug metabolism. Other research has identified alterations in metabolite profiles to illustrate pharmacokinetics and early toxicity, important in preventing adverse outcomes from drug toxicity (Winnike *et al.*, 2010). Recently, this approach has been applied to surgery, and allows for personalized pre-, intra- and post-operative care to improve patient outcomes (Kinross *et al.*, 2011; Mirnezami *et al.*, 2012). The concept of pharmacometabolomics can also be applied to outcome prediction, similar to that used in GWAS, with evidence of serum metabolite levels to be predictive of body mass following chemotherapy for breast cancer (Keun *et al.*, 2009).

Theoretically, pharmacometabolomics has advantages over pharmacogenomics in representing the phenotype resulting from multiple genetic effects. However, it is believed that a combination of approaches will provide best prediction and outcomes (Nicholson *et al.*, 2011). Given current variations in efficacy, toxicity and adverse outcomes of treatments, developing personalized medicine is imperative to provide better medical care to patients while also reducing health budget costs. Thus, the pharmacometabolomic approach is one that has potential to change the therapeutic landscape not only in oncology, but across all fields of medicine.

4.2   Metabolomics to Elucidate Biological Mechanisms

As outlined, metabolomics has been useful in displaying changes in metabolites in various healthy and pathological states. The analysis of metabolites illustrates the end product of normally functioning or disturbed cellular processes and mechanisms. Thus, analysis of changes in metabolite profiles can lead to insights about the underlying biochemical or biological mechanisms. This has been demonstrated in different areas, including but not limited to, drug toxicity, cancer and plant studies (Bylesjö *et al.*, 2007, 2008; Klenø *et al.*, 2004; Rantalainen *et al.*, 2006).

For example, metabolomics could explain how altered STAT5 signaling as a result of truncated intracellular domains of growth hormone receptor in liver tissue leads to late-onset obesity, as systemic metabolite changes were consistent with globally altered metabolism contributing to obesity (Schirra *et al.*, 2008). A similar approach was used for data obtained from a human prostate cancer xenograft model in mice measured by NMR-based metabonomics and proteomics (two dimensional difference gel electrophoresis). Pathway analysis was used to link altered protein expression to changes in amino acids, which contributed to the metabolic phenotype (Rantalainen *et al.*, 2006).

4.3   Integration with other –omics

As previously outlined, the –omics approach to sample analysis provides data sets that require complex statistical analysis to extract meaningful information. In isolation, each –omics field provides insight into that particular level of cell function, and interactions and influences causing the results are hypothesized based on previous research or logical thinking. Thus, appropriate integration of –omics datasets has become an important step in providing meaningful information in systems biology (Crockford *et al.*, 2006; Bylesjö *et al.*, 2008). This approach was e.g. used in insulin resistant mice using NMR-based metabonomics and genomics (quantitative trait locus mapping), and showed altered gut metabolites that were linked with genomic alterations (Dumas *et al.*, 2007). In both studies, large datasets were used to determine which metabolites were similarly affected by alterations in precursor compounds.

A suggested method that uses O2PLS for integration of large datasets for optimal information recovery is outlined in Figure 10 (Bylesjö *et al.*, 2008), using the example of a study that has data from transcriptomics, proteomics and metabolomics experiments. As O2PLS is able to extract information from two datasets at a time, the method for correlating multiple datasets is naturally a multi-step procedure. In the first step the joint variation between two of the three datasets (e.g. transcript and metabolite data) is extracted by O2PLS. This means using one of the datasets as X matrix in O2PLS and the other one as **Y** matrix. Note that in this case, O2PLS is effectively run as *unsupervised* analysis, because only two experimental datasets are correlated against each other, without including a set of external metadata. In the second step, the joint variation between transcript and metabolite data obtained in step 1 is then correlated with the third dataset (proteomics) in a second O2PLS, which will yield the variation common to all three datasets. In the final step, the joint variation that is common to all three datasets is deflated from the original datasets in a series of three parallel O2PLS analyses, to produce variation that is specific to each dataset.

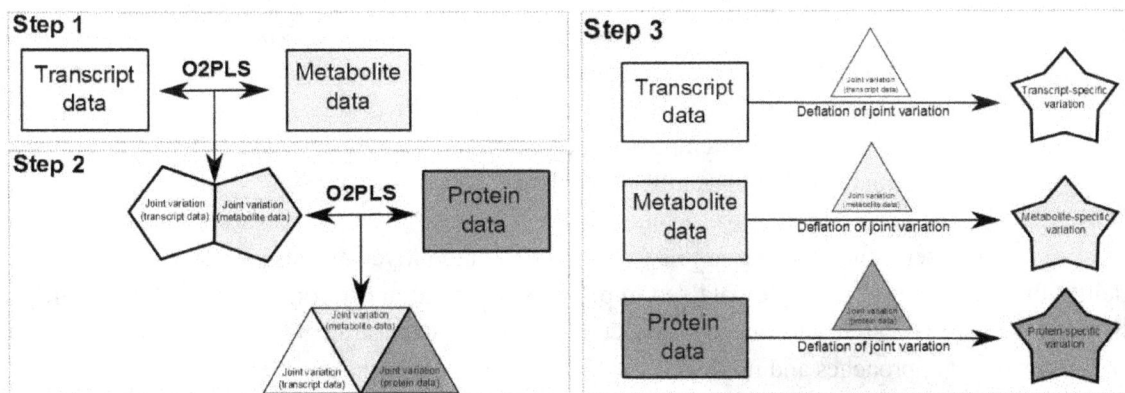

Figure 10: Graphic representation of stepwise data integration of multiple –omics datasets with O2PLS. In the first step, joint variation between two –omics datasets (e.g. transcript and metabolite data) is determined. Using O2PLS in a second step, this joint variation is then correlated with the third –omics dataset (e.g. protein data) to determine variation that is joint to all three sets of data. The third step removes the joint variation between all three individual datasets to produce variation that is specific to each dataset. This dataset-specific variation may be important in helping to address the biological question. Adapted from (Bylesjö *et al.*, 2008).

It is trivial to extend this scheme to more than three datasets by adding on further O2PLS steps between steps 2 and 3 that each time introduce a further set of experimental data into the analysis. It should also be noted that it is prudent to repeat the first two steps with different orders of combining the three datasets – e.g. transcript and metabolite data first, then including protein data, *versus* metabolite and protein data first, then including transcript data, etc. – in order to rule out that potential slight imperfections in the symmetry behavior of O2PLS might cause secondary effects on the data analysis.

4.4   Use of Computational Modeling

As is widely highlighted, the current approach to metabolomics including valid statistical analysis, metabolite identification, and biological interpretation is highly time-consuming. As such, the quest to develop computerized methods of metabolite analysis and identification is underway (Aggio *et al.*, 2011; Tulpan *et al.*, 2011). Following metabolite identification, the next step is to determine the relationship and similarities, if any, of the identified metabolites to metabolic pathways, of which some preliminary programming applications have been released to address this issue (Aggio *et al.*, 2010; Bebek & Yang, 2007; Leader *et al.*, 2011).

Even more promising is the development of genome-scale computer models of metabolic networks. Extensive work has been completed on bacteria such as *Escherichia coli*, with *in silico* simulation reported to mimic experimental changes (Edwards *et al.*, 2001). Application of these reconstructed networks is more complicated in eukaryotes, such as human cells, due to the complex cellular and organismic organisation, including intra- and extra-cellular regulation and interactions. Despite these, an initial model human cell was constructed to provide a general baseline in expression and response to biological variables (Bordbar & Palsson, 2012; Mo *et al.*, 2007). Furthermore, a reconstruction of healthy liver cells was combined with whole-body pharmacokinetics to investigate multiple levels in biological organisation and provide mechanistic insights into for various drug-induced scenarios (Krauss *et al.*, 2012). Alterations to such models to accurately reflect cancer and other pathophysiological states by incorporating known and emerging evidence will better describe the response of these cells (Jerby & Ruppin, 2012). Depending on the type of model, spatiotemporal processes and interactions within cells that may be undefinable or difficult to quantify are currently difficult to incorporate and apply to an artificial model (Materi & Wishart, 2007). Further development of these reconstructed networks may occur via integration of –omics data sets, and research in this field is continuing (Joyce & Palsson, 2006). Computational modeling by incorporating multiple data sets represents a logical and informative, yet challenging, approach to oncology research to guide pharmaceutical development strategies. The result will be better informed treatment approaches and improved treatment outcomes for these patients.

5   Conclusions

Metabolomics is a novel, modern and robust scientific approach that has shown great advances across many fields in biomedical research. The application of metabolomics to differing fields in medical science, including pathophysiology insight, drug development and *in vivo* imaging make it unique from all other approaches. Further research and collaboration to develop reconstructed networks, via integration of many terabytes of –omics data, is the next frontier in providing valuable insights to advance medical research and treatments in various human disease states.

References

Abate-Shen, C., & Shen, M. M. (2009). Diagnostics: The prostate-cancer metabolome. Nature, 457(7231), 799-800.

Adamski, J. (2012). Genome-wide association studies with metabolomics. Genome Medicine, 4(4), 34.

Aggio, R. B., Ruggiero, K., & Villas-Bôas, S. G. (2010). Pathway Activity Profiling (PAPi): from the metabolite profile to the metabolic pathway activity. Bioinformatics, 26(23), 2969-2976.

Aggio, R. B. M., Villas-Bôas, S. G., & Ruggiero, K. (2011). Metab: an R package for high-throughput analysis of metabolomics data generated by GC-MS. Bioinformatics, 27(16), 2316-2318.

Akira, K., Masu, S., Imachi, M., Mitome, H., Hashimoto, M., & Hashimoto, T. (2008). ^1H NMR-based metabonomic analysis of urine from young spontaneously hypertensive rats. Journal of Pharmaceutical and Biomedical Analysis, 46(3), 550-556.

Alum, M. F., Shaw, P. A., Sweatman, B. C., Ubhi, B. K., Haselden, J. N., & Connor, S. C. (2008). 4,4-Dimethyl-4-silapentane-1-ammonium trifluoroacetate (DSA), a promising universal internal standard for NMR-based metabolic profiling studies of biofluids, including blood plasma and serum. Metabolomics, 4(2), 122-127.

Anderson, P. E., Mahle, D. A., Doom, T. E., Reo, N. V., DelRaso, N. J., & Raymer, M. L. (2011). Dynamic adaptive binning: an improved quantification technique for NMR spectroscopic data. Metabolomics, 7(2), 179-190.

Auprich, M., Augustin, H., Budäus, L., Kluth, L., Mannweiler, S., Shariat, S. F., Fisch, M., Graefen, M., Pummer, K., & Chun, F. K. H. (2012). A comparative performance analysis of total prostate-specific antigen, percentage free prostate-specific antigen, prostate-specific antigen velocity and urinary prostate cancer gene 3 in the first, second and third repeat prostate biopsy. BJU International, 109(11), 1627-1635.

Averna, T. A., Kline, E. E., Smith, A. Y., & Sillerud, L. O. (2005). A decrease in ^1H nuclear magnetic resonance spectroscopically determined citrate in human seminal fluid accompanies the development of prostate adenocarcinoma. The Journal of Urology, 173(2), 433-438.

Balog, J., Szaniszlo, T., Schaefer, K. C., Denes, J., Lopata, A., Godorhazy, L., Szalay, D., Balogh, L., Sasi-Szabo, L., Toth, M., & Takats, Z. (2010). Identification of biological tissues by rapid evaporative ionization mass spectrometry. Analytical Chemistry, 82(17), 7343-7350.

Basu, S., Kwee, T. C., Surti, S., Akin, E. A., Yoo, D., & Alavi, A. (2011). Fundamentals of PET and PET/CT imaging. Annals of the New York Academy of Sciences, 1228, 1-18.

Bayley, J. P., & Devilee, P. (2012). The Warburg effect in 2012. Current Opinion in Oncology, 24(1), 62-67.

Bebek, G., & Yang, J. (2007). PathFinder: mining signal transduction pathway segments from protein-protein interaction networks. BMC Bioinformatics, 8:335.

Behrens, T. E. J., Johansen-Berg, H., Woolrich, M. W., Smith, S. M., Wheeler-Kingshott, C. A. M., Boulby, P. A., Barker, G. J., Sillery, E. L., Sheehan, K., Ciccarelli, O., Thompson, A. J., Brady, J. M., Matthews, P. M. (2003). Non-invasive mapping of connections between human thalamus and cortex using diffusion imaging. Nature Neuroscience. 6, 750 – 757.

Bertilsson, H., Tessem, M. B., Flatberg, A., Viset, T., Gribbestad, I., Angelsen, A., & Halgunset, J. (2012). Changes in gene transcription underlying the aberrant citrate and choline metabolism in human prostate cancer samples. Clinical Cancer Research, 18(12), 3261-3269.

Bino, R. J., Hall, R. D., Fiehn, O., Kopka, J., Saito, K., Draper, J., Nikolau, B. J., Mendes, P., Roessner-Tunali, U., Beale, M. H., Trethewey, R. N., Lange, B. M., Wurtele, E. S., & Sumner, L. W. (2004). Potential of metabolomics as a functional genomics tool. Trends in Plant Science, 9(9), 418-425.

Bloch, F., Hansen, W. W., & Packard, M. (1946). Nuclear Induction. Physical Review, 69(3-4), 127.

Bordbar, A., & Palsson, B. Ø. (2012). Using the reconstructed genome-scale human metabolic network to study physiology and pathology. Journal of Internal Medicine, 271(2), 131-141.

Brindle, J. T., Antti, H., Holmes, E., Tranter, G., Nicholson, J. K., Bethell, H. W., Clarke, S., Schofield, P. M., McKilligin, E., Mosedale, D. E., & Grainger, D. J. (2002). Rapid and noninvasive diagnosis of the presence and severity of coronary heart disease using ^1H-NMR-based metabonomics. Nature Medicine, 8(12), 1439-1444.

Broadhurst, D. I., & Kell, D. B. (2006). Statistical strategies for avoiding false discoveries in metabolomics and related experiments. Metabolomics, 2(4), 171-196.

Brown, M. V., McDunn, J. E., Gunst, P. R., Smith, E. M., Milburn, M. V., Troyer, D. A., & Lawton, K. A. (2012). Cancer detection and biopsy classification using concurrent histopathological and metabolomic analysis of core biopsies. Genome Medicine, 4:33.

Bussemakers, M. J. G., van Bokhoven, A., Verhaegh, G. W., Smit, F. P., Karthaus, H. F. M., Schalken, J. A., Debruyne, F. M. J., Ru, N., & Isaacs, W. B. (1999). DD3: a new prostate-specific gene, highly overexpressed in prostate cancer. Cancer Research, 59(23), 5975-5979.

Bylesjö, M., Rantalainen, M., Cloarec, O., Nicholson, J. K., Holmes, E., & Trygg, J. (2006). OPLS discriminant analysis: combining the strengths of PLS-DA and SIMCA classification. Journal of Chemometrics, 20(8-10), 341-351.

Bylesjö, M., Eriksson, D., Kusano, M., Moritz, T., & Trygg, J. (2007). Data integration in plant biology: the O2PLS method for combined modeling of transcript and metabolite data. The Plant Journal, 52(6), 1181-1191.

Bylesjö, M., Nilsson, R., Srivastava, V., Grönlund, A., Johansson, A. I., Jansson, S., Karlsson, J., Moritz, T., Wingsle, G., & Trygg, J. (2008). Integrated Analysis of Transcript, Protein and Metabolite Data To Study Lignin Biosynthesis in Hybrid Aspen. Journal of Proteome Research, 8(1), 199-210.

Cao, D. L., Ye, D. W., Zhang, H. L., Zhu, Y., Wang, Y. X., & Yao, X. D. (2011). A Multiplex Model of Combining Gene-Based, Protein-Based, and Metabolite-Based With Positive and Negative Markers in Urine for the Early Diagnosis of Prostate Cancer. Prostate, 71(7), 700-710.

Carroll, A. J., Badger, M. R., & Harvey Millar, A. H. (2010). The MetabolomeExpress Project: enabling web-based processing, analysis and transparent dissemination of GC/MS metabolomics datasets. BMC Bioinformatics, 11:376.

Casado-Vela, J., Cebrián, A., Gómez del Pulgar, M. T., & Lacal, J. C. (2011). Approaches for the study of cancer: towards the integration of genomics, proteomics and metabolomics. Clinical & Translational Oncology, 13(9), 617-628.

Catalona, W. J., Partin, A. W., Sanda, M. G., Wei, J. T., Klee, G. G., Bangma, C. H., Slawin, K. M., Marks, L. S., Loeb, S., Broyles, D. L., Shin, S. S., Cruz, A. B., Chan, D. W., Sokoll, L. J., Roberts, W. L., van Schaik, R. H. N., & Mizrahi, I. A. (2011). A Multicenter Study of [-2]Pro-Prostate Specific Antigen Combined With Prostate Specific Antigen and Free Prostate Specific Antigen for Prostate Cancer Detection in the 2.0 to 10.0 ng/ml Prostate Specific Antigen Range. The Journal of Urology, 185(5), 1650-1655.

Catalona, W. J., D'Amico, A. V., Fitzgibbons, W. F., Kosoko-Lasaki, O., Leslie, S. W., Lynch, H. T., Moul, J. W., Rendell, M. S., & Walsh, P. C. (2012). What the U.S. Preventive Services Task Force Missed in Its Prostate Cancer Screening Recommendation. Annals of Internal Medicine, 157(2), 137-138 & W-27.

Catto, J. W. F., Alcaraz, A., Bjartell, A. S., De Vere White, R., Evans, C. P., Fussel, S., Hamdy, F. C., Kallioniemi, O., Mengual, L., Schlomm, T., & Visakorpi, T. (2011). MicroRNA in prostate, bladder, and kidney cancer: a systematic review. European Urology, 59(5), 671-681.

Center, M. M., Jemal, A., Lortet-Tieulent, J., Ward, E., Ferlay, J., Brawley, O., & Bray, F. (2012). International Variation in Prostate Cancer Incidence and Mortality Rates. European Urology, 61(6), 1079-1092.

Chen, R., Mias, G. I., Li-Pook-Than, J., Jiang, L., Lam, H. Y. K., Chen, R., Miriami, E., Karczewski, K. J., Hariharan, M., Dewey, F. E., Cheng, Y., Clark, M. J., Im, H., Habegger, L., Balasubramanian, S., O'Huallachain, M., Dudley, J. T., Hillenmeyer, S., Haraksingh, R., Sharon, D., Euskirchen, G., Lacroute, P., Bettinger, K., Boyle, A. P., Kasowski, M., Grubert, F., Seki, S., Garcia, M., Whirl-Carrillo, M., Gallardo, M., Blasco, M. A., Greenberg, P. L., Snyder, P., Klein, T. E., Altman, R. B., Butte, A. J., Ashley, E. A., Gerstein, M., Nadeau, K. C., Tang, H., & Snyder, M. (2012). Personal omics profiling reveals dynamic molecular and medical phenotypes. Cell, 148(6), 1293-1307.

Cheng, L. L., Wu, C. L., Smith, M. R., & Gonzalez, R. G. (2001). Non-destructive quantitation of spermine in human prostate tissue samples using HRMAS ^{1}H NMR spectroscopy at 9.4 T. FEBS Letters, 494(1-2), 112-116.

Cheng, L. L., Burns, M. A., Taylor, J. L., He, W., Halpern, E. F., McDougal, W. S., & Wu, C. L. (2005). Metabolic characterization of human prostate cancer with tissue magnetic resonance spectroscopy. Cancer Research, 65(8), 3030-3034.

Chew, K. K., Gibson, N., Sanfilippo, F., Stuckey, B., & Bremner, A. (2011). Cardiovascular mortality in men with erectile dysfunction: increased risk but not inevitable. The Journal of Sexual Medicine, 8(6), 1761-1771.

Clarke, R. A., Schirra, H. J., Catto, J. W., Lavin, M. F., & Gardiner, R. A. (2010). Markers for Detection of Prostate Cancer. Cancers, 2(2), 1125-1154.

Clarke, R.A., Zhao, Z., Guo, A.Y., Roper A.K., Teng, L., Fang, Z.M., Samaratunga, H.M., Lavin M.F., Gardiner R.A. (2009). New genomic structure for prostate cancer specific gene PCA3 within BMCC1: implications for prostate cancer detection and progression. PLoS ONE, 4 (3), e4995.

Clayton, T. A., Lindon, J. C., Cloarec, O., Antti, H., Charuel, C., Hanton, G., Provost, J. P., Le Net, J. L., Baker, D., Walley, R. J., Everett, J. R., & Nicholson, J. K. (2006). Pharmaco-metabonomic phenotyping and personalized drug treatment. Nature, 440(7087), 1073-1077.

Clayton, T. A., Baker, D., Lindon, J. C., Everett, J. R., & Nicholson, J. K. (2009). Pharmacometabonomic identification of a significant host-microbiome metabolic interaction affecting human drug metabolism. Proceedings of the National Academy of Sciences, 106(24), 14728-14733.

Cloarec, O., Dumas, M. E., Trygg, J., Craig, A., Barton, R. H., Lindon, J. C., Nicholson, J. K., & Holmes, E. (2005). Evaluation of the orthogonal projection on latent structure model limitations caused by chemical shift variability and improved visualization of biomarker changes in ^1H NMR spectroscopic metabonomic studies. Analytical Chemistry, 77(2), 517-526.

Cole, L.A. (2009). Human chorionic gonadotropin and associated molecules. Expert Review of Molecular Diagnostics, 9 (1), 51-73.

Cooper, J. F., & Farid, I. (1964). The role of citric acid in the physiology of the prostate. Lactate/citrate ratios in benign and malignant prostatic homogenates as an index of prostatic malignancy. The Journal of Urology, 92, 533-536.

Cooper, J. F., & Imfeld, H. (1959). The role of citric acid in the physiology of the prostate: a preliminary report. The Journal of Urology, 81(1), 157-164.

Costello, L. C., & Franklin, R. B. (2005). 'Why do tumor cells glycolyse?': From glycolysis through citrate to lipogenesis. Molecular and Cellular Biochemistry, 280(1-2), 1-8.

Costello, L. C., & Franklin, R. B. (2006). The clinical relevance of the metabolism of prostate cancer; zinc and tumor suppression: connecting the dots. Molecular Cancer, 5:17.

Costello, L. C., & Franklin, R. B. (2009). Prostatic fluid electrolyte composition for the screening of prostate cancer: a potential solution to a major problem. Prostate Cancer and Prostatic Diseases, 12(1), 17-24.

Coy, S. L., Cheema, A. K., Tyburski, J. B., Laiakis, E. C., Collins, S. P., & Fornace, A., Jr. (2011). Radiation metabolomics and its potential in biodosimetry. International Journal of Radiation Biology, 87(8), 802-823.

Craig, A., Cloarec, O., Holmes, E., Nicholson, J. K., & Lindon, J. C. (2006). Scaling and Normalization Effects in NMR Spectroscopic Metabonomic Data Sets. Analytical Chemistry, 78(7), 2262-2267.

Crockford, D. J., Holmes, E., Lindon, J. C., Plumb, R. S., Zirah, S., Bruce, S. J., Rainville, P., Stumpf, C. L., & Nicholson, J. K. (2006). Statistical heterospectroscopy, an approach to the integrated analysis of NMR and UPLC-MS data sets: application in metabonomic toxicology studies. Analytical Chemistry, 78(2), 363-371.

Cuperlovic-Culf, M., Belacel, N., Davey, M., & Ouellette, R. J. (2010). Multi-gene biomarker panel for reference free prostate cancer diagnosis: determination and independent validation. Biomarkers, 15(8), 693-706.

Danila, D. C., Fleisher, M., & Scher, H. I. (2011). Circulating tumor cells as biomarkers in prostate cancer. Clinical Cancer Research, 17(12), 3903-3912.

Daragó, A., Sapota, A., Matych, J., Nasiadek, M., Skrzypińska-Gawrysiak, M., & Kilanowicz, A. (2011). The correlation between zinc and insulin-like growth factor 1 (IGF-1), its binding protein (IGFBP-3) and prostate-specific antigen (PSA) in prostate cancer. Clinical Chemistry and Laboratory Medicine, 49(10), 1699-1705.

De Gregori, M., Allegri, M., De, G. S., Garbin, G., Tinelli, C., Regazzi, M., Govoni, S., & Ranzani, G. N. (2010). How and why to screen for CYP2D6 interindividual variability in patients under pharmacological treatments. Current Drug Metabolism, 11(3), 276-282.

de Kok, J. B., Verhaegh, G. W., Roelofs, R. W., Hessels, D., Kiemeney, L. A., Aalders, T. W., Swinkels, D. W., & Schalken, J. A. (2002). DD3^{PCA3}, a very sensitive and specific marker to detect prostate tumors. Cancer Research, 62(9), 2695-2698.

de Lamirande, E. (2007). Semenogelin, the main protein of the human semen coagulum, regulates sperm function. Seminars in Thrombosis and Hemostasis, 33(1), 60-68.

Deepinder, F., Chowdary, H. T., & Agarwal, A. (2007). Role of metabolomic analysis of biomarkers in the management of male infertility. Expert Review of Molecular Diagnostics, 7(4), 351-358.

DeFeo, E. M., & Cheng, L. L. (2010). Characterizing human cancer metabolomics with ex vivo ^1H HRMAS MRS. Technology in Cancer Research & Treatment, 9(4), 381-391.

Delongchamps, N. B., Rouanne, M., Flam, T., Beuvon, F., Liberatore, M., Zerbib, M., & Cornud, F. (2011). Multiparametric magnetic resonance imaging for the detection and localization of prostate cancer: combination of T2-weighted, dynamic contrast-enhanced and diffusion-weighted imaging. BJU International, 107(9), 1411-1418.

DeNardo, G. L., & DeNardo, S. J. (2012). Concepts, consequences, and implications of theranosis. Seminars in Nuclear Medicine, 42(3), 147-150.

Denkert, C., Budczies, J., Kind, T., Weichert, W., Tablack, P., Sehouli, J., Niesporek, S., Könsgen, D., Dietel, M., & Fiehn, O. (2006). Mass spectrometry-based metabolic profiling reveals different metabolite patterns in invasive ovarian carcinomas and ovarian borderline tumors. Cancer Research, 66(22), 10795-10804.

Dettmer, K., Aronov, P. A., & Hammock, B. D. (2007). Mass spectrometry-based metabolomics. Mass Spectrometry Reviews, 26(1), 51-78.

Dieterle, F., Ross, A., Schlotterbeck, G., & Senn, H. (2006). Probabilistic Quotient Normalization as Robust Method to Account for Dilution of Complex Biological Mixtures. Application in ^1H NMR Metabonomics. Analytical Chemistry, 78(13), 4281-4290.

Dittrich, R., Kurth, J., Decelle, E. A., DeFeo, E. M., Taupitz, M., Wu, S., Wu, C. L., McDougal, W. S., & Cheng, L. L. (2012). Assessing prostate cancer growth with citrate measured by intact tissue proton magnetic resonance spectroscopy. Prostate Cancer and Prostatic Diseases, 15(3), 278-282.

Doyen, J., Alix-Panabières, C., Hofman, P., Parks, S. K., Chamorey, E., Naman, H., & Hannoun-Lèvi, J. M. (2012). Circulating tumor cells in prostate cancer: a potential surrogate marker of survival. Critical Reviews in Oncology/Hematology, 81(3), 241-256.

Duarte, I. F., & Gil, A. M. (2012). Metabolic signatures of cancer unveiled by NMR spectroscopy of human biofluids. Progress in Nuclear Magnetic Resonance Spectroscopy, 62, 51-74.

Duarte, N. C., Becker, S. A., Jamshidi, N., Thiele, I., Mo, M. L., Vo, T. D., Srivas, R., & Palsson, B. Ø. (2007). Global reconstruction of the human metabolic network based on genomic and bibliomic data. Proceedings of the National Academy of Sciences, 104(6), 1777-1782.

Dumas, M.E., Barton, R. H., Toye, A., Cloarec, O., Blancher, C., Rothwell, A., Fearnside, J., Tatoud, R., Blanc, V., Lindon, J. C., Mitchell, S. C., Holmes, E., McCarthy, M. I., Scott, J., Gauguier, D., & Nicholson, J. K. (2006). Metabolic profiling reveals a contribution of gut microbiota to fatty liver phenotype in insulin-resistant mice. Proceedings of the National Academy of Sciences, 103(33), 12511-12516.

Dumas, M. E., Wilder, S. P., Bihoreau, M. T., Barton, R. H., Fearnside, J. F., Argoud, K., D'Amato, L., Wallis, R. H., Blancher, C., Keun, H. C., Baunsgaard, D., Scott, J., Sidelmann, U. G., Nicholson, J. K., & Gauguier, D. (2007). Direct quantitative trait locus mapping of mammalian metabolic phenotypes in diabetic and normoglycemic rat models. Nature Genetics, 39(5), 666-672.

Dunn, W. B., Bailey, N. J. C., & Johnson, H. E. (2005). Measuring the metabolome: current analytical technologies. Analyst, 130(5), 606-625.

Dunn, W. B., & Ellis, D. I. (2005). Metabolomics: Current analytical platforms and methodologies. Trends in Analytical Chemistry, 24(4), 285-294.

Edwards, J. S., Ibarra, R. U., & Palsson, B. Ø. (2001). In silico predictions of Escherichia coli metabolic capabilities are consistent with experimental data. Nature Biotechnology, 19(2), 125-130.

Eknoyan, G. (1999). Santorio Sanctorius (1561-1636) - founding father of metabolic balance studies. American Journal of Nephrology, 19(2), 226-233.

Eriksson, L., Johansson, E., Kettaneh-Wold, N., Trygg, J., Wikström, C. & Wold, S. (2006). Multi- and megavariate data analysis. Second Edition. Umetrics AB. Umeå, Sweden.

Eriksson, L., Trygg, J., & Wold, S. (2008). CV-ANOVA for significance testing of PLS and OPLS® models. Journal of Chemometrics, 22(11-12), 594-600.

Evangelista, L., Guttilla, A., Zattoni, F., Muzzio, P. C., & Zattoni, F. (2012). Utility of Choline Positron Emission Tomography/Computed Tomography for Lymph Node Involvement Identification in Intermediate- to High-risk Prostate Cancer: A Systematic Literature Review and Meta-analysis. European Urology, 63(6), 1040-1048.

Ferlay, J., Shin, H.R., Bray, F., Forman, D., Mathers, C., & Parkin, D. M. (2010). Estimates of worldwide burden of cancer in 2008: GLOBOCAN 2008. International Journal of Cancer, 127(12), 2893-2917.

Fiehn, O. (2002). Metabolomics – the link between genotypes and phenotypes. Plant Molecular Biology, 48(1-2), 155-171.

Field, D., Sansone, S.A., Collis, A., Booth, T., Dukes, P., Gregurick, S. K., Kennedy, K., Kolar, P., Kolker, E., Maxon, M., Millard, S., Mugabushaka, A.M., Perrin, N., Remacle, J. E., Remington, K., Rocca-Serra, P., Taylor, C. F., Thorley, M., Tiwari, B., & Wilbanks, J. (2009). 'Omics Data Sharing. Science, 326(5950), 234-236.

Fitch, K. D. (2008). Androgenic-anabolic steroids and the Olympic Games. Asian Journal of Andrology, 10(3), 384-390.

Fletcher, J. W., Djulbegovic, B., Soares, H. P., Siegel, B. A., Lowe, V. J., Lyman, G. H., Coleman, R. E., Wahl, R., Paschold, J. C., Avril, N., Einhorn, L. H., Suh, W. W., Samson, D., Delbeke, D., Gorman, M., & Shields, A. F. (2008). Recommendations on the use of F-18-FDG PET in oncology. Journal of Nuclear Medicine, 49(3), 480-508.

Freeman, R. (1995). A short history of NMR. Chemistry of Heterocyclic Compounds, 31(9), 1004-1005.

Ganti, S., & Weiss, R. H. (2011). Urine metabolomics for kidney cancer detection and biomarker discovery. Urologic Oncology, 29(5), 551-557.

Gardiner, R. A., Samaratunga, M. L., Gwynne, R. A., Clague, A., Seymour, G. J., & Lavin, M. F. (1996). Abnormal prostatic cells in ejaculates from men with prostatic cancer – a preliminary report. British Journal of Urology, 78(3), 414-418.

Gates, S. C., & Sweeley, C. C. (1978). Quantitative metabolic profiling based on gas chromatography. Clinical Chemistry, 24(10), 1663-1673.

Geladi, P., & Esbensen, K. (1990). The start and early history of chemometrics: Selected interviews. Part 1. Journal of Chemometrics, 4(5), 337-354.

Giskeødegård, G. F., Bloemberg, T. G., Postma, G., Sitter, B., Tessem, M. B., Gribbestad, I. S., Bathen, T. F., & Buydens, L. M. C. (2010). Alignment of high resolution magic angle spinning magnetic resonance spectra using warping methods. Analytica Chimica Acta, 683(1), 1-11.

Goodacre, R., Broadhurst, D., Smilde, A. K., Kristal, B. S., Baker, J. D., Beger, R., Bessant, C., Connor, S., Capuani, G., Craig, A., Ebbels, T., Kell, D. B., Manetti, C., Newton, J., Paternostro, G., Somorjai, R., Sjöström, M., Trygg, J., & Wulfert, F. (2007). Proposed minimum reporting standards for data analysis in metabolomics. Metabolomics, 3(3), 231-241.

Goodwin, A. C., Jadallah, S., Toubaji, A., Lecksell, K., Hicks, J. L., Kowalski, J., Bova, G. S., De Marzo, A. M., Netto, G. J., & Casero, R. A., Jr. (2008). Increased spermine oxidase expression in human prostate cancer and prostatic intraepithelial neoplasia tissues. Prostate, 68(7), 766-772.

Griffin, J. L., & Shockcor, J. P. (2004). Metabolic profiles of cancer cells. Nature Reviews Cancer, 4(7), 551-561.

Griffiths, J. (2008). A Brief History of Mass Spectrometry. Analytical Chemistry, 80(15), 5678-5683.

Grignon, D.J., & Sakr, W.A., (1994) Zonal origin of prostatic adenocarcinoma: are there biologic differences between transition zone and peripheral zone adenocarcinomas of the prostate gland? Journal of Cellular Biochemistry, Supplement 19, 267-269.

Gu, H. W., Pan, Z. Z., Xi, B. W., Asiago, V., Musselman, B., & Raftery, D. (2011). Principal component directed partial least squares analysis for combining nuclear magnetic resonance and mass spectrometry data in metabolomics: Application to the detection of breast cancer. Analytica Chimica Acta, 686(1-2), 57-63.

Haese, A., de la Taille, A., van Poppel H., Marberger, M., Stenzl, A., Mulders, P. F. A., Huland, H., Abbou, C. C., Remzi, M., Tinzl, M., Feyerabend, S., Stillebroer, A. B., van Gils, M. P. M. Q., & Schalken, J. A. (2008). Clinical utility of the PCA3 urine assay in European men scheduled for repeat biopsy. European Urology, 54(5), 1081-1088.

Hamamah, S., Seguin, F., Barthelemy, C., Akoka, S., Le Pape, A., Lansac, J., & Royere, D. (1993). ^{1}H nuclear magnetic resonance studies of seminal plasma from fertile and infertile men. Journal of Reproduction and Fertility, 97(1), 51-55.

Hamamah, S., Seguin, F., Bujan, L., Barthelemy, C., Mieusset, R., & Lansac, J. (1998). Quantification by magnetic resonance spectroscopy of metabolites in seminal plasma able to differentiate different forms of azoospermia. Human Reproduction, 13(1), 132-135.

Han, X., Rozen, S., Boyle, S. H., Hellegers, C., Cheng, H., Burke, J. R., Welsh-Bohmer, K. A., Doraiswamy, P. M., & Kaddurah-Daouk, R. (2011). Metabolomics in early Alzheimer's disease: identification of altered plasma sphingolipidome using shotgun lipidomics. PLoS ONE, 6(7), e21643.

Henderson, R. J., Eastham, J. A., Culkin, D. J., Kattan, M. W., Whatley, T., Mata, J., Venable, D., & Sartor, O. (1997). Prostate-Specific Antigen (PSA) and PSA Density: Racial Differences in Men Without Prostate Cancer. Journal of the National Cancer Institute, 89(2), 134-138.

Hessels, D., Klein Gunnewiek, J. M. T., van Oort, I., Karthaus, H. F. M., van Leenders, G. J. L., van Balken, B., Kiemeney, L. A., Witjes, J. A., & Schalken, J. A. (2003). DD3^{PCA3}-based molecular urine analysis for the diagnosis of prostate cancer. European Urology, 44(1), 8-16.

Hoeks, C. M. A., Barentsz, J. O., Hambrock, T., Yakar, D., Somford, D. M., Heijmink, S. W. T. P. J., Scheenen, T. W. J., Vos, P. C., Huisman, H., van Oort, I. M., Witjes, J. A., Heerschap, A., & Fütterer, J. J. (2011). Prostate Cancer: Multiparametric MR Imaging for Detection, Localization, and Staging. Radiology, 261(1), 46-66.

Hoh, C. K., Schiepers, C., Seltzer, M. A., Gambhir, S. S., Silverman, D. H. S., Czernin, J., Maddahi, J., & Phelps, M. E. (1997). PET in oncology: Will it replace the other modalities? Seminars in Nuclear Medicine, 27(2), 94-106.

Holmes, E., Wilson, I. D., & Nicholson, J. K. (2008). Metabolic phenotyping in health and disease. Cell, 134(5), 714-717.

Hori, S., Blanchet, J. S., & McLoughlin, J. (2012). From prostate-specific antigen (PSA) to precursor PSA (proPSA) isoforms: a review of the emerging role of proPSAs in the detection and management of early prostate cancer. BJU International, 112(6), 717-728.

Hoult, D. I., Busby, S. J. W., Gadian, D. G., Radda, G. K., Richards, R. E., & Seeley, P. J. (1974). Observation of tissue metabolites using ^{31}P nuclear magnetic resonance. Nature, 252(5481), 285-287.

Hricak, H., Choyke, P. L., Eberhardt, S. C., Leibel, S. A., & Scardino, P. T. (2007). Imaging prostate cancer: a multidisciplinary perspective. Radiology, 243(1), 28-53.

Hyndman, M. E., Mullins, J. K., & Bivalacqua, T. J. (2011). Metabolomics and bladder cancer. Urologic Oncology, 29(5), 558-561.

Israël, M., & Schwartz, L. (2011). The metabolic advantage of tumor cells. Molecular Cancer, 10:70.

Issaq, H. J., Van, Q. N., Waybright, T. J., Muschik, G. M., & Veenstra, T. D. (2009). Analytical and statistical approaches to metabolomics research. Journal of Separation Science, 32(13), 2183-2199.

Jentzmik, F., Stephan, C., Miller, K., Schrader, M., Erbersdobler, A., Kristiansen, G., Lein, M., & Jung, K. (2010). Sarcosine in urine after digital rectal examination fails as a marker in prostate cancer detection and identification of aggressive tumors. European Urology, 58(1), 12-18.

Jerby, L., & Ruppin, E. (2012). Predicting Drug Targets and Biomarkers of Cancer via Genome-Scale Metabolic Modeling. Clinical Cancer Research, 18(20), 5572-5584.

Jones, T., & Price, P. (2012). Development and experimental medicine applications of PET in oncology: a historical perspective. The Lancet Oncology, 13(3), e116-125.

Joyce, A. R., & Palsson, B. Ø. (2006). The model organism as a system: integrating 'omics' data sets. Nature Reviews Molecular Cell Biology, 7(3), 198-210.

Kavanagh, J. P., Darby, C., & Costello, C. B. (1982). The response of seven prostatic fluid components to prostatic disease. International Journal of Andrology, 5(5), 487-496.

Keifer, P. A. (2007). High-Resolution MAS for Liquids and Semisolids. Encyclopedia of Magnetic Resonance: John Wiley & Sons, Ltd.

Kelloff, G. J., Hoffman, J. M., Johnson, B., Scher, H. I., Siegel, B. A., Cheng, E. Y., Cheson, B. D., O'Shaughnessy, J., Guyton, K. Z., Mankoff, D. A., Shankar, L., Larson, S. M., Sigman, C. C., Schilsky, R. L., & Sullivan, D. C. (2005). Progress and promise of FDG-PET imaging for cancer patient management and oncologic drug development. Clinical Cancer Research, 11(8), 2785-2808.

Keun, H. C., Sidhu, J., Pchejetski, D., Lewis, J. S., Marconell, H., Patterson, M., Bloom, S. R., Amber, V., Coombes, R. C., & Stebbing, J. (2009). Serum molecular signatures of weight change during early breast cancer chemotherapy. Clinical Cancer Research 15(21), 6716-6723.

Kinross, J. M., Holmes, E., Darzi, A. W., & Nicholson, J. K. (2011). Metabolic phenotyping for monitoring surgical patients. The Lancet, 377(9780), 1817-1819.

Kirwan, G. M., Johansson, E., Kleemann, R., Verheij, E. R., Wheelock, Å. M., Goto, S., Trygg, J., & Wheelock, C. E. (2012). Building Multivariate Systems Biology Models. Analytical Chemistry, 84(16), 7064-7071.

Klenø, T. G., Kiehr, B., Baunsgaard, D., & Sidelmann, U. G. (2004). Combination of 'omics' data to investigate the mechanism(s) of hydrazine-induced hepatotoxicity in Rats and to identify potential biomarkers. Biomarkers, 9(2), 116-138.

Kline, E. E., Treat, E. G., Averna, T. A., Davis, M. S., Smith, A. Y., & Sillerud, L. O. (2006). Citrate concentrations in human seminal fluid and expressed prostatic fluid determined via ^{1}H nuclear magnetic resonance spectroscopy outperform prostate specific antigen in prostate cancer detection. The Journal of Urology, 176(5), 2274-2279.

Koh, D.M., & Collins, D. J. (2007). Diffusion-Weighted MRI in the Body: Applications and Challenges in Oncology. American Journal of Roentgenology, 188(6), 1622-1635.

Kohl, S. M., Klein, M. S., Hochrein, J., Oefner, P. J., Spang, R., & Gronwald, W. (2012). State-of-the art data normalization methods improve NMR-based metabolomic analysis. Metabolomics, 8(1), S146-S160.

Krauss, M., Schaller, S., Borchers, S., Findeisen, R., Lippert, J., & Kuepfer, L. (2012). Integrating Cellular Metabolism into a Multiscale Whole-Body Model. PLoS Computational Biology, 8(10), e1002750.

Kurhanewicz, J., Dahiya, R., Macdonald, J. M., Chang, L. H., James, T. L., & Narayan, P. (1993). Citrate alterations in primary and metastatic human prostatic adenocarcinomas: ^{1}H magnetic resonance spectroscopy and biochemical study. Magnetic Resonance in Medicine, 29(2), 149-157.

Kurhanewicz, J., Vigneron, D. B., Nelson, S. J., Hricak, H., MacDonald, J. M., Konety, B., & Narayan, P. (1995). Citrate as an in vivo marker to discriminate prostate cancer from benign prostatic hyperplasia and normal prostate peripheral zone: detection via localized proton spectroscopy. Urology, 45(3), 459-466.

Kurhanewicz, J., Swanson, M. G., Nelson, S. J., & Vigneron, D. B. (2002). Combined magnetic resonance imaging and spectroscopic imaging approach to molecular imaging of prostate cancer. Journal of Magnetic Resonance Imaging, 16(4), 451-463.

Kwock, L., Smith, J. K., Castillo, M., Ewend, M. G., Collichio, F., Morris, D. E., Bouldin, T. W., & Cush, S. (2006). Clinical role of proton magnetic resonance spectroscopy in oncology: brain, breast, and prostate cancer. The Lancet Oncology, 7(10), 859-868.

Landers, K. A., Burger, M. J., Tebay, M. A., Purdie, D. M., Scells, B., Samaratunga, H., Lavin, M. F., & Gardiner, R. A. (2005). Use of multiple biomarkers for a molecular diagnosis of prostate cancer. International Journal of Cancer, 114(6), 950-956.

Landers, K. A., Samaratunga, H., Teng, L., Buck, M., Burger, M. J., Scells, B., Lavin, M. F., & Gardiner, R. A. (2008). Identification of claudin-4 as a marker highly overexpressed in both primary and metastatic prostate cancer. British Journal of Cancer, 99(3), 491-501.

Leader, D. P., Burgess, K., Creek, D., & Barrett, M. P. (2011). Pathos: A web facility that uses metabolic maps to display experimental changes in metabolites identified by mass spectrometry. Rapid Communications in Mass Spectrometry, 25(22), 3422-3426.

Ley, R. E., Turnbaugh, P. J., Klein, S., & Gordon, J. I. (2006). Microbial ecology: human gut microbes associated with obesity. Nature, 444(7122), 1022-1023.

Li, J., Wijffels, G., Yu, Y., Nielsen, L. K., Niemeyer, D. O., Fisher, A. D., Ferguson, D. M., & Schirra, H. J. (2010). Altered Fatty Acid Metabolism in Long Duration Road Transport: An NMR-based Metabonomics Study in Sheep. Journal of Proteome Research, 10(3), 1073-1087.

Li, X. M., Zhang, L., Li, J., Li, Y., Wang, H. L., Ji, G. Y., Kuwahara, M., & Zhao, X. J. (2005). Measurement of serum zinc improves prostate cancer detection efficiency in patients with PSA levels between 4 ng/mL and 10 ng/mL. Asian Journal of Andrology, 7(3), 323-328.

Liberati, A., Altman, D. G., Tetzlaff, J., Mulrow, C., Gøtzsche, P. C., Ioannidis, J. P. A., Clarke, M., Devereaux, P. J., Kleijnen, J., & Moher, D. (2009). The PRISMA statement for reporting systematic reviews and meta-analyses of studies that evaluate healthcare interventions: explanation and elaboration. British Medical Journal, 339, b2700.

Lilja, H. (1985). A kallikrein-like serine protease in prostatic fluid cleaves the predominant seminal vesicle protein. The Journal of Clinical Investigation, 76(5), 1899-1903.

Lim, K. S., & Tan, C. H. (2012). Diffusion-weighted MRI of adult male pelvic cancers. Clinical Radiology, 67(9), 899-908.

Lin, D., Hollander, Z., Meredith, A., Stadnick, E., Sasaki, M., Cohen Freue, G., Qasimi, P., Mui, A., Ng, R. T., Balshaw, R., Wilson-McManus, J. E., Wishart, D., Hau, D., Keown, P. A., McMaster, R., & McManus, B. M. (2011). Molecular signatures of end-stage heart failure. Journal of Cardiac Failure, 17(10), 867-874.

Lodi, A., & Ronen, S. M. (2011). Magnetic resonance spectroscopy detectable metabolomic fingerprint of response to antineoplastic treatment. PLoS ONE, 6(10), e26155.

Löfstedt, T., & Trygg, J. (2011). OnPLS-a novel multiblock method for the modelling of predictive and orthogonal variation. Journal of Chemometrics, 25(8), 441-455.

Löfstedt, T., Eriksson, L., Wormbs, G., & Trygg, J. (2012a). Bi-modal OnPLS. Journal of Chemometrics, 26(6), 236-245.

Löfstedt, T., Hanafi, M., Mazerolles, G., & Trygg, J. (2012b). OnPLS path modelling. Chemometrics and Intelligent Laboratory Systems, 118, 139-149.

Loscalzo, J., Kohane, I., & Barabasi, A. L. (2007). Human disease classification in the postgenomic era: a complex systems approach to human pathobiology. Molecular Systems Biology, 3:124.

Lu, X., Zhao, X., Bai, C., Zhao, C., Lu, G., & Xu, G. (2008). LC–MS-based metabonomics analysis. Journal of Chromatography B, 866(1–2), 64-76.

Lucarelli, G., Fanelli, M., Larocca, A. M. V., Germinario, C. A., Rutigliano, M., Vavallo, A., Selvaggi, F. P., Bettocchi, C., Battaglia, M., & Ditonno, P. (2012). Serum sarcosine increases the accuracy of prostate cancer detection in patients with total serum PSA less than 4.0 ng/ml. The Prostate, 72(15), 1611-1621.

Lughezzani, G., Lazzeri, M., Larcher, A., Lista, G., Scattoni, V., Cestari, A., Buffi, N. M., Bini, V., & Guazzoni, G. (2012). Development and internal validation of a Prostate Health Index based nomogram for predicting prostate cancer at extended biopsy. The Journal of Urology, 188(4), 1144-1150.

Lynch, M. J., Masters, J., Pryor, J. P., Lindon, J. C., Spraul, M., Foxall, P. J., & Nicholson, J. K. (1994). Ultra high field NMR spectroscopic studies on human seminal fluid, seminal vesicle and prostatic secretions. Journal of Pharmaceutical and Biomedical Analysis, 12(1), 5-19.

Lynch, M. J., & Nicholson, J. K. (1997). Proton MRS of human prostatic fluid: correlations between citrate, spermine, and myo-inositol levels and changes with disease. Prostate, 30(4), 248-255.

Ma, Y., Zhang, P., Wang, F., Liu, W., Yang, J., & Qin, H. (2012a). An integrated proteomics and metabolomics approach for defining oncofetal biomarkers in the colorectal cancer. Annals of Surgery, 255(4), 720-730.

Ma, Y., Zhang, P., Yang, Y., Wang, F., & Qin, H. (2012b). Metabolomics in the fields of oncology: a review of recent research. Molecular Biology Reports, 39(7), 7505-7511.

MacIntyre, D. A., Jiménez, B., Jantus Lewintre, E., Reinoso Martín, C., Schäfer, H., García Ballesteros, C., Ramon Mayans, J., Spraul, M., García-Conde, J., & Pineda-Lucena, A. (2010). Serum metabolome analysis by ^{1}H-NMR reveals differences between chronic lymphocytic leukemia molecular subgroups. Leukemia, 24(4), 788-797.

MacKinnon, N., Ge, W., Khan, A. P., Somashekar, B. S., Tripathi, P., Siddiqui, J., Wei, J. T., Chinnaiyan, A. M., Rajendiran, T. M., & Ramamoorthy, A. (2012). Variable Reference Alignment: An Improved Peak Alignment Protocol for NMR Spectral Data with Large Intersample Variation. Analytical Chemistry, 84(12), 5372-5379.

Marks, L. S., Andriole, G. L., Fitzpatrick, J. M., Schulman, C. C., & Roehrborn, C. G. (2006). The interpretation of serum prostate specific antigen in men receiving 5 α-reductase inhibitors: a review and clinical recommendations. The Journal of Urology, 176(3), 868-874.

Martínez-Bisbal, M. C., Martí-Bonmatí, L., Piquer, J., Revert, A., Ferrer, P., Llácer, J. L., Piotto, M., Assemat, O., & Celda, B. (2004). ^{1}H and ^{13}C HR-MAS spectroscopy of intact biopsy samples ex vivo and in vivo ^{1}H MRS study of human high grade gliomas. NMR in Biomedicine, 17(4), 191-205.

Materi, W., & Wishart, D. S. (2007). Computational systems biology in drug discovery and development: methods and applications. Drug Discovery Today, 12(7-8), 295-303.

Maxeiner, A., Adkins, C. B., Zhang, Y., Taupitz, M., Halpern, E. F., McDougal, W. S., Wu, C. L., & Cheng, L. L. (2010). Retrospective analysis of prostate cancer recurrence potential with tissue metabolomic profiles. Prostate, 70(7), 710-717.

Mazaheri, Y., Shukla-Dave, A., Hricak, H., Fine, S. W., Zhang, J., Inurrigarro, G., Moskowitz, C. S., Ishill, N. M., Reuter, V. E., Touijer, K., Zakian, K. L., & Koutcher, J. A. (2008). Prostate cancer: identification with combined diffusion-weighted MR imaging and 3D ^{1}H MR spectroscopic imaging – correlation with pathologic findings. Radiology, 246(2), 480-488.

Melamud, E., Vastag, L., & Rabinowitz, J. D. (2010). Metabolomic Analysis and Visualization Engine for LC−MS Data. Analytical Chemistry, 82(23), 9818-9826.

Menard, C., Smith, I. C., Somorjai, R. L., Leboldus, L., Patel, R., Littman, C., Robertson, S. J., & Bezabeh, T. (2001). Magnetic resonance spectroscopy of the malignant prostate gland after radiotherapy: a histopathologic study of diagnostic validity. International Journal of Radiation Oncology *Biology* Physics, 50(2), 317-323.

Mihelich, B. L., Khramtsova, E. A., Arva, N., Vaishnav, A., Johnson, D. N., Giangreco, A. A., Martens-Uzunova, E., Bagasra, O., Kajdacsy-Balla, A., & Nonn, L. (2011). miR-183-96-182 Cluster Is Overexpressed in Prostate Tissue and Regulates Zinc Homeostasis in Prostate Cells. The Journal of Biological Chemistry, 286(52), 44503-44511.

Millis, K. K., Maas, W. E., Cory, D. G., & Singer, S. (1997). Gradient, high-resolution, magic-angle spinning nuclear magnetic resonance spectroscopy of human adipocyte tissue. Magnetic Resonance in Medicine, 38(3), 399-403.

Mirnezami, R., Kinross, J. M., Vorkas, P. A., Goldin, R., Holmes, E., Nicholson, J., & Darzi, A. (2012). Implementation of molecular phenotyping approaches in the personalized surgical patient journey. Annals of Surgery, 255(5), 881-889.

Mishur, R. J., & Rea, S. L. (2012). Applications of mass spectrometry to metabolomics and metabonomics: Detection of biomarkers of aging and of age-related diseases. Mass Spectrometry Reviews, 31(1), 70-95.

Mo, M. L., Jamshidi, N., & Palsson, B. Ø. (2007). A genome-scale, constraint-based approach to systems biology of human metabolism. Molecular BioSystems, 3(9), 598-603.

Mohan, R. R., Challa, A., Gupta, S., Bostwick, D. G., Ahmad, N., Agarwal, R., Marengo, S. R., Amini, S. B., Paras, F., MacLennan, G. T., Resnick, M. I., & Mukhtar, H. (1999). Overexpression of Ornithine Decarboxylase in Prostate Cancer and Prostatic Fluid in Humans. Clinical Cancer Research, 5(1), 143-147.

Moyer, V. A. (2012). Screening for prostate cancer: U.S. Preventive Services Task Force recommendation statement. Annals of Internal Medicine, 157(2), 120-134.

Mueller-Lisse, U. G., Swanson, M. G., Vigneron, D. B., Hricak, H., Bessette, A., Males, R. G., Wood, P. J., Noworolski, S., Nelson, S. J., Barken, I., Carroll, P. R., & Kurhanewicz, J. (2001). Time-dependent effects of hormone-deprivation therapy on prostate metabolism as detected by combined magnetic resonance imaging and 3D magnetic resonance spectroscopic imaging. Magnetic Resonance in Medicine, 46(1), 49-57.

Nebert, D. W., Jorge-Nebert, L., & Vesell, E. S. (2003). Pharmacogenomics and "individualized drug therapy": high expectations and disappointing achievements. American Journal of Pharmacogenomics, 3(6), 361-370.

Neuweger, H., Albaum, S. P., Dondrup, M., Persicke, M., Watt, T., Niehaus, K., Stoye, J., & Goesmann, A. (2008). MeltDB: a software platform for the analysis and integration of metabolomics experiment data. Bioinformatics, 24(23), 2726-2732.

Ng, D. J. Y., Pasikanti, K. K., & Chan, E. C. Y. (2011). Trend analysis of metabonomics and systematic review of metabonomics-derived cancer marker metabolites. Metabolomics, 7(2), 155-178.

Nicholson, J. K., Lindon, J. C., & Holmes, E. (1999). 'Metabonomics': understanding the metabolic responses of living systems to pathophysiological stimuli via multivariate statistical analysis of biological NMR spectroscopic data. Xenobiotica, 29(11), 1181-1189.

Nicholson, J. K., & Lindon, J. C. (2008). Systems biology: Metabonomics. Nature, 455(7216), 1054-1056.

Nicholson, J. K., Wilson, I. D., & Lindon, J. C. (2011). Pharmacometabonomics as an effector for personalized medicine. Pharmacogenomics, 12(1), 103-111.

Nicholson, J. K., Everett, J. R., & Lindon, J. C. (2012). Longitudinal pharmacometabonomics for predicting patient responses to therapy: drug metabolism, toxicity and efficacy. Expert Opinion on Drug Metabolism & Toxicology, 8(2), 135-139.

Noble, W. S. (2009). How does multiple testing correction work? Nature Biotechnology, 27(12), 1135-1137.

Noworolski, S. M., Vigneron, D. B., Chen, A. P., & Kurhanewicz, J. (2008). Dynamic contrast-enhanced MRI and MR diffusion imaging to distinguish between glandular and stromal prostatic tissues. Magnetic Resonance Imaging, 26(8), 1071-1080.

Oakman, C., Tenori, L., Claudino, W. M., Cappadona, S., Nepi, S., Battaglia, A., Bernini, P., Zafarana, E., Saccenti, E., Fornier, M., Morris, P. G., Biganzoli, L., Luchinat, C., Bertini, I., & Di Leo, A. (2011). Identification of a serum-detectable metabolomic fingerprint potentially correlated with the presence of micrometastatic disease in early breast cancer patients at varying risks of disease relapse by traditional prognostic methods. Annals of Oncology, 22(6), 1295-1301.

Oberbach, A., Blüher, M., Wirth, H., Till, H., Kovacs, P., Kullnick, Y., Schlichting, N., Tomm, J. M., Rolle-Kampczyk, U., Murugaiyan, J., Binder, H., Dietrich, A., & von Bergen, M. (2011). Combined Proteomic and Metabolomic Profiling of Serum Reveals Association of the Complement System with Obesity and Identifies Novel Markers of Body Fat Mass Changes. Journal of Proteome Research, 10(10), 4769-4788.

Owen, D. H., & Katz, D. F. (2005). A review of the physical and chemical properties of human semen and the formulation of a semen simulant. Journal of Andrology, 26(4), 459-469.

Padhani, A. R. (2002). Dynamic contrast-enhanced MRI in clinical oncology: current status and future directions. Journal of Magnetic Resonance Imaging, 16(4), 407-422.

Pan, Z. Z., Gu, H. W., Talaty, N., Chen, H. W., Shanaiah, N., Hainline, B. E., Cooks, R. G., & Raftery, D. (2007). Principal component analysis of urine metabolites detected by NMR and DESI-MS in patients with inborn errors of metabolism. Analytical and Bioanalytical Chemistry, 387(2), 539-549.

Pasikanti, K. K., Ho, P. C., & Chan, E. C. Y. (2008). Gas chromatography/mass spectrometry in metabolic profiling of biological fluids. Journal of Chromatography B, 871(2), 202-211.

Pinder, U. U. B. (1506). Epiphanie Medicorum. Speculum videndi urinas hominum. Clavis aperiendi portas pulsuum. Berillus discernendi causas & differentias febrium. Sodalitas Celtica: Nuremberg.

Pinto, R. C., Trygg, J., & Gottfries, J. (2012). Advantages of orthogonal inspection in chemometrics. Journal of Chemometrics, 26(6), 231-235.

Pluskal, T., Castillo, S., Villar-Briones, A., & Orešič, M. (2010). MZmine 2: Modular framework for processing, visualizing, and analyzing mass spectrometry-based molecular profile data. BMC Bioinformatics, 11: 395.

Purcell, E. M., Torrey, H. C., & Pound, R. V. (1946). Resonance Absorption by Nuclear Magnetic Moments in a Solid. Physical Review, 69(1-2), 37-38.

Quann, P., Jarrard, D. F., & Huang, W. (2010). Current prostate biopsy protocols cannot reliably identify patients for focal therapy: correlation of low-risk prostate cancer on biopsy with radical prostatectomy findings. International Journal of Clinical and Experimental Pathology, 3(4), 401-407.

Rantalainen, M., Cloarec, O., Beckonert, O., Wilson, I. D., Jackson, D., Tonge, R., Rowlinson, R., Rayner, S., Nickson, J., Wilkinson, R. W., Mills, J. D., Trygg, J., Nicholson, J. K., & Holmes, E. (2006). Statistically Integrated Metabonomic–Proteomic Studies on a Human Prostate Cancer Xenograft Model in Mice. Journal of Proteome Research, 5(10), 2642-2655.

Rantalainen, M., Bylesjö, M., Cloarec, O., Nicholson, J. K., Holmes, E., & Trygg, J. (2007). Kernel-based orthogonal projections to latent structures (K-OPLS). Journal of Chemometrics, 21(7-9), 376-385.

Reginato, A. J., & Kurnik, B. (1989). Calcium oxalate and other crystals associated with kidney diseases and arthritis. Seminars in Arthritis and Rheumatism, 18(3), 198-224.

Reske, S. N., Blumstein, N. M., Neumaier, B., Gottfried, H. W., Finsterbusch, F., Kocot, D., Möller, P., Glatting, G., & Perner, S. (2006). Imaging prostate cancer with ^{11}C-choline PET/CT. Journal of Nuclear Medicine, 47(8), 1249-1254.

Rhee, E. P., & Gerszten, R. E. (2012). Metabolomics and cardiovascular biomarker discovery. Clinical Chemistry, 58(1), 139-147.

Roberts, M. J., Schirra, H. J., Lavin, M. F., & Gardiner, R. A. (2011). Metabolomics: a novel approach to early and noninvasive prostate cancer detection. Korean Journal of Urology, 52(2), 79-89.

Rohren, E. M., Turkington, T. G., & Coleman, R. E. (2004). Clinical applications of PET in oncology. Radiology, 231(2), 305-332.

Roobol, M. J., Schröder, F. H., Crawford, E. D., Freedland, S. J., Sartor, A. O., Fleshner, N., & Andriole, G. L. (2009). A Framework for the Identification of Men at Increased Risk for Prostate Cancer. The Journal of Urology, 182(5), 2112-2122.

Ross, A., Schlotterbeck, G., Dieterle, F., & Senn, H. (2007). Chapter 3 - NMR Spectroscopy Techniques for Application to Metabonomics. In John C. Lindon, Jeremy K. Nicholson & Elaine Holmes (Eds.), The Handbook of Metabonomics and Metabolomics (pp. 55-112). Amsterdam: Elsevier Science B.V.

Rubingh, C. M., Bijlsma, S., Derks, E. P. P. A., Bobeldijk, I., Verheij, E. R., Kochhar, S., & Smilde, A. K. (2006). Assessing the performance of statistical validation tools for megavariate metabolomics data. Metabolomics, 2(2), 53-61.

Salagierski, M., & Schalken, J. A. (2012). Molecular diagnosis of prostate cancer: PCA3 and TMPRSS2:ERG gene fusion. The Journal of Urology, 187(3), 795-801.

Salek, R. M., Maguire, M. L., Bentley, E., Rubtsov, D. V., Hough, T., Cheeseman, M., Nunez, D., Sweatman, B. C., Haselden, J. N., Cox, R. D., Connor, S. C., & Griffin, J. L. (2007). A metabolomic comparison of urinary changes in type 2 diabetes in mouse, rat, and human. Physiological Genomics, 29(2), 99-108.

Samaratunga, H., Yaxley, J., Kerr, K., McClymont, K., & Duffy, D. (2007). Significance of minute focus of adenocarcinoma on prostate needle biopsy. Urology, 70(2), 299-302.

Sansone, S. A., Rocca-Serra, P., Field, D., Maguire, E., Taylor, C., Hofmann, O., Fang, H., Neumann, S., Tong, W., Amaral-Zettler, L., Begley, K., Booth, T., Bougueleret, L., Burns, G., Chapman, B., Clark, T., Coleman, L. A., Copeland, J., Das, S., de Daruvar, A., de Matos, P., Dix, I., Edmunds, S., Evelo, C. T., Forster, M. J., Gaudet, P., Gilbert, J., Goble, C., Griffin, J. L., Jacob, D., Kleinjans, J., Harland, L., Haug, K., Hermjakob, H., Ho Sui, S. J., Laederach, A., Liang, S., Marshall, S., McGrath, A., Merrill, E., Reilly, D., Roux, M., Shamu, C. E., Shang, C. A., Steinbeck, C., Trefethen, A., Williams-Jones, B., Wolstencroft, K., Xenarios, I., & Hide, W. (2012). Toward interoperable bioscience data. Nature Genetics, 44(2), 121-126.

Savorani, F., Tomasi, G., & Engelsen, S. B. (2010). icoshift: A versatile tool for the rapid alignment of 1D NMR spectra. Journal of Magnetic Resonance, 202(2), 190-202.

Schirra, H. J., Anderson, C. G., Wilson, W. J., Kerr, L., Craik, D. J., Waters, M. J., & Lichanska, A. M. (2008). Altered metabolism of growth hormone receptor mutant mice: a combined NMR metabonomics and microarray study. PLoS ONE, 3(7), e2764.

Schouten, B. W., Bohnen, A. M., Bosch, J. L. H. R., Bernsen, R. M. D., Deckers, J. W., Dohle, G. R., & Thomas, S. (2008). Erectile dysfunction prospectively associated with cardiovascular disease in the Dutch general population: results from the Krimpen Study. International Journal of Impotence Research, 20(1), 92-99.

Schröder, F. H., van der Cruijsen-Koeter, I., de Koning, H. J., Vis, A. N., Hoedemaeker, R. F., & Kranse, R. (2000). Prostate cancer detection at low prostate specific antigen. Journal of Urology, 163(3), 806-811.

Schulz, K. F., Altman, D. G., & Moher, D. (2010). CONSORT 2010 Statement: updated guidelines for reporting parallel group randomised trials. British Medical Journal, 340:c332.

Serkova, N. J., Gamito, E. J., Jones, R. H., O'Donnell, C., Brown, J. L., Green, S., Sullivan, H., Hedlund, T., & Crawford, E. D. (2008). The metabolites citrate, myo-inositol, and spermine are potential age-independent markers of prostate cancer in human expressed prostatic secretions. The Prostate, 68(6), 620-628.

Serkova, N. J., Standiford, T. J., & Stringer, K. A. (2011). The emerging field of quantitative blood metabolomics for biomarker discovery in critical illnesses. American Journal of Respiratory and Critical Care Medicine, 184(6), 647-655.

Sevli, S., Uzumcu, A., Solak, M., Ittmann, M., & Ozen, M. (2010). The function of microRNAs, small but potent molecules, in human prostate cancer. Prostate Cancer and Prostatic Diseases, 13(3), 208-217.

Shepherd, L. V. T., Fraser, P., & Stewart, D. (2011). Metabolomics: a second-generation platform for crop and food analysis. Bioanalysis, 3(10), 1143-1159.

Shulaev, V. (2006). Metabolomics technology and bioinformatics. Briefings in Bioinformatics, 7(2), 128-139.

Siegel, R., Naishadham, D., & Jemal, A. (2012). Cancer statistics, 2012. CA: A Cancer Journal for Clinicians, 62(1), 10-29.

Simoneau, A. R., Gerner, E. W., Nagle, R., Ziogas, A., Fujikawa-Brooks, S., Yerushalmi, H., Ahlering, T. E., Lieberman, R., McLaren, C. E., Anton-Culver, H., & Meyskens, F. L., Jr. (2008). The effect of difluoromethylornithine on decreasing prostate size and polyamines in men: results of a year-long phase IIb randomized placebo-controlled chemoprevention trial. Cancer Epidemiology, Biomarkers & Prevention, 17(2), 292-299.

Simoni, R. D., Hill, R. L., & Vaughan, M. (2002). Analytical Biochemistry: the Work of Otto Knuf Olof Folin on Blood Analysis. Journal of Biological Chemistry, 277(20), e9.

Sitter, B., Sonnewald, U., Spraul, M., Fjösne, H. E., & Gribbestad, I. S. (2002). High-resolution magic angle spinning MRS of breast cancer tissue. NMR in Biomedicine, 15(5), 327-337.

Spratlin, J. L., Serkova, N. J., & Eckhardt, S. G. (2009). Clinical applications of metabolomics in oncology: a review. Clinical Cancer Research, 15(2), 431-440.

Sreekumar, A., Poisson, L. M., Rajendiran, T. M., Khan, A. P., Cao, Q., Yu, J., Laxman, B., Mehra, R., Lonigro, R. J., Li, Y., Nyati, M. K., Ahsan, A., Kalyana-Sundaram, S., Han, B., Cao, X., Byun, J., Omenn, G. S., Ghosh, D., Pennathur, S., Alexander, D. C., Berger, A., Shuster, J. R., Wei, J. T., Varambally, S., Beecher, C., & Chinnaiyan, A. M. (2009). Metabolomic profiles delineate potential role for sarcosine in prostate cancer progression. Nature, 457(7231), 910-914.

Staab, J. M., O'Connell, T. M., & Gomez, S. M. (2010). Enhancing metabolomic data analysis with Progressive Consensus Alignment of NMR Spectra (PCANS). BMC Bioinformatics, 11:123.

Stenman, K., Hauksson, J. B., Gröbner, G., Stattin, P., Bergh, A., & Riklund, K. (2009). Detection of polyunsaturated omega-6 fatty acid in human malignant prostate tissue by 1D and 2D high-resolution magic angle spinning NMR spectroscopy. Magnetic Resonance Materials in Physics, Biology and Medicine, 22(6), 327-331.

Struys, E. A., Heijboer, A. C., van Moorselaar, J., Jakobs, C., & Blankenstein, M. A. (2010). Serum sarcosine is not a marker for prostate cancer. Annals of Clinical Biochemistry, 47(3):282.

Suhre, K., Shin, S. Y., Petersen, A. K., Mohney, R. P., Meredith, D., Wägele, B., Altmaier, E., Deloukas, P., Erdmann, J., Grundberg, E., Hammond, C. J., de Angelis, M. H., Kastenmuller, G., Köttgen, A., Kronenberg, F., Mangino, M., Meisinger, C., Meitinger, T., Mewes, H. W., Milburn, M. V., Prehn, C., Raffler, J., Ried, J. S., Römisch-Margl, W., Samani, N. J., Small, K. S., Wichmann, H. E., Zhai, G., Illig, T., Spector, T. D., Adamski, J., Soranzo, N. & Gieger, C., (2011). Human metabolic individuality in biomedical and pharmaceutical research. Nature, 477(7362), 54-60.

Suzuki, T., Suzuki, K., Nakajima, K., Otaki, N., & Yamanaka, H. (1994). Metallothionein in human seminal plasma. International Journal of Urology, 1(4), 345-348.

Swanson, M. G., Vigneron, D. B., Tabatabai, Z. L., Males, R. G., Schmitt, L., Carroll, P. R., James, J. K., Hurd, R. E., & Kurhanewicz, J. (2003). Proton HR-MAS spectroscopy and quantitative pathologic analysis of MRI/3D-MRSI-targeted postsurgical prostate tissues. Magnetic Resonance in Medicine, 50(5), 944-954.

Swanson, M. G., Zektzer, A. S., Tabatabai, Z. L., Simko, J., Jarso, S., Keshari, K. R., Schmitt, L., Carroll, P. R., Shinohara, K., Vigneron, D. B., & Kurhanewicz, J. (2006). Quantitative analysis of prostate metabolites using ^{1}H HR-MAS spectroscopy. Magnetic Resonance in Medicine, 55(6), 1257-1264.

Swanson, M. G., Keshari, K. R., Tabatabai, Z. L., Simko, J. P., Shinohara, K., Carroll, P. R., Zektzer, A. S., & Kurhanewicz, J. (2008). Quantification of choline- and ethanolamine-containing metabolites in human prostate tissues using ^{1}H HR-MAS total correlation spectroscopy. Magnetic Resonance in Medicine, 60(1), 33-40.

Talesa, V. N., Antognelli, C., Del Buono, C., Stracci, F., Serva, M. R., Cottini, E., & Mearini, E. (2009). Diagnostic potential in prostate cancer of a panel of urinary molecular tumor markers. Cancer Biomarkers, 5(6), 241-251.

Tessem, M. B., Swanson, M. G., Keshari, K. R., Albers, M. J., Joun, D., Tabatabai, Z. L., Simko, J. P., Shinohara, K., Nelson, S. J., Vigneron, D. B., Gribbestad, I. S., & Kurhanewicz, J. (2008). Evaluation of lactate and alanine as metabolic biomarkers of prostate cancer using ^{1}H HR-MAS spectroscopy of biopsy tissues. Magnetic Resonance in Medicine, 60(3), 510-516.

Theodoridis, G., Gika, H. G., & Wilson, I. D. (2008). LC-MS-based methodology for global metabolite profiling in metabonomics/metabolomics. Trends in Analytical Chemistry, 27(3), 251-260.

Thompson, I. M., Pauler, D. K., Goodman, P. J., Tangen, C. M., Lucia, M. S., Parnes, H. L., Minasian, L. M., Ford, L. G., Lippman, S. M., Crawford, E. D., Crowley, J. J., & Coltman, C. A., Jr. (2004). Prevalence of Prostate Cancer among Men with a Prostate-Specific Antigen Level ≤4.0 ng per Milliliter. New England Journal of Medicine, 350(22), 2239-2246.

Thomson, J. J. (1912). Rays of positive electricity. Philosophical Magazine Series 6, 24(140), 209-253.

Thysell, E., Surowiec, I., Hörnberg, E., Crnalic, S., Widmark, A., Johansson, A. I., Stattin, P., Bergh, A., Moritz, T., Antti, H., & Wikström, P. (2010). Metabolomic Characterization of Human Prostate Cancer Bone Metastases Reveals Increased Levels of Cholesterol. PLoS ONE, 5(12), e14175.

Tombal, B., Ameye, F., de la Taille, A., de Reijke, T., Gontero, P., Haese, A., Kil, P., Perrin, P., Remzi, M., Schröder, J., Speakman, M., Volpe, A., Meesen, B., & Stoevelaar, H. (2012). Biopsy and treatment decisions in the initial management of prostate cancer and the role of PCA3; a systematic analysis of expert opinion. World Journal of Urology, 30(2), 251-256.

Tomlins, S. A., Aubin, S. M. J., Siddiqui, J., Lonigro, R. J., Sefton-Miller, L., Miick, S., Williamsen, S., Hodge, P., Meinke, J., Blase, A., Penabella, Y., Day, J. R., Varambally, R., Han, B., Wood, D., Wang, L., Sanda, M. G., Rubin, M. A., Rhodes, D. R., Hollenbeck, B., Sakamoto, K., Silberstein, J. L., Fradet, Y., Amberson, J. B., Meyers, S., Palanisamy, N., Rittenhouse, H., Wei, J. T., Groskopf, J., & Chinnaiyan, A. M. (2011). Urine TMPRSS2:ERG fusion transcript stratifies prostate cancer risk in men with elevated serum PSA. Science Translational Medicine, 3(94), 94ra72.

Trygg, J., & Wold, S. (2002). Orthogonal projections to latent structures (O-PLS). Journal of Chemometrics, 16(3), 119-128.

Trygg, J., & Wold, S. (2003). O2-PLS, a two-block (X–Y) latent variable regression (LVR) method with an integral OSC filter. Journal of Chemometrics, 17(1), 53-64.

Trygg, J., Holmes, E., & Lundstedt, T. (2007). Chemometrics in Metabonomics. Journal of Proteome Research, 6(2), 469-479.

Trygg, J., & Lundstedt, T. (2007). Chapter 6 - Chemometrics Techniques for Metabonomics. John C. Lindon, Jeremy K. Nicholson & Elaine Holmes (Eds.), The Handbook of Metabonomics and Metabolomics (pp. 171-199). Amsterdam: Elsevier Science B.V.

Tulpan, D., Léger, S., Belliveau, L., Culf, A., & Čuperlović-Culf, M. (2011). MetaboHunter: an automatic approach for identification of metabolites from ^{1}H-NMR spectra of complex mixtures. BMC Bioinformatics, 12:400.

van Asten, J. J. A., Cuijpers, V., Hulsbergen-van de Kaa, C., Soede-Huijbregts, C., Witjes, J. A., Verhofstad, A., & Heerschap, A. (2008). High resolution magic angle spinning NMR spectroscopy for metabolic assessment of cancer presence and Gleason score in human prostate needle biopsies. Magnetic Resonance Materials in Physics, Biology and Medicine, 21(6), 435-442.

van der Graaf, M., Schipper, R. G., Oosterhof, G. O., Schalken, J. A., Verhofstad, A. A., & Heerschap, A. (2000). Proton MR spectroscopy of prostatic tissue focused on the detection of spermine, a possible biomarker of malignant behavior in prostate cancer. Magnetic Resonance Materials in Physics, Biology and Medicine, 10(3), 153-159.

van der Greef, J., & Smilde, A. K. (2005). Symbiosis of chemometrics and metabolomics: past, present, and future. Journal of Chemometrics, 19(5-7), 376-386.

Vargas, H. A., Wassberg, C., Akin, O., & Hricak, H. (2012). MR Imaging of Treated Prostate Cancer. Radiology, 262(1), 26-42.

Vollmer, R. T. (2004). Race and the linkage between serum prostate-specific antigen and prostate cancer: a study of American veterans. American Journal of Clinical Pathology, 122(3), 338-344.

Wagner, S., Scholz, K., Donegan, M., Burton, L., Wingate, J., & Völkel, W. (2005). Metabonomics and Biomarker Discovery: LC–MS Metabolic Profiling and Constant Neutral Loss Scanning Combined with Multivariate Data Analysis for Mercapturic Acid Analysis. Analytical Chemistry, 78(4), 1296-1305.

Wang, Z., Klipfell, E., Bennett, B. J., Koeth, R., Levison, B. S., DuGar, B., Feldstein, A. E., Britt, E. B., Fu, X., Chung, Y. M., Wu, Y., Schauer, P., Smith, J. D., Allayee, H., Tang, W. H. W., DiDonato, J. A., Lusis, A. J., & Hazen, S. L. (2011). Gut flora metabolism of phosphatidylcholine promotes cardiovascular disease. Nature, 472(7341), 57-63.

Warburg, O. (1956). On the origin of cancer cells. Science, 123(3191), 309-314.

Weckwerth, W. (2011). Unpredictability of metabolism–the key role of metabolomics science in combination with next-generation genome sequencing. Analytical and Bioanalytical Chemistry, 400(7), 1967-1978.

Wei, J., Xie, G., Zhou, Z., Shi, P., Qiu, Y., Zheng, X., Chen, T., Su, M., Zhao, A., & Jia, W. (2011). Salivary metabolite signatures of oral cancer and leukoplakia. International Journal of Cancer, 129(9), 2207-2217.

Weiss, R. H., & Kim, K. (2012). Metabolomics in the study of kidney diseases. Nature Reviews Nephrology, 8(1), 22-33.

Westerhuis, J. A., Hoefsloot, H. C. J., Smit, S., Vis, D. J., Smilde, A. K., van Velzen, E. J. J., van Duijnhoven, J. P. M., & van Dorsten, F. A. (2008). Assessment of PLSDA cross validation. Metabolomics, 4(1), 81-89.

Wiklund, S., Johansson, E., Sjöström, L., Mellerowicz, E. J., Edlund, U., Shockcor, J. P., Gottfries, J., Moritz, T., & Trygg, J. (2008). Visualization of GC/TOF-MS-based metabolomics data for identification of biochemically interesting compounds using OPLS class models. Analytical Chemistry, 80(1), 115-122.

Wilson, I. D., Plumb, R., Granger, J., Major, H., Williams, R., & Lenz, E. M. (2005). HPLC-MS-based methods for the study of metabonomics. Journal of Chromatography B, 817(1), 67-76.

Wilson, I. D. (2009). Drugs, bugs, and personalized medicine: Pharmacometabonomics enters the ring. Proceedings of the National Academy of Sciences, 106(34), 14187-14188.

Winnike, J. H., Li, Z., Wright, F. A., Macdonald, J. M., O'Connell, T. M., & Watkins, P. B. (2010). Use of pharmaco-metabonomics for early prediction of acetaminophen-induced hepatotoxicity in humans. Clinical Pharmacology and Therapeutics, 88(1), 45-51.

Wishart, D. S. (2008). Quantitative metabolomics using NMR. Trends in Analytical Chemistry, 27(3), 228-237.

Wishart, D. S., Knox, C., Guo, A. C., Eisner, R., Young, N., Gautam, B., Hau, D. D., Psychogios, N., Dong, E., Bouatra, S., Mandal, R., Sinelnikov, I., Xia, J. G., Jia, L., Cruz, J. A., Lim, E., Sobsey, C. A., Shrivastava, S., Huang, P., Liu, P., Fang, L., Peng, J., Fradette, R., Cheng, D., Tzur, D., Clements, M., Lewis, A., De Souza, A., Zuniga, A., Dawe, M., Xiong, Y., Clive, D., Greiner, R., Nazyrova, A., Shaykhutdinov, R., Li, L., Vogel, H. J., & Forsythe, I. (2009). HMDB: a knowledgebase for the human metabolome. Nucleic Acids Research, 37, D603-D610.

Wright, A. J., Buydens, L. M. C., & Heerschap, A. (2012). A phase and frequency alignment protocol for ^{1}H MRSI data of the prostate. NMR in Biomedicine, 25(5), 755-765.

Wu, C. L., Jordan, K. W., Ratai, E. M., Sheng, J., Adkins, C. B., Defeo, E. M., Jenkins, B. G., Ying, L., McDougal, W. S., & Cheng, L. L. (2010). Metabolomic imaging for human prostate cancer detection. Science Translational Medicine, 2(16), 16ra18.

Xia, J., Mandal, R., Sinelnikov, I. V., Broadhurst, D., & Wishart, D. S. (2012). MetaboAnalyst 2.0—a comprehensive server for metabolomic data analysis. Nucleic Acids Research, 40(W1), W127-W133

Xie, B., Waters, M. J., & Schirra, H. J. (2012). Investigating potential mechanisms of obesity by metabolomics. Journal of Biomedicine and Biotechnology, 2012, Article ID 805683, 1-10.

Yong, W. P., Innocenti, F., & Ratain, M. J. (2006). The role of pharmacogenetics in cancer therapeutics. British Journal of Clinical Pharmacology, 62(1), 35-46.

Zaichick, V. Y., Sviridova, T. V., & Zaichick, S. V. (1996). Zinc concentration in human prostatic fluid: normal, chronic prostatitis, adenoma and cancer. International Urology and Nephrology, 28(5), 687-694.

Zhang, A., Sun, H., Wang, P., Han, Y., & Wang, X. (2012). Modern analytical techniques in metabolomics analysis. Analyst, 137(2), 293-300.

Prostate Cancer, Hormone Treatment and Bone Health: Present Management and Future Directions

Evan Kovac
Department of Surgery, Division of Urology
McGill University, Montreal, Quebec, Canada

Yosh Taguchi
Department of Surgery, Division of Urology
McGill University, Montreal, Quebec, Canada

1   Introduction

Prostate cancer is the most common organ cancer in men, with more than two million American men currently living with the disease. Approximately 16% of all men will be diagnosed with this malignancy during their lifetime. Most cancers are low grade (Gleason grade 6 or less) and carry a thirty percent chance of progression, some intermediate (Gleason grade 7) with those designated 4+3 being worse than those designated 3+4, and the remainder high grade (Gleason grade 8-10) with a high likelihood of life-threatening morbidity. Treatments for prostate cancer range from simply following the disease, as in watchful waiting or active surveillance, potentially curative treatments like surgery or radiotherapy, and palliative hormonal therapy.

Androgen deprivation therapy (ADT) has become the accepted treatment for patients whose cancer has spread beyond the gland or who have recurrent disease, after surgery or radiotherapy. ADT lowers the body's ability to make and to respond to the male sex hormone, testosterone. Since testosterone is the most potent promoter of prostate cancer, regulating its production and limiting its effects on a cellular level are essential to controlling the progression of prostate cancer.

Side effects of ADT include hot flashes, anemia, and cognitive dysfunction, but what are most serious are the deleterious effects on bone health. ADT may lead to osteoporosis, predisposing castrated men to fractures and, ultimately, decreased survival.

This chapter will discuss the epidemiology, screening, diagnosis and treatment options of prostate cancer and its association with osteoporosis.

2   Epidemiology

Prostate cancer is the most common non-cutaneous malignancy in the United States. According to the American Cancer Society, men have a 16.7% lifetime risk of developing the disease, while the lifetime risk of death is approximately 2.6% (American Cancer Society, 2008).

African Americans are at higher risk than Caucasians, with a relative incidence of 1.6 (American Cancer Society, 2008). Family history is also a contributing factor.

Prostate cancer incidence peaked in 1992, and mortality has fallen steadily after the introduction of the blood test, prostate-specific antigen (PSA). PSA alone, however, does not fully explain the reduction in mortality from the disease during the last 30 years. Many clinicians believe that the reduction in mortality is due largely to the more aggressive treatment since the 1980s (Walsh, 2000). While rates of hormone therapy and observation strategies have remained stable since the 1980s, the rates of radical prostatectomy and radiation treatment have increased over the same time period (Stephenson, 2005). Today, the 5-year disease-specific survival for localized disease approaches 100%, and is 34% for men diagnosed with metastatic disease (American Cancer Society, 2008).

There is wide variation in the incidence of this malignancy among men of different nationalities. The incidence is higher in men who have immigrated to America compared to men who have stayed in their native country where the disease is less frequent. For example, Asian men living in the United States have a lower incidence than Caucasians, but their incidence is higher than age-matched men in Asia. These findings implicate environmental factors (Haenszel & Kurihara, 1968; Yu et al., 1991).

Many reasons have been proposed to account for the varying incidence among different population groups. Certain genes contribute towards tumor initiation, promotion and/or progression. Higher intake of animal fat, higher body mass index (BMI), lower socioeconomic status and higher testosterone levels are all recognized factors. Differences in medical practice, like access to health care, rectal examinations, and PSA screening are all factors that influence the incidence of prostate cancer.

The lowest rate of prostate cancer is seen in the Far East and on the Indian subcontinent, while the highest rates occur in North America, Australia and Western Europe. Prostate cancer is the 5th most common malignancy worldwide, and second most common in men (Parkin *et al.*, 2002). Mortality from prostate cancer is highest in the Caribbean nations (28 per 100,000 per year) and lowest in Southeast Asia, China and North Africa (<5 per 100,000 per year) (Parkin *et al.*, 2002).

The strongest risk factor for prostate cancer is age. Prostate cancer is rare in men younger than age 50 (2% of all cases). The median age at diagnosis is 68 years, with 63% of all prostate cancers diagnosed after the age of 65, and the vast majority of mortalities occur in this age group (Ries *et al.*, 1975-2007). Despite the widespread use of PSA, the average age of prostate cancer related death has remained stable since the late 1970s.

3   Screening

Screening for prostate cancer refers to the testing of healthy, asymptomatic men for the possibility of disease. For a screening test to be effective the disease entity must be prevalent in the general population, the test must be specific, sensitive, and cost effective. Furthermore, effective treatments must exist to affect outcomes. The goal of screening, after all, is to improve the overall health of the patient population by earlier diagnosis and earlier treatment

For prostate cancer, routine screening consists of regular rectal examinations and a PSA blood test.

The benefits of screening for prostate cancer, however, are uncertain. Many studies have shown that screening reduces the number of men diagnosed at an advanced stage (van der Cruijsen-Koeter, 2006; Aus *et al.*, 2007). However, the harm associated with treatments must be considered against the potential benefits.

3.1   PSA

Prostate specific antigen is a member of the human glandular kallikrein family, known as human glandular kallikrein 3 (hK3). It, along with kallikrein 2, is one of the most widely studied members of the kallikrein family. So far, 15 functional kallikrein genes have been identified and extensive study of these markers has helped to improve the utilization of these markers. Other markers show promise and may improve on PSA as a screening tool for prostate cancer.

Mortality from prostate cancer has declined since the introduction of widespread PSA testing, with an absolute reduction of 32.5% since the early 1990s (SEER database) and a 75% reduction in the proportion of advanced disease at diagnosis. Two randomized trials that looked at prostate cancer-specific mortality in relation to PSA screening have been published, with contradictory results.

The European Randomized Trial of Prostate Cancer Screening (ERSPC) carried out PSA testing every 4 years and biopsied men with PSA counts over 4 ng/ml. This study reported a 20% reduction in prostate cancer-specific mortality in the screened population. Their screened cohort also had less high-grade cancer, less locally advanced cancer and less metastatic disease. The Prostate, Lung, Colon and Ovary (PLCO) study of the National Cancer Institute (NCI) in the United States initiated its study in 1993. Screening consisted of annual PSA testing, with PSA readings over 4 ng/ml triggering a prostate biopsy. This study did not show any difference in prostate cancer specific mortality in the screened and unscreened population. It has been speculated that the unscreened population may have had PSA testing more often than admitted, contaminating the results. Despite the survival advantage of PSA screening demonstrated by the ERSPC trial, the study did show that 1410 men needed to be screened and 48 men treated to prevent one prostate cancer-related death (de Koning *et al.*, 2002; Schroder *et al.*, 2009; Andriole *et al.*, 2009).

These two large trials have contributed important information regarding screening, such as frequency of testing and PSA cut-offs. Clearly, screening has led to a stage migration towards organ-confined disease and a reduction in patients diagnosed with advanced cancers. Unfortunately, these trials have also exposed the perils of screening, such as the overdetection of inconsequential disease and, possibly, overtreatment of prostate cancer. Information gathered from the prostate cancer prevention trial (PCPT) has shed light on the sensitivity and specificity of PSA screening in healthy men (Table 1).

PSA	Cancer versus no cancer		Aggressive cancer versus all others
	Sensitivity	Specificity	Sensitivity
1.1	83%	39%	93%
2.6	40%	81%	67%
4.1	20%	94%	40%

Table 1: Sensitivity and specificity of PSA values in detecting prostate cancer (Thompson et al., 2004)

The National Comprehensive Cancer Network and the U.S. Preventive Services Task Force have published guidelines for prostate cancer screening. They concluded that PSA screening is inappropriate for men 75 years or older. More recently, advocates of screening have recommended screening for patients with at least a 10-year life expectancy (Lim & Sherin, 2008).

PSA cutoff values as an indication for prostate biopsy have changed to a more dynamic, spectrum-based practice. For example, the average annual increase of serum PSA ranges from 0.1 to 0.5 ng/ml in men with benign prostatic hyperplasia, related to a prostate growth of 1.8 ml/yr (Bonilla & McConnell, 1995).

The use of PSA escalation, or velocity, as an indication for biopsy has improved diagnostic accuracy. A PSA velocity that exceeds 0.75 ng/ml per year is associated with a higher rate of prostate cancer (Carter *et al.*, 1992). Unfortunately, PSA velocity is not cancer-specific and varies significantly from day to day.

PSA density is the ratio of PSA value in relation to prostate volume, as measured by transrectal ultrasound (Benson *et al.*, 1992). Normal prostatic epithelium contributes 0.1 ng/ml PSA per gram of tissue to the serum PSA level. That number jumps to 0.3 ng/ml for BPH (benign prostatic hyperplasia) tissue, and 3.5 ng/ml for prostate cancer epithelium. Variations in prostate volume measurement by different examiners and the variability between machines limit the accuracy of PSA density. In addition, the ratio of prostate stroma to epithelium varies from gland to gland (Partin *et al.*, 1990). To date, the use of PSA density has not gained widespread acceptance as a screening tool.

Free to total serum PSA ratio has become an adjunctive assessment tool in determining the probability of cancer. PSA is either freely circulated in serum, or bound or complexed to protease inhibitors, notably, antichymotripsin (ACT) and macroglobulin (MG) (Christensson *et al.*, 1993; Lilja, 1993; Stenman *et al.*, 1994). Approximately 70% of serum PSA is bound to proteins. Free and total PSA can be detected through immunoassays. Prostate cancer cells do not produce more PSA, per gram, than benign prostatic tissue. However, in the cancerous state, malignant cells may greatly outnumber those of benign stroma, while the PSA produced by malignant cells escapes proteolytic processing. Therefore, men with prostate cancer have a greater ratio of protein bound PSA and a lower percentage of free PSA, and can present with elevated levels of total PSA. The role of %fPSA is more applicable to PSA levels less than 10 ng/ml. A cutoff of <18% free/total ratio (0.18) improves the ability to diagnose cancer than total PSA readings (Christensson *et al.*, 1993).

PSA is strongly affected by androgens (Young *et al.*, 1991). However, PSA readings can be elevated by BPH, prostatitis, recent instrumentation, metabolic factors, and medications. The 5-alpha-reductase inhibitors can lower PSA by 50% after one year of use (Roehrborn *et al.*, 2002). Medical treatments for prostate cancer, such as antiandrogens and luteinizing hormone releasing hormone (LHRH) agonists can profoundly reduce PSA levels. Surgery for BPH can reduce PSA levels, as well (Shingleton *et al.*, 2000).

3.2   Digital Rectal Exam (DRE)

The addition of PSA to screening protocols has largely supplanted DRE as a prostate cancer screening test. DRE can miss many early cancers, and is seldom reproducible, even by experienced physicians (Catalona *et al.*, 1997). Improved detection occurs when DRE and PSA are combined (Catalona *et al.*, 1991) as the two tests detect different cancers (Okotie *et al.*, 2007). Thus, DRE and PSA are considered complementary, and both tests should be offered simultaneously to screen for prostate cancer.

3.3   PCA-3

A unique non-coding RNA gene on chromosome 9, termed PCA-3, has been identified (Bussemakers *et al.*, 1999). This protein, found in high concentrations in prostate tissue, is highly expressed in 95% of prostate cancers. Through PCR assays, investigators have found a 66-fold upregulation of this protein in prostate cancer tissue, compared to benign prostatic tissue samples. Additionally, the marker has been shown to be detectable in tissue samples with a paucity of cancerous tissue in a background of normal acini (de Kok *et al.*, 2002). Thus, PCA-3 represents a potentially highly sensitive and specific biomarker for detecting prostate cancer. Sensitivities of up to 67% and specificities of up to 83% have been reported (Hessels *et al.*, 2003).

With a negative predictive value of 90%, this test shows potential for reducing unnecessary and invasive biopsies and other costly diagnostic procedures. Unlike PSA, PCA-3 levels are unaltered by vigorous prostate massage or instrumentation. Thus the assay is performed on a urine sample collected after prostate massage. Finally, PCA-3 levels do not correlate directly with prostate volume, but have correlated well to prostate tumor volume (Whitman *et al.*, 2008). PCA-3 shows promise by potentially removing the hazard of background biomarker elevation due to BPH or other benign processes, as is the case for PSA.

4   Diagnosis

Trans rectal ultrasound (TRUS) of the prostate was introduced in 1955 and was made popular in the 1970s (Watanabe *et al.*, 1968). Then, in the 1980s, ultrasound-guided, spring-loaded needle biopsy of the prostate was introduced (Lee *et al.*, 1989). A sextant biopsy template has largely been replaced by the more extensive 10-16 biopsy template, reducing the undersampling and understaging of disease (Hodge *et al.*, 1989; Stamey, 1995; Presti *et al.*, 2003).

TRUS not only guides the needle into the desired area of the prostate to be sampled, but also provides information regarding prostate size, shape and tumor localization. Mild complications of TRUS biopsy of the prostate include hematuria and hematospermia, which usually resolve within 3-7 days (Rodriguez & Terris, 1998).

Antibiotic prophylaxis is mandatory to prevent serious infectious complications, but the choice of antibiotics and duration of coverage are controversial. A 3-day course of oral fluoroquinolone was shown to be no better than a single dose regimen (Kapoor *et al.*, 1998; Sabbagh *et al.*, 2004; Wolf *et al.*, 2008). Despite antibiotic prophylaxis, post-biopsy infection rates vary between 0.7% and 4% (Webb *et al.*, 1993; Aus *et al.*, 1993).

The indications for recommending a prostate biopsy are controversial. Rather than classifying PSA values as "normal" or "abnormal", the current view is that the risk of harboring prostate cancer is continuous as PSA values increase (Thompson *et al.*, 2005). Even if a PSA value is deemed suspicious or elevated by the clinician, the PSA should be re-measured due to daily fluctuations in PSA levels.

4.1 MRI

Magnetic resonance imaging is gaining popularity when PSA readings are suspicious before invasive measures like needle biopsies are advised. The test is costly due to the special training that is required for accurate interpretation of the images.

5   Treatment

A comprehensive description of management strategies for localized, locally advanced and metastatic prostate cancers is beyond the scope of this chapter. We will discuss different treatment modalities their respective indications, risks and benefits.

5.1 Conservative Management

Historically, conservative management, that is, watchful waiting and active surveillance, are reserved for patients with life expectancies of more than 10 years and with low-risk features (i.e. low Gleason Grade, small volume disease, PSA<10). The term 'watchful waiting' refers to delayed treatment of disease until it manifests clinically, with little to no intervening follow-up. Active surveillance, on the other hand, mandates close follow-up and constant re-evaluations. This consists of PSA testing every 6 months and an annual biopsy. Active surveillance has been advised for younger patients with low to intermediate grade cancer in recent times. While attempts to better define aggressive and non-aggressive disease are ongoing (Epstein *et al.*, 1994; Epstein *et al.*, 1998; Kattan, 2003), several observation protocols have been suggested, but consensus is lacking (Zietman *et al.*, 2004; Choo *et al.*, 2002; Klotz, 2004; Patel *et al.*, 2004; Dall'Era *et al.*, 2008).

Watchful waiting has been reserved for patients who are too unwell to undergo definitive management, or have medical comorbidities and/or projected lifespan of less than 10 years. Two recent studies randomized patients to watchful waiting or radical prostatectomy, with conflicting results (Bill-Axelson *et al.*, 2008; Wilt *et al.*, 2012).

Prostate cancer commonly follows an indolent course. The median time from PSA failure after radical prostatectomy to bone metastases is 8 years, and the time to the development of bone metastases and death is another 5 years (Pound *et al.*, 1999). Thus, watchful waiting or active surveillance are considered valid options for select patients.

5.2   Radical Prostatectomy

Radical prostatectomy was first reported by the German, Kuchler in 1866 (Kuchler, 1866), then by Young in 1905 (Young, 1905), and remains the gold standard for the treatment localized prostate cancer, with cure rates exceeding those obtained by radiation, castration or chemotherapy.

Since the widespread utilization of PSA as a screening test, more patients are being diagnosed with localized disease, thus improving the efficacy of radical prostatectomy (Moul *et al.*, 2002).

Radical prostatectomy has evolved, with the open retropubic and perineal technique challenged by the minimally invasive (laparoscopic and robotic) techniques. In skilled hands, radical prostatectomy can be curative regardless of approach, with minimal damage to surrounding tissues (Hull *et al.*, 2002). Radical prostatectomy involves the complete removal of the prostate gland along with the regional lymph nodes in selected cases with higher grades and elevated PSA.

The advantages of surgery are numerous, and include:

- Accurate tumor staging because the pathologist can examine the entire gland.

- PSA values after radical prostatectomy should fall to undetectable levels. Any rise in PSA postoperatively denotes disease recurrence.

- Patients with residual or recurrent disease can be treated with radiotherapy (Trock *et al.*, 2008).

Disadvantages to radical prostatectomy include:

- The need for hospitalization and a significant recovery period.

- Erectile dysfunction, depending on the degree of nerve-sparing

- Urinary incontinence

- Failure to cure

- Risk of rectal injury

There has been a major shift towards the robotic-assisted approach in the past decade. This has occurred with little scientific data to support it and represents a major marketing success story. Different studies reported no advantages to the robotic approach (Smith, 2004; Wood *et al.*, 2007), while another suggested higher recurrence with this novel technique (Hu *et al.*, 2008).

Radical prostatectomy is a viable option in patients who have failed radiation or focal therapy. Surgery in this setting, though, is associated with increased technical difficulty and higher complication rates (Sanderson *et al.*, 2006). Ideally, candidates for radical prostatectomy should be in good health, have a life expectancy of over 10 years and have significant cancer that can be completely removed.

5.3   Radiation Therapy

Radiotherapy is an effective and less invasive method to treat prostate cancer. Several forms of radiation therapy have been described, and different modalities are currently used worldwide. External beam radiotherapy involves gamma radiation directed at the prostate. Three dimensional conformal radiotherapy (3D-CRT) and intensity modulated radiation therapy (IMRT) are sophisticated methods for aiming radiation at complex geometric structures while sparing surrounding tissues, thus minimizing side effects of the treatment.

Adequate cancer control after radiation treatment is more difficult to define because not all prostate cells are eliminated and undetectable PSA readings are not expected. Despite the differences in outcome assessment, cancer control rates are comparable between radiation and radical prostatectomy (Gretzer *et al.*, 2002). 76 to 80 Gray are commonly used, and this dose escalation has been shown to improve cancer control (Pollack *et al.*, 2000).

Side effects from radiation treatment arise when surrounding structures absorb radiation. Specifically, the bladder, rectum, urinary striated sphincter and urethra are most commonly affected. Urinary incontinence is uncommon, but approximately 50% of treated patients develop erectile dysfunction after radiotherapy. For those patients with high risk or locally advanced disease at the time of diagnosis, several studies show a benefit from combined radiation therapy and androgen deprivation therapy (Bolla *et al.*, 2002).

Assessing the success of cancer control can be challenging. PSA levels gradually decrease up to 2 to 3 years after the completion of radiation treatment. Inflammatory flares in the gland during the first two years after treatment can produce spikes in PSA values, called the PSA "bounce", and complicate interpretation of post-radiation PSA values (Critz *et al.*, 2000).

The American Society of Therapeutic Radiology and Oncology (ASTRO) define 3 consecutive PSA increases at 6-month intervals as a recurrence of disease. Cancer progression is defined as the halfway date between the PSA nadir and the first rising PSA reading. More recently, the Phoenix criterion, defined as a PSA rise of 2 ng/ml above nadir, has proven to be a more robust marker of post-radiotherapy biochemical recurrence and long-term survival (Abramowitz et. al., 2008).

5.4   Brachytherapy

Brachytherapy involves the implantation of radioactive "seeds" or needles directly into the prostate gland. Under ideal conditions, this method delivers a high dose of extremely localized radiation, with minimal effect to surrounding structures. Seeds of the radioactive isotopes Iodine-125 and Palladium-103 are used; iodine for the less aggressive cancers and Palladium for the more aggressive malignancies.

While potentially efficacious, the treatment is less successful in patients with high prostate gland volumes because seed implantation is more difficult in larger glands. Often, patients with large glands are treated with ADT prior to seed implantation. Cancer control is excellent with this modality, using the ASTRO criteria (Ragde *et al.*, 2001). Urinary side effects and erectile dysfunction are more common with brachytherapy than with external beam radiotherapy. However, rectal injury and proctitis are less with brachytherapy.

5.5   Adjuvant Radiotherapy Post Radical Prostatectomy

Surgery, followed by radiation is used for patients with adverse findings on the radical prostatectomy specimen, such as positive margins or capsular involvement. Radiotherapy is recommended, as well, for PSA recurrence, that is, PSA readings over 0.2 ng/ml after radical prostatectomy and rising (Leibovitch *et al.*, 2000; Trock *et al.*, 2008). Patients with seminal vesicle involvement and/or positive lymph nodes may also benefit from adjuvant radiation treatment (Cozzarini *et al.*, 2004).

5.6   Cryoablation

When tissues are frozen the cells die. Cryoablation uses this principle to destroy prostate tissue, specifically, prostate cancer cells. Current technology freezes the entire gland using argon gas passed through hollow needles inserted directly into the prostate. Warm helium gas is passed through the urethra to protect the urethral mucosa during the procedure.

Cryoablation is used as primary treatment or as a salvage procedure for patients who have failed other treatments. ASTRO criteria are used to assess the success of cryoablation. There is, however, no consensus on the definition of biochemical failure after cryotherapy (Long *et al.*, 2001). Current practice involves two cycles of freezing/thawing the prostate to -40^0 Celsius. The cytotoxic and antineoplastic effects of cryotherapy occur via several mechanisms:

- Mechanical – ice crystal formation and shear stress on cell membranes

- Biochemical – pH changes, osmolarity and electrolyte concentration changes

- Ischemic – blood stasis and thrombosis, disrupting blood supply

- Apoptotic – programmed cell death in injured but not killed cells

- Immunologic – antitumor immune response through the release of antigens

The advantages of cryoablation are that it is minimally invasive, it can be effectively repeated, there is no ionizing radiation involved and potency can be (although rarely is) preserved (Asterling & Greene, 2009). The most common complication is urinary incontinence (Pisters *et al.*, 1999).

Long-term data regarding the efficacy, survival and quality of life outcomes of patients undergoing primary or salvage cryoablation are not yet available.

5.7   High-Intensity Focused Ultrasound (HIFU)

HIFU involves heating, rather than cooling the prostate (as in cryoablation) in order to destroy prostate tissue. Temperatures can reach as high as 100^0 Celsius. Cell death occurs days to months after the initial treatment through coagulative necrosis (Chapelon *et al.*, 1999). The rectum is cooled during the procedure to minimize collateral damage from the heating probes. The most common complication is erectile dysfunction, and urinary retention. Patients often have a suprapubic catheter inserted before or during the procedure. Initial results are promising, but, as with cryoablation, long-term data is lacking.

6   Hormone Therapy for Prostate Cancer

Since the landmark research by Huggins in the 1940s, ADT remains one of the most durable treatment modalities for any known cancer. The development, growth and maintenance of the prostate gland are dependent on androgens. The arrival of androgens into the circulation begins with the secretion of gonadotropin-releasing hormone (GnRH) from the hypothalamus in a pulsatile manner. The next step in the cascade is the release of luteinizing hormone (LH) and follicle-stimulating hormone (FSH) from the anterior pituitary gland. LH acts directly on the Leydig cells in the testis to synthesize testosterone.

Testosterone circulates in the blood, largely bound to sex-hormone binding globulin (SHBG) and to albumin. Testosterone is also bound to corticosteroid-binding globulin, but with much less affinity. Approximately 97% of circulating testosterone is protein bound, while less than 3% is unbound. However, it is the unbound form of testosterone that is bioavailable (Debes & Tindall, 2002).

Once in the prostate, testosterone is converted to the more biologically active dihydrotestosterone through the enzymatic action of 5-alpha-reductase (5-AR). Of the two types of 5-AR, type 2 is the isoform that is in greatest concentration in the prostate. The testis produces more than 95% of circulating androgens. Androgens are also produced by the adrenal glands, but they are considered to be inconsequential to the growth and maintenance of prostatic tissue. On the receptor end of the equation lies the androgen receptor (AR). The AR is a cytoplasmic monomer, that when bound to DHT, dimerizes and translocates to the nucleus, acting as a transcription factor.

Androgens and the AR are essential to the regulation of apoptosis in prostate tissue. The presence of the androgen inhibits the enzymatic cascade that leads to programmed cell death, and up-regulates the antiapaptotic pathways (Kimura et al., 2001; Lu et al., 1997). In addition, castration limits angiogenesis by inhibiting both vascular endothelial growth factor (VEGF) and basic fibroblast growth factor (bFGF) (Joseph et al., 1997). Thus, inhibitions of androgens through either upstream (hypothalamic) or downstream (AR) targets are recognized mechanisms for inhibiting the growth and progression of prostate cancer. All current forms of ADT reduce the ability of androgens to activate the AR. However, when mutated, the AR can escape the normal, regulatory influences of the hormonal milieu. In prostate cancer, AR mutations can lead to androgen independent prostate cancer growth and progression, despite castration.

6.1   Mechanisms of Androgen Blockade

There are four methods of androgen blockade that are in clinical use:

1. Androgen source ablation

2. Inhibition of androgen synthesis

3. Androgen receptor blockade

4. Inhibition of the hypothalamic/pituitary axis

Side effects of castration are common to all of the above methods, including loss of libido, erectile dysfunction, decreased energy, gynecomastia and hot flushes. The development of osteopenia and osteoporosis as a result of castration and fractures associated with bone metastases will be discussed later.

1. Androgen Source Ablation

Bilateral orchiectomy is a quick and effective method for removing all biologically active androgens from the circulation. Within 24 hours of bilateral orchiectomy, serum testosterone levels are reduced by over 90% (Maatman et al., 1985). However, testosterone that is produced by the prostate, itself is not halted by orchiectomy, and is a potential contributor to eventual prostate cancer progression in this setting.

2. Inhibition of Androgen Synthesis

Several compounds halt the body's production of endogenous testosterone. Ketoconazole is a broad-spectrum antifungal agent. However, it also inhibits a key enzymatic step in steroid production by preventing the conversion of lanosterol to cholesterol. As cholesterol is the building block for all steroid hormones, blocking this enzymatic step is extremely effective at rapidly lowering testosterone levels. The response is not durable, with testosterone levels rebounding to normal ranges within 5 months of therapy (Vanuytsel *et al.*, 1987). Ketokonazole is effective during bony pain crises in men with castrate resistant prostate cancer, but its long-term durability as a sustainable treatment is limited.

Abiraterone inhibits the enzyme cytochrome P17, a key and early enzyme in sex hormone synthesis. In addition to suppressing sex hormone synthesis, the compound also suppresses mineralcorticoids such as aldosterone, and glucocorticoids, such as cortisol. Accordingly, concurrent administration of exogenous steroids (e.g. prednisone) is prescribed when commencing abiraterone therapy.

3. Androgen Receptor Blockade

Cyproterone acetate, one of the first antiandrogens described and lowers testosterone levels by 70%-80% (Jacobi *et al.*, 1980; Barradell & Faulds, 1994). Its use is limited, however, because of severe cardiovascular complications in 10% of patients (de Voogt *et al.*, 1986).

Non-steroidal antiandrogens are widely used in current clinical practice. The common drugs in clinical use are Flutamide, Bicalutamide and Nilutamide. Because these compounds block the AR, the normally active negative feedback loop to the hypothalamus is disrupted. Thus, men treated with any of the above drugs have elevations in serum testosterone. This is clinically important, as men treated with these drugs are theoretically able to preserve potency. However, clinical trials have failed to demonstrate meaningful preservation of erectile function compared to patients undergoing orchiectomy (Schröder *et al.*, 2000).

Bicalutamide is the most extensively studied non-steroidal antiandrogen, and at doses of 150 mg daily, has been shown to improve survival in men with metastatic prostate cancer comparable to bilateral orchiectomy (Wirth *et al.*, 2005; McLeod *et al.*, 2005).

4. Inhibition of the hypothalamic/pituitary axis

The use of an LH-RH agonist seems counterintuitive, as the product will stimulate androgen production, in what has been called the androgen flare (Waxman *et al.*, 1985). However, with continued activation, the LH-RH receptors become desensitized, halting the production of LH, which leads to castrate levels of testosterone. There are 4 widely studied LH-RH analogues: Leuprolide, Goserelin, Triptorelin and Histrelin. In a meta-analysis, patients who received an LH-RH analogue had similar outcomes as patients undergoing orchiectomy (Seidenfeld *et al.*, 2000).

To offset the initial rise in serum testosterone after initiating an LH-RH agonist, an anti-androgen is prescribed for 2 weeks prior to the administration of the agonist (Schultz & Senge, 1990). To avoid the negative consequences of the androgen flare, LH-RH antagonists (e.g. Abarelix, Degarelix) have been developed. These compounds competitively bind the LH-RH receptor in the pituitary and their administration precipitates a rapid decline in LH and circulating testosterone within 72 hours.

6.2 The Androgen Withdrawal Phenomenon

The androgen withdrawal phenomenon is a clinical observation when patients are treated with concurrent LH-RH agonist and an antiandrogen. Patients with a rising PSA despite combination therapy maybe benefit with a PSA decline of approximately 50% when the antiandrogen is withdrawn. This phenomenon is observed in approximately 15%-30% of patients (Kelly & Scher, 1993; Small & Srinivas, 1995).

6.3 Bone-Related Complications of Androgen Blockade

Androgen deprivation therapy (ADT) is associated with multiple adverse events, including hot flashes, gynecomastia, sexual dysfunction, decline in cognitive function, increased BMI and, most importantly, mortality from cardiovascular disease. This chapter, however, will focus on bone-related events associated with metastatic prostate cancer and medical castration, which is a source of major morbidity to the patient.

7   Bone Metastases in Advanced Prostate Cancer

There are two major cells that determine the strength and regulation of bone turnover: osteoclasts and osteoblasts. The primary function of the osteoclast is to break down bone, while the osteoblast functions to form new bone. Together, their concerted functions continuously remodel and reshape the skeleton. Osteoclasts migrate to an area of bone, resorb it, initiate apoptosis and allow for new bone formation by osteoblasts.

Prostate cancer preferentially spreads to bone, forming mainly osteoblastic lesions. Post-mortem studies have found that more than 80% of men who die from prostate cancer have bone metastases at autopsy (Harada *et al.*, 1992). Typically, Patients with bone metastases present with pain. With advanced metastatic disease, vertebral lesions can compress the spinal cord, leading to nerve root compression, or cauda equina syndrome. Pathological fractures to the vertebrae are common consequences of metastatic disease. Finally, ADT contributes to osteoclast activity in men with prostate cancer, accelerating bone turnover and leading to an increased risk of fractures.

7.1   Androgen Deprivation Therapy (ADT) and Osteoporosis

As men age, they become pre-disposed to bone mineral loss and pathological fractures. In the patient with locally advanced or metastatic prostate cancer, ADT can intensify the process of bone loss and worsen the risk of fracture in an already vulnerable patient population. ADT leads to decreased bone mineral density (BMD) and, eventually, patients receiving ADT develop osteopenia – a decrease in BMD compared to an age-matched mean, or osteoporosis – defined as more than 2.5 standard deviations below an age-matched mean. Depending on the castration strategy and the patient population, bone mineral loss occurs at about 3% to 5% in the first year on ADT. Osteoporosis is common after 4 years of ADT (Wei *et al.*, 1999). Other studies have shown that after 15 years, the cumulative incidence of pathological fractures was 40% in men treated with ADT, and 19% in non-castrated men (Melton *et al.*, 2003). As our understanding of the short and long-term effects of ADT has grown, so has our need to develop countermeasures to preserve bone health in men receiving ADT.

8   Prevention of fractures

8.1   Recognition

BMD is the measuring stick for bone health in both men and women. While the gold standard for assessing BMD is histomorphometry (Humadi *et al.*, 2010), several imaging techniques are available to estimate the BMD in men with hormone treated prostate cancer. These modalities include quantitative computerized tomography (CT), quantitative radiography, single x-ray absorptiometry and ultrasound. However, dual energy x-ray absorptiometry (DEXA) has become the most common measuring tool because of several advantages. Firstly, scores are reported as World Health Organization T-scores. Secondly, DEXA predicts future fracture risks. Finally, DEXA can accurately determine response to treatment (Blake & Fogelman, 2010). All men on long term ADT should undergo baseline and follow-up BMD testing (Bae & Stein, 2004; Diamond *et al.*, 2004).

9   Current Prevention and Treatment Strategies

Bone fractures are a major source of morbidity and can lead to mortality in men treated with ADT. Accordingly, preventative measures, such as supplemental calcium and vitamin D, are recommended by the National Institute of Health (Michaelson *et al.*, 2008). Bisphosphonates are a class of medications that have been long-used in the prevention of fractures in post-menopausal women with osteoporosis. Recent evidence suggests that the bisphosphonates offer protection to men on ADT, as well by reducing bone resorption through inhibiting osteoclast activity. The bisphosphonates pamidronate and alendronate showed increased prevention of osteoporosis compared to a placebo and even reversed bone loss in men on ADT (Smith *et al.*, 2001; Greenspan *et al.*, 2008).

Zoledronic acid is an intravenously administered bisphosphonates with potent anti-osteoclastic properties. In 2002, it was approved for the treatment of hypercalcemia and osteopenia in women (Green & Rogers, 2002). In 2004, the drug was approved for use in men on ADT and with bony metastases, and has been shown to prevent skeletal-related adverse events in this patient population (Saad *et al.*, 2004).

Patients treated with zoledronic acid can experience fatigue, anemia, weakness, mild renal dysfunction and myalgia. Additionally, patients receiving this drug are at risk for developing osteonecrosis of the mandibular bone, called osteonecrosis of the jaw (ONJ). Thus patients are advised to undergo a dental evaluation before starting this treatment, especially those with a history of dental disease or poor overall dentition.

Another class of drugs, the receptor activator of nuclear factor $_kB$ ligand (RANKL) inhibitors, interacts with the microenvironment of bone marrow to suppress osteoclasts. RANK is a receptor found on the cell surface of osteoclasts, and RANKL is its ligand. Inhibition of RANKL by the monoclonal antibody denosumab has been evaluated in several phase 3, placebo-controlled trials. Results showed superiority over zoledronic acid in delaying skeletal-related events in men with castration-resistant prostate cancer (CRPC) (Lipton *et al.*, 2012).

As with zoledronic acid, denosumab produced side effects, including fatigue, nausea, hypocalcemia and ONJ. Men receiving zoledronic acid or denosumab should receive supplemental calcium and vitamin D. While denosumab does not require periodic renal function monitoring, serum calcium must be tested regularly.

9.1   Estrogens

Since the landmark study of Charles Huggins in 1941 (Huggins & Hodges, 1941), estrogens have had a longstanding role in the treatment of advanced prostate cancer. A direct correlation between serum levels of estrogen and bone density in men has been established (Slemenda *et al.*, 1997). Ironically, though, the exact mechanism of action of estrogen on prostatic tissue is unknown. Estrogens act centrally, inhibiting LHRH secretion from the hypothalamus, halting testicular production of testosterone. At higher concentrations, estrogens competitively block prostate cancer androgen receptors. Historically, the most commonly used and studied estrogen is the synthetic estrogen, diethylstilbestrol (DES)

DES is a synthetic ethinyl estrogen. It exerts a negative feedback effect on the hypothalamus, decreasing LH secretion and, consequently, decreases androgen secretion by the testis. In addition, DES indirectly upregulates the secretion of sex hormone binding globulin and stimulates pituitary prolactin secretion. Thus, DES is very effective at shutting down testicular androgen secretion and causes castration (Robinson & Thomas, 1971; Malkowicz, 2001). Recent evidence suggests that DES exhibits high affinity for the AR and could modulate the course of prostate cancer (Wang et al., 2010).

In early studies in the 1970s by the Veterans Administration Cooperative Urological Research Group (VACURG), daily administration of 5 mg of DES was as effective as orchiectomy at achieving castrate levels of testosterone. Unfortunately, as this dose, a large number of patients experienced significant cardiovascular complications (Blackard et al., 1970).

Estrogen replacement has been used to prevent osteoporosis in women for decades. For men receiving ADT, the use of estrogen might seem an intuitive answer to combat pathological fractures. However, due to cardiac and thromboembolic complications, estrogen as a treatment for prostate cancer and as a preserver of bone health has fallen out of favor in urologic practice. While 5 mg of DES daily may carry significant cardiovascular and thromboembolic risks, other studies, using lower doses of DES, have shown promising results with less associated morbidity.

In the late 1990s, Smith and colleagues conducted a small pilot study, consisting of 21 men and administered 1 mg of DES daily to men with advanced prostate cancer. No blood thinners were used. Adverse thromboembolic events were observed in only 1 patient (Smith et al., 1998).

Jazieh and colleagues placed 14 men with advanced, castrate resistant prostate cancer on 3 mg of daily DES. They also administered warfarin concurrently in sufficient doses to achieve an international normalized ratio (INR) between 1.8-2.0. Interestingly, no thromboembolic events were noted in any of the study participants (Jazieh et al., 1994). Then, a phase 1-2 study conducted by Klotz and colleagues enrolled 32 men with advanced prostate cancer to receive both 2-3 mg daily of DES plus 1 mg warfarin, a commonly used blood thinner. While the outcomes of the study were geared towards PSA response to estrogen therapy, 28% of the study participants experienced a thromboembolic event (Klotz et al., 1999). However, warfarin doses were not titrated to an international normalized ratio (INR) between 2 to 3, which is considered to be an acceptable therapeutic range.

Researchers have found conclusive evidence that estrogens help to preserve bone density in men (Vandenput & Ohlsson, 2009). While zoledronic acid and denosumab are promising medications to prevent adverse bone events in men with advanced prostate cancer, they are expensive, require intravenous or subcutaneous injections, and can cause significant side effects. Estrogen can be taken orally and is inexpensive. In addition, there has been resurgence in research geared towards estrogen as a potential treatment for advanced prostate cancer. It is our belief that estrogen replacement therapy warrants further investigation as a potential adjunct for men on ADT in order to preserve and promote bone health, despite castration.

Alternative estrogen-related treatments for prostate cancer are the selective estrogen receptor modulators (SERMs). These compounds act as either estrogen receptor agonists or antagonists, depending on the biochemical milieu and presence of certain co-regulators. One of the SERMs, Toremifene, has been shown to decrease circulating testosterone levels by suppressing the hypothalamic-pituitary axis (Taneja et al., 2006). Perhaps the most interesting potential application of Toremifene is for chemoprevention of prostate cancer. High-grade prostatic intraepithelial neoplasia (PIN) is considered by many to be a premalignant precurser to prostate cancer, and this patient population could be an attractive target for chemoprevention strategies. In a multicentered, double-blind study, 514 men with high grade PIN and no evidence of cancer on TRUS biopsy were given 20 mg of daily oral Toremifene, taken for 6-12 months. Results showed a significant reduction in the incidence of prostate cancer in the treatment group, compared with placebo (Price *et al.*, 2006). However, in a larger double-blind study, involving 1590 men, 20 mg of daily Toremifene showed no overall risk reduction of developing prostate cancer, and no disease-specific survival benefit (Taneja *et al.*, 2013).

Since the initial studies of Huggins and the VACURG, effective blood thinners have been approved and are prescribed to millions of North Americans for the prevention of thromboembolic events. The future of DES, other synthetic estrogens and SERMs in the context of ADT for advanced prostate cancer will likely prompt randomized controlled trials comparing low dose DES in combination with an effective blood thinner, such as warfarin, acetylsalicylic acid (ASA) and/or clopidogrel, to currently approved medications, such as alendronate, zoledronic acid and denosumab.

If the safety and efficacy of estrogen can be demonstrated, it could become, once again, another weapon in the urologist's armamentarium against the morbidity associated with advancing prostate cancer and its therapies.

10   Summary

Prostate cancer is a common disease among older men. While most low-grade cancers display an indolent, non life-threatening course, other, higher-grade cancers are more aggressive and can be life threatening without treatment.

Screening for prostate cancer is controversial. However, mortality from prostate cancer has plummeted since the introduction of PSA into mainstream practice. The downside of PSA screening is over-diagnosis and over-treatment of some cancers.

Therapeutic options for prostate cancer range from non-invasive radiotherapy, to minimally invasive surgical procedures. In most instances, cure rates are high for localized disease. Should prostate cancer extend beyond the gland, or recur after definitive therapies such as surgery or radiotherapy, ADT is considered and initiated. Side effects of ADT are not benign, and osteoporotic fractures are a major source of morbidity in this patient population.

While estrogen was once considered a first line hormonal therapy for prostate cancer, its use has fallen out of favour due to the high incidence of thromboembolic events associated with its use. Fortunately, new blood thinners could re-ignite the use of low dose estrogen for the prevention of ADT-related fractures. More studies are necessary to determine the safety and efficacy of low dose estrogen to preserve bone health in men with advanced prostate cancer receiving ADT.

References

American Cancer Society. American Cancer Society : Cancer facts and figures 2008. 2008

Walsh, 2000. Walsh PC: Cancer surveillance series: Interpreting trends in prostate cancer—part I: evidence of the effects of screening in recent prostate cancer incidence, mortality, and survival rates. J Urol 2000; 163:364-365.

Stephenson, 2005. Stephenson RA: Prostate cancer overdiagnosis and overtreatment: analysis of US mortality and SEER incidence. Trends in the PSA and pre-PSA eras. In: Klein EA, ed. Management of prostate cancer, Totowa (NJ): Humana Press; 2005:3-13.

Haenszel W, Kurihara M. Studies of Japanese migrants. I. Mortality from cancer and other diseases among Japanese in the United States. J Natl Cancer Inst 1968;40:43-68.

Yu H, Harris RE, Gao YT, et al. Comparative epidemiology of cancers of the colon, rectum, prostate and breast in Shanghai, China versus the United States. Int J Epidemiol 1991;20:76-81.

Parkin DM, Bray F, Ferlay J, Pisani P: Global cancer statistics, 2002. CA Cancer J Clin 2005; 55:74-108.

Ries LAG, Melbert D, Krapcho M, et al: SEER cancer statistics review, 1975-2007.

van der Cruijsen-Koeter IW, Roobol MJ, Wildhagen MF, et al: Tumor characteristics and prognostic factors in two subsequent screening rounds with four-year interval within prostate cancer screening trial, ERSPC Rotterdam. Urology 2006; 68(3):615-620.

Aus G, Bergdahl S, Lodding P, et al: Prostate cancer screening decreases the absolute risk of being diagnosed with advanced prostate cancer—results from a prospective, population-based randomized controlled trial. Eur Urol 2007; 51(3):659-664.

Koning HJ, Auvinen A, Berenguer Sanchez A, et al: Large-scale randomized prostate cancer screening trials: program performances in the European Randomized Screening for Prostate Cancer trial and the Prostate, Lung, Colorectal and Ovary cancer trial. Int J Cancer 2002; 97(2):237-244.

Schroder FH, Hugosson J, Roobol MJ, et al: Screening and prostate-cancer mortality in a randomized European study. N Engl J Med 2009; 360(13):1320-1328.

Andriole GL, Grubb 3rd RL, Buys SS, et al: Mortality results from a randomized prostate-cancer screening trial. N Engl J Med 2009; 360(13):1310-1319.

Lim LS, Sherin K: Screening for prostate cancer in U.S. men ACPM position statement on preventive practice. Am J Prev Med 2008; 34(2):164-170.

Bonilla JRC, MC Connel JD. Patterns of prostate growth observed in placebo treated patients in the PLESS trial over four years [Abstract]. J Urol 1995;159(Suppl 5):301A.

Carter HB, Morrell CH, Pearson JD, et al. Estimation of prostatic growth using serial prostate-specific antigen measurements in men with and without prostate disease. Cancer Res 1992;52:3323-3328

Benson MC, Whang IS, Olsson CA, et al. The use of prostate specific antigen density to enhance the predictive value of intermediate levels of serum prostate specific antigen. J Urol 1992;147:817-821.

Partin AW, Carter HB, Chan DW, et al. Prostate specific antigen in the staging of localized prostate cancer: influence of tumor differentiation, tumor volume and benign hyperplasia. J Urol 1990;143:747-752.

Christensson A, Bjork T, Nilsson O, et al: Serum prostate specific antigen complexed to alpha 1-antichymotrypsin as an indicator of prostate cancer. J Urol 1993; 150(1):100-105.

Lilja H: Significance of different molecular forms of serum PSA. The free, noncomplexed form of PSA versus that complexed to alpha 1-antichymotrypsin. Urol Clin North Am 1993; 20(4):681-686.

Stenman UH, Hakama M, Knekt P, et al: Serum concentrations of prostate specific antigen and its complex with alpha 1-antichymotrypsin before diagnosis of prostate cancer. Lancet 1994; 344(8937):1594-1598.

Catalona WJ, Smith DS, Ornstein DK: Prostate cancer detection in men with serum PSA concentrations of 2.6 to 4.0 ng/mL and benign prostate examination. Enhancement of specificity with free PSA measurements. JAMA 1997; 277(18):1452-1455.

Catalona WJ, Smith DS, Ratliff TL, et al: Measurement of prostate-specific antigen in serum as a screening test for prostate cancer. N Engl J Med 1991; 324(17):1156-1161.

Okotie OT, Roehl KA, Han M, et al: Characteristics of prostate cancer detected by digital rectal examination only. Urology 2007; 70(6):1117-1120.

Young CY, Montgomery BT, Andrews PE, et al: Hormonal regulation of prostate-specific antigen messenger RNA in human prostatic adenocarcinoma cell line LNCaP. Cancer Res 1991; 51(14):3748-3752.

Roehrborn CG, Boyle P, Nickel JC, et al: Efficacy and safety of a dual inhibitor of 5-alpha-reductase types 1 and 2 (dutasteride) in men with benign prostatic hyperplasia. Urology 2002; 60(3):434-441.

Shingleton WB, Terrell F, Kolski J, et al: Prostate specific antigen measurements after minimally invasive surgery of the prostate in men with benign prostatic hypertrophy. Prostate Cancer Prostatic Dis 2000; 3(3):200-202.

Bussemakers MJ, van Bokhoven A, Verhaegh GW, et al: DD3: a new prostate-specific gene, highly overexpressed in prostate cancer. Cancer Res 1999; 59:5975-5979.

de Kok JB, Verhaegh GW, Roelofs RW, et al: DD3(PCA3), a very sensitive and specific marker to detect prostate tumors. Cancer Res 2002; 62:2695-2698.

Hessels D, Klein Gunnewiek JM, van Oort I, et al: DD3(PCA3)-based molecular urine analysis for the diagnosis of prostate cancer. Eur Urol 2003; 44:8-15.discussion 15–16

Whitman EJ, Groskopf J, Ali A, et al: PCA3 score before radical prostatectomy predicts extracapsular extension and tumor volume. J Urol 2008; 180(5):1975-1978.discussion 1978–9

Watanabe H, Kato H, Kato T, et al. Diagnostic application of ultrasonotomography to the prostate. Nippon Hinyokika Gakkai Zasshi 1968;59: 273-279.

Lee F, Torp-Pedersen ST, Carroll JT, et al. Use of transrectal ultrasound and prostate-specific antigen in diagnosis of prostatic intraepithelial neoplasia. Urology 1989;34:4-8.

Hodge KK, McNeal JE, Terris MK, et al. Random systematic versus directed ultrasound guided transrectal core biopsies of the prostate. J Urol 1989;142:71-74; discussion 74-75.

Stamey TA. Making the most out of six systematic sextant biopsies. Urology 1995;45:2-12.

Presti JC Jr, O'Dowd GJ, Miller MC, et al. Extended peripheral zone biopsy schemes increase cancer detection rates and minimize variance in prostate specific antigen and age related cancer rates: results of a community multi-practice study. J Urol 2003;169:125-129.

Rodriguez LV, Terris MK. Risks and complications of transrectal ultrasound guided prostate needle biopsy: a prospective study and review of the literature. J Urol 1998;160:2115-2120.

Kapoor DA, Klimberg IW, et al: Single-dose oral ciprofloxacin versus placebo for prophylaxis during transrectal prostate biopsy. Urology 1998; 52(4):552-558.

Sabbagh R, McCormack M, et al: A prospective randomized trial of 1-day versus 3-day antibiotic prophylaxis for transrectal ultrasound guided prostate biopsy. Can J Urol 2004; 11(2):2216-2219.

Wolf Jr JS, Bennett CJ, et al: Best practice policy statement on urologic surgery antimicrobial prophylaxis. J Urol 2008; 179(4):1379-1390.

Webb JA, Shanmuganathan K, McLean A. Complications of ultrasound-guided transperineal prostate biopsy. A prospective study. Br 1993;72:775-777.

Aus G, Hermansson CG, Hugosson J, et al. Transrectal ultrasound examination of the prostate: complications and acceptance by patients. Br 1993;71:457-459.

Thompson IM, Ankerst DP, et al: Operating characteristics of prostate-specific antigen in men with an initial PSA level of 3.0 ng/ml or lower. JAMA 2005; 294(1):66-70.

Epstein JI, Walsh PC, Carmichael M, Brendler CB: Pathologic and clinical findings to predict tumor extent of nonpalpable (stage T1c) prostate cancer. JAMA 1994; 271:368-374.

Epstein JI, Chan DW, Sokoll LJ, et al: Nonpalpable stage T1c prostate cancer: prediction of insignificant disease using free/total prostate specific antigen levels and needle biopsy findings. J Urol 1998; 160:2407-2411.

Kattan MW: Nomograms are superior to staging and risk grouping systems for identifying high-risk patients: preoperative application in prostate cancer. Curr Opin Urol 2003; 13:111-116.

Zietman AL, Chung CS, Coen JJ, Shipley WU: 10-year outcome for men with localized prostate cancer treated with external radiation therapy: results of a cohort study. J Urol 2004; 171:210-214.

Choo R, Klotz L, Danjoux C, et al: Feasibility study: watchful waiting for localized low to intermediate grade prostate carcinoma with selective delayed intervention based on prostate specific antigen, histological and/or clinical progression. J Urol 2002; 167:1664-1669.

Klotz L: Active surveillance with selective delayed intervention: using natural history to guide treatment in good risk prostate cancer. J Urol 2004; 172:S48-S50.discussion S50–S1

Patel MI, DeConcini DT, Lopez-Corona E, et al: An analysis of men with clinically localized prostate cancer who deferred definitive therapy. J Urol 2004; 171:1520-1524.

Dall'Era MA, Konety BR, Cowan JE, et al: Active surveillance for the management of prostate cancer in a contemporary cohort. Cancer 2008; 112:2664-2670.

Bill-Axelson A, Holmberg L, Filen F, et al: Radical prostatectomy versus watchful waiting in localized prostate cancer: the Scandinavian prostate cancer group-4 randomized trial. J Natl Cancer Inst 2008; 100:1144-1154.

Wilt TJ, Brawer MK, Jones KM, Barry MJ, Aronson WJ, Fox S, Gingrich JR, Wei JT, Gilhooly P, Grob BM, Nsouli I, Iyer P, Cartagena R, Snider G, Roehrborn C, Sharifi R, Blank W, Pandya P, Andriole GL, Culkin D, Wheeler T; Prostate Cancer Intervention versus Observation Trial (PIVOT) Study Group. Radical prostatectomy versus observation for localized prostate cancer. N Engl J Med. 2012 Jul 19;367(3):203-13.

Pound CR, Partin AW, Eisenberger MA, et al: Natural history of progression after PSA elevation following radical prostatectomy. JAMA 1999; 281:1591-1597.

Kuchler, 1866. Kuchler H: Uber prostatavergrossgrugen. Deutsch Klin 1866; 18:458.

Young, 1905. Young HH: The early diagnosis and radical cure of carcinoma of the prostate. Johns Hopkins Hosp Bull 1905; 16:315-321.

Moul JW, Wu H, Sun L, et al: Epidemiology of radical prostatectomy for localized prostate cancer in the era of prostate-specific antigen: an overview of the Department of Defense Center for Prostate Disease Research national database. Surgery 2002; 132:213-219.

Hull GW, Rabbani F, Abbas F, et al: Cancer control with radical prostatectomy alone in 1,000 consecutive patients. J Urol 2002; 167:528-534.

Trock BJ, Han M, Freedland SJ, et al: Prostate cancer-specific survival following salvage radiotherapy vs observation in men with biochemical recurrence after radical prostatectomy. JAMA 2008; 299:2760-2769.

Smith Jr JA: Robotically assisted laparoscopic prostatectomy: an assessment of its contemporary role in the surgical management of localized prostate cancer. Am J Surg 2004; 188:63S-67S.

Wood DP, Schulte R, Dunn RL, et al: Short-term health outcome differences between robotic and conventional radical prostatectomy. Urology 2007; 70:945-949.

Hu JC, Wang Q, Pashos CL, et al: Utilization and outcomes of minimally invasive radical prostatectomy. J Clin Oncol 2008; 26:2278-2284.

Sanderson KM, Penson DF, Cai J, et al: Salvage radical prostatectomy: quality of life outcomes and long-term oncological control of radiorecurrent prostate cancer. J Urol 2006; 176:2025-2031.discussion 2031–2

Gretzer MB, Trock BJ, Han M, Walsh PC: A critical analysis of the interpretation of biochemical failure in surgically treated patients using the American Society for Therapeutic Radiation and Oncology criteria. J Urol 2002; 168:1419-1422.

Pollack A, Zagars GK, Smith LG, et al: Preliminary results of a randomized radiotherapy dose-escalation study comparing 70 Gy with 78 Gy for prostate cancer. J Clin Oncol 2000; 18:3904-3911.

Bolla M, Collette L, Blank L, et al: Long-term results with immediate androgen suppression and external irradiation in patients with locally advanced prostate cancer (an EORTC study): a phase III randomised trial. Lancet 2002; 360:103-106.

Critz FA, Williams WH, Benton JB, et al: Prostate specific antigen bounce after radioactive seed implantation followed by external beam radiation for prostate cancer. J Urol 2000; 163:1085-1089.

Abramowitz MC[1], Li T, Buyyounouski MK, Ross E, Uzzo RG, Pollack A, Horwitz EM. The Phoenix definition of biochemical failure predicts for overall survival in patients with prostate cancer. Cancer. 2008 Jan 1;112(1):55-60.

Ragde H, Grado GL, Nadir BS: Brachytherapy for clinically localized prostate cancer: thirteen-year disease-free survival of 769 consecutive prostate cancer patients treated with permanent implants alone. Arch Esp Urol 2001; 54:739-747.

Leibovich BC, Engen DE, Patterson DE, et al: Benefit of adjuvant radiation therapy for localized prostate cancer with a positive surgical margin. J Urol 2000; 163:1178-1182.

Trock BJ, Han M, Freedland SJ, et al: Prostate cancer-specific survival following salvage radiotherapy vs observation in men with biochemical recurrence after radical prostatectomy. JAMA 2008; 299:2760-2769.

Cozzarini C, Bolognesi A, Ceresoli GL, et al: Role of postoperative radiotherapy after pelvic lymphadenectomy and radical retropubic prostatectomy: a single institute experience of 415 patients. Int J Radiat Oncol Biol Phys 2004; 59:674-683.

Long JP, Bahn D, Lee F, et al: Five-year retrospective, multi-institutional pooled analysis of cancer-related outcomes after cryosurgical ablation of the prostate. Urology 2001; 57:518-523.

Asterling S, Greene DR: Prospective evaluation of sexual function in patients receiving cryosurgery as a primary radical treatment for localized prostate cancer. BJU Int 2009; 103:788-792.

Pisters LL, Perrotte P, Scott SM, et al: Patient selection for salvage cryotherapy for locally recurrent prostate cancer after radiation therapy. J Clin Oncol 1999; 17:2514-2520.Chapelon et al, 1999.

Chapelon JY, Ribault M, Vernier F, et al: Treatment of localised prostate cancer with transrectal high intensity focused ultrasound. Eur J Ultrasound 1999; 9:31-38.

Debes JD, Tindall DJ. The role of androgens and the androgen receptor in prostate cancer. Cancer Lett 2002;187:1-7.

Kimura K, Markowski M, Bowen C, et al. Androgen blocks apoptosis of hormone-dependent prostate cancer cells. Cancer Res 2001;61:5611-5618.

Lu S, Tsai SY, Tsai MJ. Regulation of androgen-dependent prostatic cancer cell growth: androgen regulation of CDK2, CDK4, and CKI p16 genes. Cancer Res 1997;57:4511-4516.

Joseph IB, Nelson JB, Denmeade SR, et al. Androgens regulate vascular endothelial growth factor content in normal and malignant prostatic tissue. Clin Cancer Res 1997;3:2507-2511.

Maatman TJ, Gupta MK, Montie JE: Effectiveness of castration versus intravenous estrogen therapy in producing rapid endocrine control of metastatic cancer of the prostate. J Urol 1985; 133:620-621.

GH, Altwein JE, Kurth KH, et al: Treatment of advanced prostatic cancer with parenteral cyproterone acetate: a phase III randomized trial. Br J Urol 1980; 52:208-215.

Barradell LB, Faulds D: Cyproterone: a review of its pharmacology and therapeutic efficacy in prostate cancer. Drugs Aging 1994; 5:59-80.

de Voogt HJ, Smith PH, Pavone-Macaluso M, et al: Cardiovascular side effects of diethylstilbestrol, cyproterone acetate, medroxyprogesterone acetate and estramustine phosphate used in the treatment of advanced prostatic cancer: results from the European Organization for Research on Treatment of Cancer trials 30761 and 30762. J Urol 1986; 135(2):303-307.

Schröder FH, Collette L, de Reijke TM, et al: Prostate cancer treated by antiandrogens: is sexual function preserved?. Br J Cancer 2000; 82:283-290.

Wirth M, Tyrekk C, Delaere K, et al: Bicalutamide (Casodex) 150 mg in addition to standard care in patients with nonmet-astatic prostate cancer: updated results from a randomized double-blind phase III study (median follow-up 5.1 y) in the early prostate cancer programme. Prostate Cancer Prostatic Dis 2005; 8:194-200.

McLeod DG, Iversen P, See WA, et al: Bicalutamide 150 mg plus standard care vs standard care alone for early prostate cancer. BJU Int 2005; 97:247-254.

Waxman J, Man A, Hendry WF, et al: Importance of early tumour exacerbation in patients treated with long acting ana-logues of gonadotrophin releasing hormone for advanced prostate cancer. BMJ 1985; 291:1387-1388.

Seidenfeld J, Samson DJ, Hasselblad V, et al: Single-therapy androgen suppression in men with advanced prostate cancer: a systematic review and meta-analysis. Ann Intern Med 2000; 132:566-577.

Schultz H, Senge T: Influence of different types of antiandrogens on luteinizing hormone-releasing hormone analogue-induced testosterone surge in patients with metastatic carcinoma of the prostate. J Urol 1990; 144:934-941.

Vanuytsel L, Ang KK, Vantongelen K, et al: Ketoconazole therapy for advanced prostatic cancer: feasibility and treatment results. J Urol 1987; 137:905-908.

Kelly WK, Scher HI: Prostate specific antigen decline after antiandrogen withdrawal: the flutamide withdrawal syn-drome. J Urol 1993; 149:607-609.

Small EJ, Srinivas S: The antiandrogen withdrawal syndrome. Experience in a large cohort of unselected patients with advanced prostate cancer. Cancer 1995; 76:1428-1434.

Harada M, Iida M, Yamaguchi M, et al. Analysis of bone metastasis of prostatic adenocarcinoma in 137 autopsy cases. Adv Exp Med Biol 1992; 324:173-182.

Wei JT, Gross M, Jaffe CA, et al: Androgen deprivation therapy for prostate cancer results in significant loss of bone den-sity. Urology 1999; 54:607-611.

Melton LJ, Aalothman KL, Khosia S, et al: Fracture risk following bilateral orchiectomy. J Urol 2003; 169:1747-1750.

Humadi A, Alhadithi RH, Alkudiari SI. Validity of the DEXA diagnosis of involutional osteoporosis in patients with femoral neck fractures. Indian J Orthop. 2010 Jan;44(1):73-8.

Blake GM, Fogelman I. An update on dual-energy x-ray absorptiometry. Semin Nucl Med. 2010 Jan;40(1):62-73. Review.

Bae DC, Stein BS: The diagnosis and treatment of osteoporosis in men on androgen deprivation therapy for advanced carcinoma of the prostate. J Urol 2004; 172:2137-2144.

Diamond TH, Higano CS, Smith MR, et al: Osteoporosis in men with prostate carcinoma receiving androgen-deprivation therapy: recommendations for diagnosis and therapies. Cancer 2004; 100:892-899.

Michaelson MD, Cotter SE, Gargollo PC, et al: Management of complications of prostate cancer treatment. Ca Cancer J Clin 2008; 58:196-213.

Smith MR, McGovern FJ, Zietmen AL, et al: Pamidronate to prevent bone loss during androgen-deprivation therapy for prostate cancer. N Engl J Med 2001; 345:948-955.

Greenspan SL, Nelson JB, Trump DL, et al: Skeletal health after continuation, withdrawal, or delay of alendronate in men with prostate cancer undergoing androgen-deprivation therapy. J Clin Oncol 2008; 26:4426-4434.

Green JR, Rogers MJ: Pharmacologic profile of zoledronic acid: a highly potent inhibitor of bone resorption. Drug Dev Res 2002; 55:210-224.

Saad F, Gleason DM, Murray R, et al: Long-term efficacy of zoledronic acid for the prevention of skeletal complications in patients with metastatic hormone-refractory prostate cancer. J Natl Cancer Inst 2004; 96:879-882.

Lipton A, Fizazi K, Stopeck AT, Henry DH, Brown JE, Yardley DA, Richardson GE, Siena S, Maroto P, Clemens M, Bilyn-skyy B, Charu V, Beuzeboc P, Rader M, Viniegra M, Saad F, Ke C, Braun A, Jun S. Superiority of denosumab to *zoledronic acid for prevention of skeletal-related events: A combined analysis of 3 pivotal, randomised, phase 3 trials. Eur J Cancer. 2012 Nov;48(16):3082-92.*

Huggins C, Hodges CV. Studies on prostatic cancer I. The effect of castration, of estrogen and of androgen injection on serum phosphatases in metastatic carcinoma of the prostate. Cancer Res 1941;1:193-197

Slemenda, C. W., Longcope, C., Zhou, L. et al: Sex steroids and bone mass in older men. J Clin Invest, 100: 1755, 1997

Malkowicz SB . The role of diethylstilbestrol in the treatment of prostate cancer . Urology 2001 ; 58 : 108 – 13.

Robinson MR , Thomas BS . Effect of hormonal therapy on plasma testosterone levels in prostatic carcinoma . B MJ 1971; 4 : 391 – 4.

Wang H, Li J, Gao Y et al . Xenooestrogens and phyto-oestrogens are alternative ligands for the androgen receptor . Asian J Androl 2010 ; 12 : 535 – 47

Blackard, C. E., Doe, R. P., Mellinger, G. T., and Byar, D. P.: Incidence of cardiovascular disease and death in patients receiving diethylstilbestrol for carcinoma of the prostate. Cancer 26:249-256,1970.

Smith DC, Redman BG, Flaherty LE, et al. A Phase 11 Trial of Oral DES as a second-line Hormonal Agent in Advanced Prostate Cancer. Urology 1998;52:257-60.

Jazieh AR, Munshi NC, Muirhead M, et al. Clinical efficacy of Diethylstilbestrol treatment in post-orchiectomy progressive prostate cancer. Proc AACR 1994;35:233.

Klotz L, McNeil I, Fleshner N. A Phase 1-2 trial of diethylstilbestrol plus low dose warfarin in advanced prostate carcinoma. J Urol 1999;161:169-72.

Vandenput L, Ohlsson C. Estrogens as regulators of bone health in men. Nat Rev Endocrinol 2009;5:437-43.

Taneja SS, Smith MR, Dalton JT, Raghow S, Barnette G, Steiner M, et al. Toremifene--a promising therapy for the prevention of prostate cancer and complications of androgen deprivation therapy. Expert Opin Investig Drugs. 2006;15(3):293–305.

Price D, Stein B, Sieber P, Tutrone R, Bailen J, Goluboff E, et al. Toremifene for the prevention of prostate cancer in men with high grade prostatic intraepithelial neoplasia: results of a doubleblind, placebo controlled, phase IIB clinical trial. J Urol. 2006; 176(3):965–970.

Taneja SS, Morton R, Barnette G, Sieber P, Hancock ML, Steiner M. Prostate Cancer Diagnosis Among Men With Isolated High-Grade Intraepithelial Neoplasia Enrolled Onto a 3-Year Prospective Phase III Clinical Trial of Oral Toremifene. J Clin Oncol. 2013 Jan 7. [Epub ahead of print]

Thompson IM, Pauler DK, Goodman PJ, Tangen CM, Lucia MS, Parnes HL, Minasian LM, Ford LG, Lippman SM, Crawford ED, Crowley JJ, Coltman CA Jr. Prevalence of prostate cancer among men with a prostate-specific antigen level < or =4.0 ng per milliliter. N Engl J Med. 2004 May 27;350(22):2239-46.

www.ingramcontent.com/pod-product-compliance
Lightning Source LLC
Chambersburg PA
CBHW071957220326
41599CB00032BA/6104